RECLAIMING NATURAL
MOVEMENT

Reclaiming Natural Movement
Practical and Effective Therapy for Ataxic Movements due to Neurodegenerative Disorders and Other Causes
Second Edition, Abridged

For information about this title or to order other books and/or electronic media, contact the publisher:

Reclaiming Natural Movement with TLC, Inc.
ReclaimingNaturalMovement.com
tom@reclaimingnaturalmovement.com

ISBNs
978-1-7348734-3-6 (hardcover)
978-1-7348734-4-3 (softcover)
978-1-7348734-5-0 (eBook)

Printed in the United States of America

Cover and Interior design: 1106 Design
Editing assistance: Robert Hartmann

Publisher's Cataloging-In-Publication Data

Names: Clouse, Thomas L., author.
Title: Reclaiming natural movement : practical and effective therapy for ataxic movements due to neurodegenerative disorders and other causes / Thomas L. Clouse, M.D.
Description: Second edition, abridged. | [Zellwood, Florida] : Reclaiming Natural Movement with TLC, Inc., [2021]
Identifiers: ISBN 9781734873436 (hardcover) | ISBN 9781734873443 (softcover) | ISBN 9781734873450 (eBook)
Subjects: LCSH: Movement disorders--Physical therapy. | Posture disorders--Physical therapy. | Nervous system--Degeneration--Rehabilitation.Classification: LCC RC376.5 .C56 2021 (print) | LCC RC376.5 (ebook) | DDC 616.83--dc23

Notice

This book is intended as a reference volume only, not as a medical manual. The information, advice, and exercise instruction in this book are not a substitute for any treatment or therapy your doctor may have prescribed. You should seek your doctor's approval before beginning any therapy or exercise program.

The information in this book is meant to supplement, not replace, proper exercise and rehabilitation training. All forms of exercise pose some inherent risks. The author, editors, and publisher advise readers to take full responsibility for their safety and to know their limits. If attempting the activities described in this book, be sure that you use sturdy support when needed, and do not take risks beyond your level of fitness.

This work is dedicated to my children, especially my two daughters. Unbeknown to me at the time of their birth, I had an unrecognized neurodegenerative disorder which they inherited. I lacked the knowledge of my evolving situation when I held and protected them during their childhood, and then was powerless to protect them in their adult life when the effects of the disorder I had passed to them became evident.

This book describes in detail how I learned to help myself have a better life with the problems associated with our shared disorder. Thus, it also empowers my daughters with the best help I can now offer them, as is also the case for a multitude of other people with the same and similar disorders and conditions. It is with utmost hope that they, as well as any other person requiring it, will use this resource wisely in their efforts to maintain a productive, fulfilling and happier life.

This work is also dedicated to my grandchildren, who hopefully are not harboring this mutation within, and to all future generations.

TABLE OF CONTENTS

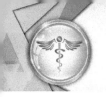

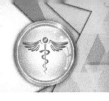

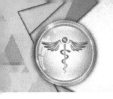

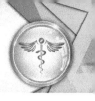

INTRODUCTION

by Michael C. Clouse

I *have to begin this by saying* that my dad is my hero. He set within me the examples of fatherhood that I try every day to live by when dealing with my four children. In good moments and bad, I constantly refer back to his examples in my younger years to determine which path I'll follow as I grow as a parent.

From those early years, I jump forward to the present and see further examples in Dad that I hope to emulate someday in my own life. I see him reaching out to help others who are in situations similar to his own. He has become a role model to me and his grandchildren. I don't think they quite understand all this yet, but in time they will.

To put things in perspective, I must go back a couple of decades to a time when I was absorbed in my own life and issues. I was raising two very young children and, to be honest, I lost track of what was going on with Dad. I heard rumblings and some concerns but never really paid much attention. Figuring that everything would work itself out somehow, I didn't bother asking too many questions.

Then the day came when I received a call that Dad had to quit practicing medicine entirely. That got my attention. I knew there was something medically going on that had prevented him from continuing his career in his chosen field of surgery. I was caught totally off guard when I learned of his actual diagnosis. Dad did his best to explain what it meant, but at that point in my life it did not really sink in. My response was more or less, "Well, that sucks!" and I continued on with things as usual.

Fast-forward to today, with the clear images in the rearview mirror, and I see things that I missed. I don't know if my involvement then would have changed things, but after seeing the struggle and darkness my dad went through in dealing with the "demon in his head," I honestly did not know how to help. Either way, Dad had to find himself in that darkness and pull himself out on his own. He found the way to do that. His accomplishments during that grueling process resulted in this book.

Dad rediscovered in himself the desire that had driven him into the medical field so many years before. He wanted to help people and make a positive difference. That mission has not changed in him to this day. His tireless efforts in working with people with movement issues are proof of that.

The transformation I have seen in Dad in the past decade is remarkable. If you would have told me fifteen years ago that my dad would still be out on the links playing golf today, I would have scoffed, because he was already losing that ability back then. On the contrary, I would have believed it if I had

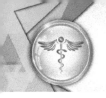

been told he would be in a wheelchair right now, unable to do most things on his own. But he is not in a wheelchair and does not need a cane or walker, and he still plays golf regularly.

He altered his fate when he decided to step out of his comfort zone and try something new. That something new, something he had never done before, namely taking dance lessons, was the first step out of the darkness and into the light I now see him in every day. From that beginning resurrection, the rest of the story is revealed in his words in this book.

Dad will be the first person to tell anyone following him down the road in their quest to recover lost movement abilities that it is not going to be an easy process. He will also tell them that there are no promises or guarantees within these pages as to exactly how anything will work for them. They must first learn how to apply what he has written. However, there is a standing promise and guarantee that the information is truthful.

This book is a guide to finding yourself again, to regaining parts of you that seem lost. It is about finding the courage within yourself to step out of your comfort zone and into a world that is better and brighter. It is about wanting and working to have more than you have right now. It is about a better quality of life not only for you, but also for your loved ones. These things can only come from you. How you choose to use this guide will, in large part, determine your future.

When I began reading and doing some editing of this book, I really did not expect it to have anything to do with me. After all, Dad wrote this for people with problematic movement issues, especially those caused by neurological problems. That is not me. I do not have his disorder. My movements are still very natural and normal, or so I thought. That was a huge mistake.

As I read, I began to see "crutches" I had already started to implement within my own body. I deal with recurring back problems and had just found out I had arthritis in my right knee. When I started considering what Dad had written with respect to my situation, I was amazed to realize that I was already beginning to do some "guarding" within my own body and compensating with restricted movements. So, I then started consciously incorporating some of the techniques he describes in this book into my daily life. Within a very short time, I realized that I felt better. My movements had become easier and a little quicker. Much of the time, my pain and stiffness were less, and my posture improved.

Many times throughout the book, he reminds you about how you learned to do all these basic things when you were just a toddler. Well, as fate would have it, I happen to have a toddler at home. I spent many hours and afternoons watching this little guy getting around. I was repeatedly surprised to see the examples listed in the book play out before my eyes. My son had no idea what he was doing or why. He was only two, but many times I saw him doing exactly what Dad has laid out for you in this book. Dad, I couldn't help but chuckle.

So, holding this book in your hands, why should you buy this book? It is the heart and desire of Dad, with the blood, sweat, and tears he has poured into teaching himself and others with movement problems how to regain a part of themselves they thought they had lost forever. But, more importantly, it contains factual information about our movements that I have not seen or heard of anywhere else. It is the simple and basic information that explains exactly what we do in our movements, both the right and the wrong.

I have talked with Dad and spent countless hours with him over the past few years. I have seen a wonderful transformation in him. I have seen the drive and the hope in his eyes. He wants you to know and feel the same, knowing there is a light at the end of your darkened tunnel. But ultimately it is you who must find that light. To find it, you must first have the desire to search and reach for it, and then continue the learning process until you step out from the shadows.

    Fill the hopes of your desire by putting forth the time and effort to help yourself. When you honestly do that, you will see a difference.

    That is all he really wants.

■ ■ ■

CHAPTER 1

SAME BODY, SAME FUNCTION

WE CAN ALL DO BETTER.

Do you remember the day you were told of your diagnosis? Can you recall the emotions and bewilderment that quickly filled your mind? Of course, you can. I doubt that you or I shall ever forget that fateful day. Never again would anything be the same. Our hopes, our dreams, our future aspirations suddenly stopped at an idle as we struggled to understand. What is to come of me? What will I do? How do I live with this?

On that day we were given a label (diagnosis), and it came with a set of instructions. Simply stated, we were informed, "You can't change or control your condition, and there isn't much of anything you can do that will make much of a difference. It will only get worse. Hopefully, with time you will learn to accept it."

The doom and gloom of our new reality was thrust upon us with a thunderous numbing thud. Hearing the meaning of our diagnosis spoken, we sat stunned in confusion. Our voices muted. In an instant our life was stripped of dreams and aspirations. It happened to me too, and for years I also lived according to the label and instructions we were given on that day. And just as it has been for nearly everyone with this fate, I believed what I was told and what I had read in the academic literature—until the day I woke up.

Very unexpectedly, I discovered I could do a few things better than I had been. This opened my eyes and my mind. As I continued exploring and pushing my abilities envelope, additional unrecognized opportunities came into focus. I was making improvements in my physical fitness and with it my movement abilities improved. I was not as clumsy. Life became good again, and my quality of life improved substantially. All of these things led me to share what I was finding with the world, so other people could enjoy the same benefits.

The bottom line. Most people with movement issues, including those with degenerative disorders, can do much better than they presently are. "How much," many of you are asking? In large part it depends on the relative ability and/or inability circumstances of the individual, with respect to their physical fitness level and the characteristics of their condition and/or disorder.

We can all do better. Knowing how to go about it is the key, and much of that information is provided within the pages of this book.

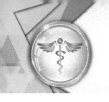

Another important tip is, the ultimate control over you resides within you. You choose how you will live your life. You choose what your expectations and motivations will be. For example, upon awakening each morning you have a choice. Will you choose to be happy and optimistic or would you rather be grumpy and depressed?

Our mind is our most powerful tool. It can bring us up or pull us down in the time it takes our heart to beat but once. Negative thoughts and attitudes fill us with doubt and indecision, and can pull us into the deepest pit of despair when we allow them to control us. Free yourself. Use an optimistic mind to discover your positive potential.

The Same.

The most important common link we share in our natural movement abilities is the fact that, without deformity or damaged nerve issues, the basic structure and function of every person's body is the same. Man or woman, young or old, in all the very different people throughout the world, our bodies are of the same design. The same bones, muscles, nerves, and organs are all in the same places and functioning the same way.

Naturally every person born with a full set of limbs has the same externally moving body parts, with the only differences being in how they are proportioned. Therefore, how and why our movements work as they do are the same for each and every one of us. It doesn't matter where we were born, where we live, or what condition, disorder, or complaint any person has. Every person's natural movements work per the design of the human body, and therefore according to the same basic principles of function. The same is true for our collective movement inabilities and disabilities.

Yes, there is variability in our movements when comparing individuals. But the observed variability is not with differing anatomical gross movements or function. The observed variability is due to the unique physical stature, or build, of any person, such as tall versus short, heavy versus thin, and other physical traits.

Basically, the quality of our natural movements is determined by how well our external moving body parts cooperatively function. To many of you, this will read as intuitively obvious and unnecessarily spoken. But it is also too often overlooked, and, in large part, remains misunderstood.

When everything about us works per natural design, our movements are great. But when something does not work per our natural design, we have problems. Then, as the inciting issues persist, problem movements tend to become bigger problems that show resistance to correction.

To understand our movement abilities, it is extremely important to consider things from a practical external use perspective. Individually, the functioning cooperativity of our feet, legs, arms, and body (how we use our body to make our natural movement ability possible), is overlooked by most people—but this is where the realism of understanding movement begins.

Early in our life we physically learned how to do our natural movements. But because we were so young we formed no memory, or intellectual understanding, of what we physically learned. This explains why there are misconceptions and misunderstandings in our knowledge of our natural movements in our adult life.

Now consider the implications. We struggle with verbally describing how our natural movements work. Physically, what happens? How do we do the things we do, without thought every day? Without understanding this basic knowledge, we are unable to provide factual and reasonable answers to the people who are struggling with problem and unnatural movements. And this is especially true for those with a neurodegenerative disorder.

This issue led to the writing of this book. How? I couldn't find answers when I needed help. Due to my neurodegenerative disorder, I was losing natural abilities and no one could help me change any of it. No person, nor any source, could provide me with meaningful and helpful answers. This is the plight people with problem movements repeatedly encounter; which also means they are on their own to figure out how best to deal with their situation. But stubbornly, I was determined to find answers that would help me preserve as much of my natural ability as possible. For that selfish reason, I continued working until the helpful answers became clear and proven to myself. And as I learned to apply what I was learning, my movements improved substantially. The next step was to share this life altering knowledge with others.

During the long process of discovery and improvement, I documented the lengthy details. These answers and explanations of how our body works to provide us with our natural movement abilities fill the pages of this book. And now it is in your hands. You are holding the factual answers to previously unanswered questions about our natural movements.

What about problem movements? This book also contains answers and explanations to the unanswered questions of why people develop problem and unnatural movements. In detail, the involved physical and postural issues are explained and shown with examples. And very importantly, the rationale and effective methods for correcting many of these problem issues are explained and demonstrated.

■ ■ ■

CHAPTER 2

UNTREATABLE MOVEMENT CONDITIONS

Is the disorder untreatable,
or is it partially misunderstood with the treatable parts going unrecognized?

I *have a degenerative neurological disorder*, and because of it I have balance and coordination movement issues. That's the bad news.

The good news. I learned how to correct or diminish many of my balance and movement problems. I did this by gaining a practical understanding of how our body makes our movements happen, and learned to re-adapt to more natural postures and movement patterns. This was the key to my success. Gaining the knowledge of how our body naturally functions to produce our movements gave me the information I needed to understand what I was, or was not doing, to physically cause or exacerbate my movement problems. This is a simple concept.

Let's clarify that last sentence. Is it necessary to know what happens under our skin, and have a working knowledge of how our body structure and systems function internally? No. Understanding how we work internally does not help the person with movement problems. In fact, it only complicates their movement efforts when their focus is directed to the internal functioning of their body. What they need to understand and use is the opposite; which is how our external body parts cooperatively function to create our easy to do movements. We then use that knowledge to make sense of our body posture and movements that have become difficult. For example. What am I physically doing that is different from how the movement is naturally done? Knowing this, what I need to do to make my problem movements less of a problem is more easily understood. So, and most importantly, first we must understand how our body works to make natural movements, to then understand what is physically wrong with problem and "unnatural" movements.

Let's take this concept one step further. It is often said that many of the problem/ataxic/unnatural movements caused by many movement disorders, and some conditions, are difficult to treat, or are untreatable. But, after living many years with the increasing negative effects of my disorder (spinocerebellar atrophy), I have repeatedly demonstrated that this is not categorically true. Through my

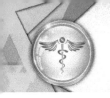
own efforts I discovered how to improve my balance and coordination, and my movement ability improved and remains improved. When I worked with other people, their problem movements also improved. This is proof that many of our problem movements are not categorically un-treatable. So, how do we know when a problem movement is treatable or untreatable? In truth, the amount of treatability is very relative to the individual and the nature of their issues. The following is what I have come to understand.

1. With few exceptions, the individual person with the disorder does not have the ability to alter or control anything with respect to the cause or progression of the neurodegenerative disorder that is within their brain.

2. With few exceptions, they also have no ability to alter or control any of the direct effects that the disorder causes.

3. With few exceptions, it is also true that the medical community is powerless to alter or control the direct effects of many neurodegenerative disorders.

4. Therefore, with few exceptions, the person with the disorder can, indeed, be seen as a victim of the disorder when referring *ONLY* to the disorder's direct effects.

5. However, many of the people with neurodegenerative disorders are for the most part not powerless victims. The same is true of many people with other disorders and conditions that cause problematic movements. Whether practitioners and patients realize it or not, many of these people absolutely do have choices they can act on that would likely improve their movement ability.

Showing what these choices are and describing how to implement them is a primary purpose of this book. Each chapter addresses these issues in detail with a descriptive understanding and the application thereof. Thus, it is a detailed resource of practical basic instruction in natural movement that empowers the readers to help themselves; to effect positive changes in their lives by simply improving their basic movement abilities.

Direct vs Indirect Issues

For any person with movement problems, there are at least two contributing causative factors. These are the direct and indirect effects. The direct effects are those changes the disorder or condition create.

The indirect effects comprise postural changes the affected person consciously or subconsciously makes that negatively affect their movement ability. For example, a person modifies his or her posture in an attempt to compensate for a problem caused by a direct effect, yet this self-induced modification (indirect effect) further complicates and/or restricts their movements. This is very common.

Since indirect effects are created by the individual in response to the issues caused by the direct effects, indirect effects can be referred to as optional. Consider what this means. When the person

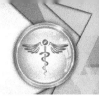

realizes how they are making their movements more of a problem, and then learns how to stop doing it, their movement ability improves. In this process they are correcting self-induced postural changes, and this allows their body to function more naturally. This is where affected people are treatable and can be helped.

So yes, we can correct and/or improve our personal stability and movement ability by working to undo the indirect effects we have acquired. It is also important to understand that this correction is made without the need to change anything about the condition. And now the crucial message. Focusing only on the positives of those things they can change, the affected person is working to reduce, correct, or eliminate indirect effects. Importantly, this more practical approach is not limited in any way by any condition or disorder, because, per the design of our body, everyone has the same natural body function that creates our natural movement ability.

However, I must openly admit that in the advanced stages of neurodegenerative disorders, corrections and improvements to the affected movements are frequently very difficult to achieve, are often fleeting, and sometimes are not achievable. The reason for this is the extreme nature of the direct effects afflicting that person, in addition to the deeply ingrained indirect effects which are difficult or impossible to work on because of the advanced direct effects.

For those with a milder presentation of their condition or disorder, the opportunity to achieve corrections and improvements to their stability and movement ability is characteristically high. This is because their direct effects are limited. In this case, what is or is not possible to alter and improve in their problem movements lies largely within that person's determination and efforts. However, there are at least two issues that will help them be more successful. The first is, many of them will benefit from improving their level of fitness. The second, many of them require thorough and knowledgeable instruction in how to go about making these positive changes.

■ ■ ■

CHAPTER 3

Maladaptive Behavior

To fix something that is not working properly, you need to understand how it correctly works.
Otherwise you will likely not recognize what needs fixing.

To correct the problem and unnatural movements many people develop,
the practical mechanics of our natural movements must be understood.

Direct effects: These are the changes that happen to posture and movements as a direct result of the disorder or condition the person is afflicted with.

Indirect effects: In response to the direct effects, these are the changes the person creates in their posture and movements.

Indirect effects accumulate slowly. Reacting to the developing direct effects of their disorder, people make small adjustments to their posture. This is an attempt to compensate for the gradual and subtle mishaps and uncoordinated changes they are beginning to experience in their movements. These postural adjustments may be small, but they are also additive. This is because each newly added adjustment requires an additional adjustment to counter the effects of the previous one(s). This slowly evolving process begins on a subconscious level and later involves conscious choices.

The affected person intends for these changes to be adaptive adjustments, to help correct awkwardness, clumsiness, instability, postural guarding, and stiffness. But as the small adjustments accumulate, they merge into larger changes that become maladaptive behaviors and habits that further complicate and hinder that person's movements. For many, *these accumulated maladaptive reactionary adjustments are the more significant cause of their observed unnatural movements.* However, this important realization has largely gone unrecognized. One reason for this is an overriding misperception that these observed changes are due entirely to the direct effects of the disorder. Then follows the belief that nothing can be done to alter what is being observed, because the disorder, or causitive condition, cannot be altered.

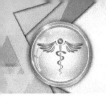

This belief gathers further reinforcement from the fact that nearly everyone with these disorders has or eventually will have these same postural and movement issues. As the disorder advances, this commonality of necessitated loss of function and ability is a primary focus that is used to gain an understanding of what is happening to these people, and is used as a prognostic indicator. Thus, a medical professional's opinion of the severity of each person's disorder is highly dependent upon their observations of an individual's posturing, behavior and movements. This is why it is extremely important to understand the true extent to which the correctable indirect effects have changed each person's movement abilities, and then work to correct them. When they remain unrecognized and uncorrected, indirect effects have an enormous and devastating negative impact on their quality of life.

An individual with these direct and indirect movement problems believes, "My disorder caused these problems I have. The only thing I can do is wait and hope the doctors can find a cure or treatment for my disorder." So, what happens? Slowly and without resistance, natural movement abilities devolve into unnatural movement *inabilities*. This is very sad, and more so because of the unrealized positive things the individual could be doing to help retard and restrict this downward-spiraling pattern. The truth for many people is, the accumulation of unnecessarily acquired maladaptive postural adjustments is causing an exaggeration of the direct-effect changes. The ramifications of this are staggering.

In the early stages of a disorder's physically expressed direct effects, the indirect-effect postural adjustments are primarily used to preserve and control small changes in *fine motor skills.*

Then, later, as the direct effects of the degenerative process increase in number or expression, the use of indirect-effect postural adjustments also increases. As both effects increase, the person relies more and more on indirect-effect adjustments to preserve and control *gross motor skills.*

People make adjustments (modifications) in an effort to adapt to their changing situation and improve their situation. But how can these modifications be adaptive when the end effect is detrimental? The answer is that most of them are *not* adaptive. Their use undermines the body's natural cooperative functioning and destroys natural movement. Thus, the indirect-effect postural adjustments and modifications *quickly become maladaptive.*

Maladaptive modifications exist in a self-perpetuating process from two sources:

1. Direct effects trigger indirect responses. Due to the direct effects caused by the disorder's progressively degenerative nature, movements become increasingly uncoordinated.

2. Acquired indirect postural modifications also cause increasing movement dyscoordination and clumsiness, forcing additional indirect postural modifications to be added.
   For very many affected people, the accumulation of maladaptive indirect effects explains the accelerated increase in movement clumsiness, dyscoordination, and inabilities commonly documented and attributed to the direct effects, and progression of the disorder.

3. The same pattern of accumulating maladaptive indirect effects is also seen with *nondegenerative* conditions.

STIFFNESS

There are two components, *physio*logical stiffness and *psycho*logical stiffness.

- The physiological component is a direct effect of the disorder and can only be partially controlled by the individual.

- The psychological component is an indirect component, and it can be controlled, corrected, and eventually released by the individual.

The **psychological** component of their stiffness largely consists of maladaptive behaviors. As a person's dyscoordination and clumsiness increase, the mishaps, falls, and injuries they experience also multiply. Growing apprehension and fear quickly follow.

The truth is, the *learned* psychological stiffness is, in large part, responsible for many of the unnatural postural changes they acquire and use. As clumsiness increases, they attempt to control it with postural guarding and stiffness. But this does not work, because it invariably creates additional postural instability, guarding, and stiffness, which create additional clumsiness. Thus, postural guarding and stiffness can only make movements worse, because the person is replacing a cooperative posture with a restrictive one. This is a self-perpetuating and escalating maladaptive behavioral cycle that contributes to a higher likelihood of mishaps and falls.

Each added adjustment/modification to the posture induces another cycle of guarding and/or stiffening. Each cycle adds another maladaptive layer, even though each added layer is intended to be adaptive, to compensate for the previous layer's effects. Each added layer further restricts movement and brings greater fear. The burgeoning fear brings about more caution and apprehension, which prompts another layer of postural guarding and stiffening. This is their self-induced perpetual cycle.

Think this process through. Test it by doing some of it yourself. Feel it. Hold varying amounts of guarding in your body, arms and legs, as you do simple movements. Pay attention to how the simple becomes challenging. As you add more guarding or tightening to your posture, note how you are also paying more attention to the movement. Feel how your balance and coordination are not as good, forcing you to think about what you are doing. Now consider how different your life would be if you had to cope with these issues every day.

With fearful minds filled with hesitation and doubt, people who have lapsed into these uncooperative stiffened postures must think very carefully about each movement they would *like* to make. At this heightened level of fear and instability, every movement is "preplanned." However, the preplanning is seldom effective. Why? It is not effective because the person has no clue what they should be physically preplanning.

The anxiety in their thoughts about the next movement is not about the movement. It is about the fear of the movement. Instead of reasoning out how they should adjust their posture for the movement they want to do, their thoughts are filled with anxiety about past problems and a potential fall. Their mind is preoccupied with incoherent thoughts that do not address potential solutions, because their focus is on the disaster they are expecting. Thus, they are physically totally unprepared for any movement.

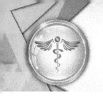

Instability, dyscoordination, clumsiness, and falls increase, with the heightened level of fear in their minds ensuring they will continue this pattern. The attention they devote to their every movement becomes total. They constantly look to hold on to or lean on something while praying nothing interferes with their slow, deliberate, and awkward progress. Under the assumed rules of the disorder, this becomes their daily life. However, this cascade of cause and effect often stems only *minimally* from the disorder. Rather, it is often largely the result of the indirect effects that their maladaptive reactions to postural changes have created.

It starts at the bottom. In the beginning, only the feet tense to intermittent mild instability and clumsiness. With added instability and concern, the stiffening in the feet increases and extends into the knees. As the knees tense, postural instability increases more quickly, causing concerns to become anxiety. As the anxiety and instability continue, the cycles of increasing generalized postural guarding and stiffening always follow. Eventually, even the neck and face are involved, but the guarding and stiffening always remain strongest where they began, in the feet.

Can these destructive cycles be interrupted and reversed? Yes. *But that will happen **only** when **natural stability returns**.* Only the individual can break and reverse this cycle, and only when he or she develops the renewed ability to confidently reproduce his or her own self-made natural stability. Just as importantly, this is also the only way they will have the ability to reduce and release their fear. Yes, this self-perpetuating process also works in reverse. With every cycle of physically improved stability, a portion of the fear in their mind retreats and is released. Then another layer of renewed ability is created as postural tensing and stiffening diminish.

The **physiological** component of stiffness **is** a *direct effect* of the disorder, and/or the environment, and has at least two subcomponents. One is temporary and manageable by the person. The other is rather permanent, or at least persistent and largely unmanageable by the person.

Many people with neurodegenerative disorders have a stiffening response to relatively cool or cold temperatures, standing or sitting too long, or becoming overly tired or fatigued. Fortunately, the stiffening reaction from these causes fades away as we warm from being chilled, or as we begin to "loosen up" and then carefully move after standing or sitting too long.

Some also experience a stiffening sensation of the hands when exercising. Along with the temporary, reactionary stiffening episodes mentioned above, I have also experienced this exercise-induced stiffening of the hands. The onset is gradual and makes my fingers feel "thickened" and sluggish, but there is no visible difference in them. This issue was very concerning until I realized that it correlates directly with my level of exertion, and it is directly relative to my physical conditioning and stamina. As I begin to tire, the thickening feeling comes.

When I'm walking or exercising, this feeling will fade away if I rest for a bit. I've also found that it dissipates if I continue to walk or exercise at an easy pace. Then a surprising discovery came. As I became more physically fit, the feeling of thickness did not occur as often and did not stay as long. Then it seldom came at all.

This was a very important learning point. *By improving my conditioning and endurance*, I have the ability to control it. So, now I use this feeling as a personal fitness guide in a positive way. No longer is it a negative reminder of: "Oh my God! I have to stop because of my disorder." The bigger observation

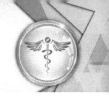

is what this implies for many other things we deal with. *For example, we can learn to control, limit, and release some of our physiological stiffness* by using some common sense in dealing with it. Thus, we do not need to be as badly off as most assume.

In cold weather my posture stiffens rapidly, but *only* when I'm not appropriately dressed for it. Therefore, when I know I'll be out in the cold or even in cool weather, I dress in clothing that will keep me warm. This prevents most and sometimes all of the stiffness. When I do this, my movements are minimally altered and sometimes not altered at all. One downside is the combination of cooler temperatures and sitting or standing too long. This causes an exaggerated stiffening response that takes longer to resolve.

Some people have a residual background stiffness that is very resistant to individual efforts to diminish it. I have worked with individuals with this issue and have noted only minimal fluctuations in their ability to reduce it through postural stability and relaxation. Keeping it reduced is also very problematic for them. Many of them require medication to help this condition.

Fear

The number of maladaptive behaviors any person will eventually develop is proportional to their degree of impairment and their personal reaction to that impairment. However, overall, every person's physical and psychological responses are *very* similar compared with those of all people affected with problematic movements, with similar or dissimilar disorders or conditions.

Some degree of postural guarding and stiffness is very common, but the proportion of direct and indirect effects varies widely. What is this saying? For one, the psychological reaction of any one individual (driving the indirect effects) does not necessarily correlate to the severity of the disorder's direct effects. I have worked with many people who had a great amount of fear in their movements. Interestingly, though, the actual physical severity of the movement impairments in this group ranged from mild to severe. Then, in all these people, when their fear level decreased as they built up their standing stability, their impairment improved. Thus, an individual's personal interpretation, experiences, and mindset greatly affect their observed appearance and movement ability. In short, they unknowingly make themselves worse.

This is important to understand, because, in large part, it is their personal appearance that determines the ultimate scoring of their "disorder." Therefore, it is very important that those who are charged with evaluating and helping these people be able to differentiate between the indirect and direct effects on an individual basis. Also realize that many people with these disorders *do* live according to what their treating physician and therapist tell them. When told their disorder has advanced, many will physically and psychologically live and act accordingly. In so doing, they will succumb to depression, fear, and inactivity. Then, what very commonly happens? Their "disorder" quickly advances. What is the evidence used to support this? Their physical appearance. In too many ways for too many people, this becomes a self-fulfilling prophecy.

Fear drives outcomes. The fear of falling is consistently the *big* factor in the mix that ensures the continued accumulation of additional maladaptive behaviors, postural guarding, stiffening, and dysfunctional movements.

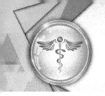

Learned responses develop gradually. The more often the "danger" alert happens, the more their physical and psychological reaction becomes a conditioned response to just the hint of danger. This reactionary response happens slowly and becomes extremely deep seated. As the situation that triggers the fear response happens more often, that person becomes less likely to relax between the occurrences. Their posture remains guarded, and then stiffened, because they are constantly anticipating what they fear: the prospect of instability and falling with each movement they attempt.

In a short amount of time, these people learn and accept all of what they fear, because for them their fear is very real—and it happens on a daily basis. This is why their postural changes remain. The adjustments are consistently reinforced and used, even though they make the person's movement situation worse. They do this because *they do not know how not to*, and they believe they are forced to because the disorder is directly causing it.

The following is a very common reply when asked about their stiffening posture. "*The stiffness protects me. It helps me because without it, I can't stand. My body is different now, and the stiffness keeps me from falling as much. I hate it. I am constantly afraid. But I can't function without it.*" In reality, this is valid to only a very small degree, with physical qualifications. Therefore, overall it is very much *invalid*. This will be discussed in many areas throughout many chapters of this book.

You will never know how much you can improve until you try.

■ ■ ■

CHAPTER 4

ADAPTIVE BEHAVIOR

Many people want to be special, but few want the responsibility that comes with it.

An *adaptive behavior is something* we do that improves our situation. A maladaptive behavior is something we do that makes our situation more difficult.

Throughout this book, images and details of multiple people with neurodegenerative disorders are used to illustrate reactive postures and maladaptive behaviors. However, this does not imply that the information in this book applies only to a group of people with neurodegenerative disorders. Actually, *it is intended to show exactly the opposite*, **and highlights the applicability to EVERYONE.**

Consider this. Neurodegenerative disorders are the most difficult movement issues to treat. And, this book documents how people suffering from these disorders are improving their postures and movement abilities. Now imagine the possibilities for the other people in the world who do not have a degenerative cause for their movement problems. Their positive results often come quicker with less work. So again, this book applies to everyone because it uses our body's natural function to describe and understand the problem, unnatural postures and movements many people develop.

Thus, the information in this book will help any person understand, create, and use adaptive behaviors in their posture and movements when it is properly applied. The only caveat is that each person must have the physical ability to remain stable while they are standing on their feet, with or without assistance.

In a discussion of natural and unnatural movements, it is *critically more important to understand our common functioning and postural responses* than it is to understand any specific situation, condition, disease process, or disorder. The rationale for this is the following. With some exceptions, *the function of our natural movements is altered more by maladaptive behaviors than by a disorder, condition, or situation.* Therefore, the therapy provided to any person with problem movements should rightfully focus on restoring natural movement by correcting the maladaptive behaviors and postures that person is using.

NATURAL REACTIONS

From the very beginning of our lives, we are genetically programmed to physically respond to certain things in the same manner. Then, as we mature, through our experiences we learn to modify these basic responses.

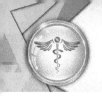

For example, every neurologically intact normal newborn will react to a sudden stimulus with the same startled response. It is called the Moro reflex. In this normal reflex, the baby suddenly opens its hands with arms spread outward when startled. Seconds later the baby will relax its arms and hands and settle back into a relaxed posture.

Now consider this. How many people of any age have you seen reacting in a very similar manner when they are on the receiving end of a great Halloween-type prank or scare? Even in adulthood, many people throughout this world still share the same startle responses. We all began our lives the same. We learn the same basic movement skills and abilities doing the same things, and during the same age span. So again, *we are more alike than we are different.* And, very importantly, virtually everything we know about our movements, we learned entirely on our own by trial and error.

From a baby to a toddler and young child, no one *taught* us anything related to our movements. Our natural development and adaptive nature allowed us to acquire increasing ability. We wanted to go and do, so we practiced until we did. In the beginning we had difficulties. But we kept trying until we could, until we moved to where we wanted to go. We found a way. We gained the natural ability as our neurological and musculoskeletal systems continued developing. Because of our youth, we knew little about fear, so we never stopped trying. The concept of fear only came to us later as experiences and controlling thoughts accumulated in our minds.

So, in our adult life, through the addition of decades of accumulated experiences and memories, our personal concept of fear is driven by the multitude of thoughts that, in part, creates our version of reality. Based on our thoughts, learned experiences, and concerns, we adjust our present and future actions and reactions accordingly. Much of what we use in this capacity is essential to our well-being and is adaptive. However, some is not, and is maladaptive.

■   ■   ■

CHAPTER 5

Finding Your Feet

Anything is possible.
However, we must do the work to reveal our possibilities.

*I*n the practical-use sense, every person with natural ability is a masterful movement expert. However, almost every person is also intellectually ignorant in understanding how they are an expert. Walking, running, going about any activity, our movements just naturally happen. We want to do something, and we do it. Our naturally cooperative body and relaxed posture make this possible.

But what about the people whose natural movements no longer happen easily, because their balance and movements have become a problem? Their naturally easy ability has been modified, and now their movements are challenging. When this happens, that's when it matters a great deal that they do not understand the basics of how their former natural movement ability was created by their body. But what if they did? If they did have an understanding of how their body works in natural movement, they then would have a better ability to work out what they are now having problems with.

To understand how nearly everyone is in the same unknowing situation, ask yourself and others these questions. How do we walk across the floor? Our body does it, but what does it actually do that provides us with our natural movement ability? When asked these questions, a good half of the people do not mention their feet in their answers. The other half say something like, "By putting one foot in front of the other, I guess? And when questioned further, the collective replay is, "I really do not know." Truthfully, we honestly have a very limited practical understanding of many of the common things we have been doing since our lives began.

1. We know quite well what we can and cannot do in our movements, yet we know next to nothing about how we do them.

2. We are intimately familiar with what feels right and wrong during our movements, yet we don't understand what it is that tells us: "this is right and this is wrong."

3. We can demonstrate what our correct way is, but we lack the intellectual understanding to explain how we physically do it, or why it is correct.

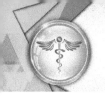

How Do We Know What Is Right and Wrong?

A vast amount of the information we use in knowing precisely the right and wrong in our movements comes from our feet.

Down on the floor, your feet, the only parts of you that are in contact with the floor, provide you with a wealth of information. In your feet and so very far removed from your mind, this is where the useful, practical, basic, and precise information about your posture and movements originates. Therefore, to answer the previous questions, you must understand the information your feet are providing. But how do we know what information is coming from our feet? What is it and how do we interpret it?

1. The information coming from our feet is the feeling of the various pressures. This describes how they are in contact with floor.

2. To recognize and understand what you are *physically* feeling in your feet, you must learn how to focus your undivided attention to them.

   What you are **not** searching to feel is, "What am I supposed to be feeling?" This is the exact opposite of where you want to be, and is something you are making up. It is simply you thinking about what the feeling might be. Therefore, a thought about the feeling tells you nothing about what is physically happening.

3. *You are searching to feel the purity of the physical feeling. This will come to you as: "I feel . . ."* That is the actual feeling you will learn to use because it tells you a great deal of what you need to know about your posture and movements.

4. When you understand how to easily feel and interpret the pressure, these once seemingly unimportant feelings in your feet will instantly and exactly tell you what is right or wrong with your posture and movements.

Mind versus Feet

1. People with natural movement ability control their movements with their feet, with a cooperative posture. There is very little input from their thinking minds. *Most often there is no conscious input.*

2. When easy movements become challenging movements, these affected people will typically adjust their posture and control their movements with increasing amounts of thought.

   The transition from thought-free movements to thought-filled movements creates the exact opposite of what is intended. The person's intent is to be more careful to prevent mishaps. Instead, this thinking complicates their movements and makes mishaps more likely to occur.

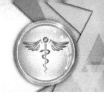

So, what are these people thinking about with their excessive thoughts? They think about their worsening difficulties, embarrassment, fear of falling, future and past injuries, and how they want to avoid experiencing these troubles again. But another problem is, they do not have a knowledgeable understanding of how to avoid any of these things. Simply put: It is impossible for anyone to change or control any physical part of a physical situation using just thought. To change and/or control a physical action, physical input is required.

Disclaimer:

Do not trust any of what you are reading
UNTIL you feel it and can readily reproduce it for yourself.

You can believe everything in this book. The information is factual and accurate to the best of my ability and understanding. All of the information presented is what I have learned to use every day. It is the same information I have taught to many others. However, *do not **trust** any of it until you have proven it to be true in your use of it.* Just as it has always been, you must have the ability to trust yourself in your movements, and your trust can only come from you—not me or anyone else. For this simple reason, you must prove everything by doing your movements your way, using the same basic skills we all share. The other ingredient is to be critically honest during the process.

The reason for this is simple. None of this information will make a difference for you until you combine the intellectual part with the physical part and learn to use both. Only when you understand and can reproduce what you are feeling without ambiguous, rampant thought, only then will you have the capacity to use and trust any of it. In order for your mind to relax and release fear, you must have trust in your physical ability. Only then will your body be able to relax and function more naturally.

OUR FEET

In practical and simple terms, our feet serve three basic purposes:

1. They are the platforms we stand on. If all we did was stand in one spot, then our feet would only need to be like inflexible pieces of thick wood.

2. Our natural movement ability is dependent on our feet remaining flexible.

3. Our feet have fantastic sensors within them, and the information coming from them provides us with a wealth of information.

Naturally, we pay very little conscious attention to our feet until something is wrong with them. This is for good reason. Imagine how life would be if you were consciously aware of everything that happened to your feet during every second of every day. Your mind would be overloaded with too much input.

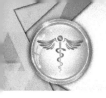

To avoid this mental overload, pressure sensors in your skin quickly adapt to constant pressure and effectively zero it out. For example, when you put on a shirt, you feel it for a few seconds, and then quickly you don't. You stop feeling it because the sensors in your skin effectively reset so as not to register the constant pressure. As you continue wearing the shirt, you will feel part of it only when something causes a part of it to apply increased pressure in an area. This same thing happens in your feet. This is why we're only alerted to what we feel in our feet when we feel something different, and then we are very aware of it.

So, feeling discomfort in our feet makes us acutely aware that something is not right, and we can also feel when our shoes become loose on our feet. Consider the wider meaning of this. If we have the ability to be so keenly aware of what we feel in our feet during times of discomfort and when our shoe is loosely fitting, we certainly also have the ability to become keenly aware of what we feel in our feet when they are comfortable. The key to doing this is quieting your mind enough to physically focus on feeling.

For movement purposes, consider your feet as "Mama" of your body. An old saying within families is: *"If Mama's not happy, nobody's happy."* We all understand how this statement holds a great deal of truth. Now apply that same reasoning to your body. Keeping your feet happy means keeping them comfortable and secure. We do this by applying, holding, and using the correct pressure in our feet.

For any posture or movement, when the pressure in our relaxed feet is correct, the rest of our relaxed body will be exactly where it is supposed to be. This foundation provides comfort and stability, and allows the movements we intend to be doing to happen.

When the pressure in our feet is not correct, our posture will not be where it needs to be, and the resulting movement will not be what we had intended. Discomfort and instability are the results.

When we're standing on our feet, the correct pressure in our feet
determines and controls our movements and abilities.

POSTURE AND MOVEMENT

With a relaxed posture our body cooperatively aligns, balances and sets the pressure in our feet, using nothing more than *this feels right*. In our natural movements, the pressures we create in our feet direct the movement of our body without conscious thought or effort. This is *relaxed postural control.*

In our natural postures and movements, our body cooperatively adjusts itself to be aligned how and where it must be, as if it were on autopilot. In many ways this is exactly what is happening. And in that sense, the autopilot setting that we use is the pressure that is required in the foot or feet for the movement we intend to do. So, naturally speaking, the reflexive and cooperative movements of our relaxed body set the required pressure in the feet, and then maintain that pressure throughout the movement. Thus, using relaxed and flexible feet, these freely flowing cooperative and counterbalancing bodily movements provide us with the *thoughtless movement ability* we enjoy.

Impaired and problematic movements often use varying amounts of nonreflexive, uncooperative and restricted counterbalancing bodily movements. Simply stated, tensed muscles restrict the body from moving as it otherwise naturally would. The result is complicated, unintended movements and instability.

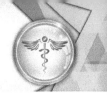

Because of this, thought-free movements are replaced with thought-*filled* movement attempts. In a short time, these movements often become more problematic, and then become a self-perpetuating cause and effect in the downward spiral of increasing movement disability and inability.

STABILITY FIRST, THEN FEELING

To gain the ability to focus on what you feel happening in your feet, you must first have the ability to stabilize your body on your feet. Without a stable foundation and a sense of well-being to quiet your mind, you will always be thinking about and reacting to your instability. And it doesn't take much instability to force added thoughts.

For many people with impaired movements, stabilizing on their feet is not an easy task. With only a slight amount of body sway when standing, the location of the pressure in their feet is constantly changing. This is the source of the instability they feel.

If this mild instability happens to you, touch or lightly hold on to something to help you stop swaying. Typically, a light touch is all that is required. What is so special about this that makes such a big difference? Basically, the answer is *nothing*, because the stabilizing effect is, for the most part, not coming from what you're touching. Instead it is coming from what you're doing. When touching or lightly holding on to something, you gain some reassurance, and then you begin to relax. This small amount of *postural relaxation is the primary reason you become more stable.* This is totally what you are doing for yourself and *not* what the object is doing for you.

To have the ability to control your movements, you must be able to relax your body enough to have control of the pressure in your feet. Thus, it is necessary to stabilize your body first, to then have the ability to relax it, before you will have the ability to set and control the required pressure in your feet.

We are about to do an exercise to begin the process of feeling pressure in the feet. If you are having problems holding your body steady while standing, please use something to help you stabilize. This can be your walker, a piece of furniture, or a countertop, for example. The object really doesn't matter, as long as it is sturdy and stable and you are not overly dependent on it. Just try not to hold on to it too tightly or lean on it too much. Another point: How far apart should your feet be on the floor? It doesn't matter. Have them where you want or need them to be in order to feel comfortable.

Standing as balanced as you can on both feet, allow your body to relax as much as you're able. Then try to focus on what is happening in your feet. There's no need to describe it yet. Simply allow the physical feeling to be what it is. This is different from what you think the feeling might be, or should be. So, stop thinking about it. Thinking always takes you farther away from understanding the physical feeling.

Do your best to *ignore the noise in your head and the voices* of any other people in the room. Focus only on what your body is telling you. Simply *feel what you feel.* Next, **slowly** move your body to feel what changes in your feet. Then, after you have practiced and have become comfortable with it, do this same thing while looking at yourself in a mirror; full length works best. This is important. It allows you to compare what you are feeling in your feet with what you see of your posture. Feel the changing pressure in your feet while watching the very small and slow movements of your body. Look for the correlation of body position to where you feel the pressure in your feet.

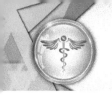

Practice and learn this well, because it is the first skill you must understand to proceed through the process of understanding and improving your posture and movements. Everything depends on it. This is the required fundamental skill natural movement is based on.

The feeling in your feet describes the pressure in your feet,
and the amount and location of that pressure describes your posture.

Standing in a comfortable posture, your next focus is to feel where the increased pressure is located on the bottom of your feet. Then, *slightly and gently* move your shoulders from side to side, and forward and back, to feel how these small movements move the location of the pressure in your feet. Feel the cause and effect. And importantly, with the direction of movement of your shoulders, where does the pressure move in your feet?

For those who are unable to stand and remain stable, do the following experiments while sitting. But you must be aware that it will be more of a challenge to feel the pressure in your feet because there will not be as much of it. So, sit forward in the chair with your feet firmly and completely on the floor and then proceed.

Now try this. With both arms hanging loosely at your sides, begin to slowly lower only one shoulder. What changes in your feet? Repeat this with the other shoulder.

With your right shoulder lowered you should feel a small amount of extra pressure in the right side of your body, and some of you will feel a change in the right lower back area. This happens because your rib cage is tilting down and inward on the right side, causing the lower ribs to apply pressure into that area of your body.

Now feel the pressure this is putting into your right hip, right leg, and right foot. Feel how the right side of your body feels slightly heavier and different from the left side. What else do you feel? Feel the tendency for your body to move to the right. Also, do you feel how you are holding or bracing it from moving?

Now focus only on feeling the pressure in your right foot. With your right shoulder held down, the outside part of the right foot will have increased pressure, and the inside part of the right foot has less pressure. Next, do the same experiment on the left side. Feeling these pressures in your feet is often difficult for some people, and there are usually two basic reasons for this. One, you did not move your shoulder low enough to cause enough change to the location of the pressure. Two, you are focusing too much on your instability or what your body is doing. Any extra focus points, and the thinking that typically goes with them, will interfere with your ability to feel the pressure in your feet.

Now experiment with moving your shoulder upward. Standing comfortably with your body centered over your feet, slowly move your shoulders up (shrug them) as high as you can, and feel the pressure changes in your feet. This may cause some of you to feel slightly unstable, and that is because the pressure slightly decreases in your feet. This small pressure change may be difficult for some to feel. If this applies to you, carefully exaggerate shrugging your shoulders upward to make the change more obvious.

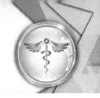

Be careful. Some of you may feel that the location of the pressure in your feet moves, and that happens when you also move your shoulders a small amount forward or backward as you move them upward. Be very careful of this because you may change the location of the pressure enough that you begin to tip forward or backward. So, anyone with a stability issue should begin these experiments with feet flat on the floor, and practice carefully moving their shoulders straight upward so the pressure in their feet does not move.

Use a mirror, and full length is best! This is very important. You need to know exactly what you are doing in these movements, and how it correlates with the pressure changes in your feet.

Feel the changes happening in your feet to the body movements you see in the mirror. When standing, take note of how a little body movement makes a big difference in the location and amount of pressure in your feet.

These are important to do, feel and understand, because it is the beginning to understanding the correlation of how you adjust your posture, to set and adjust the pressure in your feet, to control your stability and movements.

Now that you are beginning to realize how the movement of the upper body changes the location of the pressure in the feet, experiment with how to stabilize the pressure and your body. To do this, you are to center your body over your feet to put an equal amount of pressure in both feet. For improved stability you should also adjust the pressure so it is equal in the heel areas and the ball areas of both feet.

Please remember to use very slow and gentle movements of your body to do this. When you feel equal pressure in both feet stop moving your body, then relax as much as you are able while not moving the pressure in the feet. While you are doing this, it may be helpful to watch your posture in the mirror to compare what you feel.

For example:

1. When your body is relaxed, or close to it, with the pressure equal in both feet, your posture will be upright and relatively straight with shoulders level.

2. When the pressure is not equal in both feet you will see that your body is not centered between your feet, such as a lowered shoulder and possibly the body offset to that side.

3. When your body is not relaxed your posture will likely be too upright and the shoulders may or may not be level. With a too-upright posture the pressure in your feet will be slightly less than it is when your posture is relaxed.

AREAS OF THE FOOT

Standing stable on your feet, shift your focus to the pressure you feel in the heels and the ball areas of your feet, as shown in Figure 5.1. Feel the difference when the pressure is equal (the same) in the heel and ball area of both feet. With this stable foundation you feel more comfortable, stable and it is easier to relax. These are your feet physically "flat on the floor."

Your first goal is to become very skilled and comfortable with creating and staying on "flat feet" while standing still. Learn to relax into the stability and the comfort you are creating. This is a very important prerequisite to all your advancing/improving movement abilities. If you **do not** have this ability to control the pressure in your feet and relax your body when standing still, you will **not** have control of them during movements. Why is this important? Our natural movements require it.

Relaxing your body into flat and stabilized feet on the floor creates two very important effects:

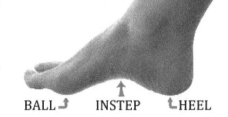

BALL↴   INSTEP↑   ↳HEEL

FIGURE 5.1: Areas of the foot.

1. It allows flexible and reflexive cooperative body movements.

2. The postural relaxation allows the knees and hips to flex more easily. This contributes to improved functioning of the muscles in the legs and improved foot pressure creation and use.

MAJOR PARTS OF THE BODY

Pertaining to natural movement, the basic function of the body is divided into three parts:

1. From the waist up, the **upper body** *adjusts and maintains* the location of the pressure in the feet.

2. From the waist down to the ankles, the **lower body** (legs) supports the body and generates additional pressure to be used in the feet.

3. The function of the **feet** is to use the pressure to move the body. The location of the increased pressure in the feet is set by the upper body, and that pressure determines the direction the body will move when it is used. The additional pressure from the functioning leg muscles serves to improve the body's stability and movement ability.

4. In summary, in our basic natural movements, the upper body only supports the movement. The lower body supports the body, and initiates and powers the movement. The flexing feet do the movement.

5. This natural arrangement of function for the body, is compromised in those with problem movements, and has been altered in people with unnatural movements.

OUR FOUNDATION STANCES

To reach your goal of improving your movements, there are six basic stances you must have the ability to do. These are the foundation stances that all our natural basic movements are based on, and they are the very same ones we all learned so well while we were in diapers. So again, you will not be constructing a new way of movement using anything presented in this book. You will simply be learning how to return to more natural movements.

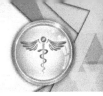

The sequence of these six stances is reviewed in the natural order in which we learn our movements as toddlers. First, we learn to stand, then squat, walk sideways, and eventually walk forward. Then we quickly learn that we can run, jump, throw things, kick, climb, and explore our expanding world with unlimited anticipation.

Thus, the sequence we have watched every child progress through as they come out of the crawling stage is the same sequence we adults must use to correct our problem movement issues, to improve our movement ability. What is true in our early years has the same truth and application in our adult years.

1. If you're unstable while standing, you will be more unstable when you attempt to move or walk.

2. If you can't remain stable while standing on two feet, then you *do not* have the ability to be stable when standing on one foot.

3. Big *HINT*: What is it you do every time you walk anywhere? You stand on one foot and then transition to the other foot. So, to become more stable in your movements, you must have the ability to stabilize, even for only a second or two, on just one foot.

Just like any child, you must have the ability to do the first stance before you will have the ability to do the second. It continues that same way all the way through to the sixth stance and beyond. The six stances are:

1. **Standing upright** with feet flat on the floor.

2. Standing in the **ready stance** with stabilized feet and a steady, comfortable posture. (The ready stance is the stance we use to move into and out of nearly every movement.)

3. **Simple squat** to touch the fingertips of both hands to the floor just in front of the toes, and return to the ready stance or standing upright while keeping both feet stabilized with a steady, comfortable posture.

4. **Sideward stride**

5. **Forward stride**

6. **Forward stride squat**

Could it be that simple? Yes. These six basic stances are the foundation of all our movements, for everything we do standing on and moving using our feet.

■ ■ ■

CHAPTER 6

First Stance: Standing Upright

Personal limits are arbitrary and imaginative creations from speculative minds.

For the many things we will be doing throughout the chapters, when you are feeling unsteady, I suggest you practice these things on a hard and smooth floor. The flat and firm surface will provide you with more stability. However, a carpeted floor is fine provided it is not too textured and has minimal padding under it. When the carpet is thick and/or has a good deal of padding under it, it often is challenging for movement impaired people because it is too spongy.

Shoes. If you are comfortable standing without shoes on, that is perfectly fine. But if you feel better while wearing them, securely fitting shoes will provide you with more support and stability. Ill-fitting footwear often cause added difficulties. This is especially true with loose-fitting house slippers, sandals, and "flip-flop"–type footwear, because your feet can shift or slip on or in them. Pay attention. Unwanted movement of your feet will add to the instability and clumsiness you feel.

For those living in a culture where shoes are almost always worn, it is more typical for people with movement impairments to be more unstable when they're not wearing shoes. In large part this is because their shoes provide more surface area for support. Another reason. Their feet flex more easily without the shoes, and they have difficulty controlling that added movement in their feet.

For those with movement issues who are accustomed to *not* wearing shoes, wearing them tends to increase their instability because the shoes hinder the flexing of their feet.

Relative to the size of the foot, the sole of the shoe provides a larger area of support on the floor. Those with moderately to significantly impaired movements frequently require the stiffer and wider platform the shoes provide. However, many people with mildly impaired movements will often find that a stiffer shoe restricts their movements more than it helps.

Another issue: The visual input from our eyes is an important part of our equilibrium that many people require for stable standing and walking. Thus, many people with problem movements have difficulties with balance when they're in an area that is poorly lighted. Getting out of bed at night in the darkness is a good example. They become clumsier because that visual input is missing. So, to help avoid

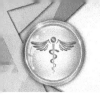

darkened nighttime misadventures and prevent stubbed toes and bruised noses, use night-lights. The soft light will help them avoid some of the issues they encounter.

ASSISTIVE DEVICES

The simple object so many people put their unconditional trust in for their safety and well-being is too often abused and improperly used. As an example, they do not realize that the way they use a walker is creating additional movement and instability problems. A common issue is leaning forward and pushing upper-body weight into their hands and into the walker. This applies angled pressure into the walker, making both it and the person less stable, because the non-wheeled walker is designed to have equal pressure applied into the four legs. Further, it is **NOT** meant to be used as primary support, and many people do use it for too much support. This topic will be covered in detail throughout the book.

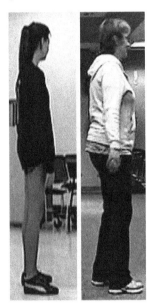

FIGURE 6.1: Standing upright, in the first stance.

The first stance is merely standing upright on your own with stability and balance, as shown in Figure 6.1. For those who sway like a tree in the wind when standing without touching anything, use your binky (an assistive device—yes, I sometimes refer to them by the name some people use for a baby's pacifier) or another object.

If you need to use external support, use it. This could involve standing behind a heavy chair, in front of the kitchen countertop, or facing anything heavy, stable, and about the height of your waist. The goal is to have your hands, but more preferably your fingers only, on it to provide the extra stability you require without leaning on it for primary support. This means the pressure in your hands and fingers should be rather light. This is not cheating. It is merely using a tool to help you learn the required skill, so later you'll have the ability not to need that tool.

When you overuse, lean on, or push excessively on what you're using, this will cause problems and prevent you from accomplishing the goal of the stance. When you use this type of excessive upper-body dependency, your posture will be restricted and the pressure in your feet will be altered. In this overdependent posture, when the object you're using for support moves, unpleasant consequences are the result.

Suppose you're using a chair that moves without much effort. If you push straight down toward the floor equally through all its legs, it most likely will not move, or will move only slightly. But when you lean against the movable chair at an angle, you will push more pressure into one or two of its legs, and it will move very easily. Hint: The same happens with your walker.

So, what typically happens when a person with problem movements has difficulty standing, and then leans on something? When that object moves, their body moves with it, *but their feet do not*. Then the scary stuff happens as they react to the sudden unexpected movement. To prevent this, do not lean or push on objects at an angle. Use your feet and legs for more support than you are and stand with a more upright posture. This is common sense. However, trusting and understanding how not to lean or push on something while keeping your body stable is challenging for many movement-impaired people, and for those with weakened leg strength.

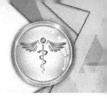

Beware when using a walker—your binky. They are lightweight. Without wheels, they can be easily tipped. With wheels, they can be easily pushed away. Yes, many of them have brakes. But for many people, this just means they will lean on and abuse the walker even more, necessitating an excessive use of the hand brakes to stop the walker's forward movement.

An "assistive device" is intended to provide partial support, not total support. It is *not* a replacement for your legs and feet. It is *not* something that is designed to save you from yourself. By design, it is only meant to be a tool to help you stabilize your posture using your feet and legs. When you use it properly, it allows you to help yourself better than you could without it. But when you use it *improperly*, the problems you create force you to become more dependent on it, and that makes your movements deteriorate further.

Consider these two questions. How intelligent are the inanimate assistive devices people use? The answer is, not at all. And how much can those objects do on their own? Absolutely nothing.

So then, exactly how are these objects supposed to keep you safe and prevent you from falling? By themselves, they simply cannot. You are using these objects *to help YOU keep yourself safe*. Therefore, you—not your binky, or anything or anyone else—you are responsible for your own stability and safety. So, to those of you who have surrendered this part of your responsibility, now is the time for you to begin the process of taking it back.

What am I *not* saying here? I am not saying you should stop using these things for support when you clearly need them. If you need them, use them. But use them more appropriately, with common sense. Use them, but do not abuse them or yourself. Do not surrender your responsibility, because you need it to reach your movement ability goals.

To recover *any* natural movement ability, you must have the independent ability to stand with stability on your feet. Some of you will say, "But I don't have a choice. I can't do that on my own." This is true for some, but for many it is not. Many people have the physical ability to stand stable on their feet but don't know how to make it possible.

What is behind the "I can't" statement? Is it inadequate strength or coordination, shaky legs, lack of trust, or flat-out fear? For many, all these things play some role. For others, only a few of them apply. How these physical and psychological issues affect anyone is a guess until each person learns the truth about themselves. This requires an honest examination.

Adjusting the Location of the Pressure in Your Feet

In Chapter 5, the emphasis was on creating and standing with feet flat on the floor. Do that now. Feel the stability of having equal weight (pressure) on the heel and ball areas of both feet, with the same amount of pressure going into each foot. Now remind yourself how small and slow shoulder movements change the distribution (the location) of the pressure in your feet.

Stand with your feet flat on the floor and make yourself as comfortable and stable as you can. How far apart are they? Most likely you have them where they feel right to you, and for now that is where they need to be. What is the point? When standing in place, it does not matter how far apart or how close your feet are positioned. The only thing that matters is you are stable and comfortable. However, when you begin a movement it matters a great deal how your feet are on the floor.

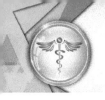
Now get as comfortable as you can while standing upright, and keeping your feet flat on the floor with knees relatively straight. Next, feel where the pressure is in your feet. It should be evenly distributed between both feet, and equal in the ball area and heel of each foot. If it is not, get it as close to this as you can before we begin experimenting with upper body movements. For those feeling unstable, you should lightly hold onto something secure that will help you relax and stabilize.

Begin by **slightly and very slowly** moving your shoulders backward. As you *slowly* move them *only slightly* backward, the pressure in the heels of your feet increases, and the pressure in the ball areas decreases. It is very important that you feel this pressure change happening. And at the same time, what do you feel happening with your stability and posture?

Now reverse it. Begin with your feet flat, equal pressure in the ball areas and heels, then **slightly and very slowly** move your shoulders forward until you *begin* to feel the pressure increase in the ball areas. As your shoulders move forward, the pressure increases in the ball areas and decreases in the heels. Repeat these small shoulder movements to more easily recognize and feel the small pressure changes in your feet. If you are anxious or unstable, you'll have a difficult time with this. The more comfortable and relaxed you are, the easier it will be to feel.

With guarding and stiffness in their posture, many people with impaired movements frequently stand with straightened knees, as do many with balance issues and generalized weakness. With straightened knees, smaller movements of the shoulders create larger pressure changes in the feet, and the change happens more quickly. The suddenness of this change often becomes difficult to control and creates increasing instability. So, what creates the suddenness? Rapid and excessive shoulder movements. This issue must be recognized and corrected. Otherwise, improving stabilized standing and movements will not happen.

You must play with this to understand it. Make both feet flat on the floor. *Slowly* move your shoulders to move the pressure in your feet so it is evenly spread between the ball and heel areas of both feet. You'll know they're flat by feeling that your body is more stable, and also feel how you are better able to relax. Now pay very close attention to how stable, steady, and relaxed the rest of your body is in this more balanced posture. Seeing it happening in a mirror helps. You see the movement and feel the result in your feet. When the pressure *begins to increase* in the ball or heel areas, stop moving your shoulders and feel what has happened to your posture and stability. Then slowly move your shoulders back toward a better feeling of flat feet, to where it's easier to keep your body relaxed. It is important to pay very close attention to how little your shoulders physically move to make a big difference in the pressure you feel in your feet.

Now, *carefully and slowly* see how much farther your shoulders move forward before you begin to feel unsteady on the ball areas and toes. Then do the same with shoulders moving back to feel the unsteadiness developing in your heels.

In each direction, how far did your shoulders move before you felt your body tipping? The answer: not much. With straightened knees, the distance your shoulders move is very small before you go from flat and stable feet to tipping off the front or back of your feet. *From being unsteady in the front to unsteady in the back, the distance your shoulders physically move is surprisingly small.* Carefully repeat doing this until you completely understand and convince yourself of what you feel in your feet.

1. In an upright posture, as you move your shoulders forward past your knees, the pressure in the forward part of your feet increases.

2. In an upright posture, as you move your shoulders backward past your knees, the pressure in your heels increases.

Got it? You **must** know, feel, and fully understand this before what is to come will make sense.

TO THE SIDE

Next, we'll repeat this same exercise moving your shoulders slowly from side to side, to shift the pressure from side to side in your feet. BUT, before you begin, I must offer a word of **caution**. Do this *very slowly. Stop* the sideward movement of your shoulders when you feel a small amount of pressure change in the sides of your feet. Too fast or too much sideward movement of the shoulders can quickly cause you to tip and fall to the side they're moving toward.

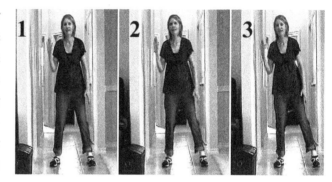

FIGURE 6.2: Standing beside a wall is a good idea. When you move your shoulders too far, the wall will stop your tipping body. A hallway provides that support on both sides at the same time.

Therefore, please take precautions. Stand with your feet approximately shoulder width apart. Also, stand beside a wall on the side you're leaning toward, to stop a tipping fall if it should happen. Begin with the shoulder nearest the wall approximately one of your foot lengths away from the wall, and then adjust that distance according to your comfort level, as shown in Figure 6.2. Then, to practice in the other direction, simply turn around to face the opposite direction. An easier option is standing in a hallway that's about four feet wide. This provides you with a wall on both sides.

Keeping your knees relatively straight, very carefully and **very slowly** move your shoulders toward the right wall and feel the pressure *increasing on the outside half of your right foot*. At the same time, feel the total pressure in your left foot decreasing, as the pressure moves toward the inside of the left foot.

Now **very slowly** move your shoulders back to center your body over flattened feet, where you feel balanced and more stable. Stop here for a moment to feel it and to again relax your posture. Next, **very slowly** move your shoulders toward the wall on the left. The pressure increases in the outside half of the left foot, as the total pressure decreases in the right foot and moves toward the inside of the right foot.

When you become comfortable with this, it's time to experiment with additional shoulder movement. **Slowly** move your shoulders toward the foot nearest the wall until you begin to feel the pressure increasing on the outside of that foot, pause, and then continue moving your shoulders **very slowly** toward the wall. As your shoulders move farther, pay special attention to the increasing pressure on the outside of the foot next to the wall. As this pressure continues to increase, your comfort level is going, going, and

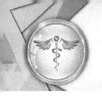

suddenly gone. As you continue with the shoulder movement, suddenly your body is forced to tip to the wall. While this is happening, also pay very close attention to how quickly the other foot loses pressure and eventually is pulled off the floor.

There is a critical point of no return as you continue moving your shoulders to the side. That is what you are feeling in your foot. The point of no return is when the increasing pressure in the outside of your foot reaches the point where that increasing and concentrating pressure quickly pushes your body to the side. Your tipping body suddenly becomes fast-moving, and is too often unstoppable. This is why those with impaired movements need the wall beside them. This is why they complain they suddenly fall during the day. "One second I'm okay, and the next I'm on the floor!" Now, about that comment. Note that your body *did not fall* into the wall as you were practicing. It was pushed into the wall.

Staying in an upright posture while allowing your shoulder to tip and then push you into the wall is showing you something important happening in your feet. In this example, you began using the entire surface area (100 percent) of the bottoms of *both feet*. Then, when the pressure in the outside of one foot forced the shoulder to tip to the wall, you were using only about half of the surface area of *one foot*. At the point of no return, your body is being supported by just the outside of one foot, which is approximately 25 percent of the total surface area of both feet. The important point: You *destroy your foundation and stability with excessive shoulder (upper-body) movement*. This is an issue many people with balance and movement problems create for themselves every day, and it is mostly preventable.

Excessive upper-body movement causes two of the scariest situations these people live with: feeling they are *falling to the side* and *falling backward*. But no, they are not falling. They push themselves to the side and have nothing but an outstretched arm to help stop their fall. Then, by straightening and moving their shoulders backward, they frequently also tip backward when they overreact to the scary tipping-sideways feeling. With increasing pressure in the outside of the foot, this also is why the resulting *pushing* accident is commonly to the back corner. They suddenly and violently push themselves into a situation with no ability to recover, and do not understand why it keeps happening.

Practice all these controlled shoulder-movement exercises, including the excessive movement, and absolutely prove the effects to yourself. Also, hold your knees straight on purpose to feel the more sudden effects of shoulder movements. Know what is happening and why it's happening. Feel how a small amount of upper-body movement on straight knees quickly creates unpleasant results. Understand the good and not-so-good feelings of the pressure in your feet, and learn how to control where the pressure needs to be.

PRESSURE IN THE HEEL AREA

Let's move on to the big problem of increased heel pressure. Many people with balance and movement problems, especially those with a neurodegenerative cause, stand and walk with increased heel pressure: unknowingly setting themselves up for added problems.

Doing the following heel-pressure exercise in a hallway is a great idea because then you will also have a wall in front of you if you need it. The rationale for this comes from a common reaction to the feeling of tipping and falling backward. In an attempt to stop the backward "fall," many people with balance

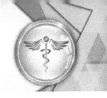

and movement problems will push themselves forward in a reactionary, quickened, and excessive forward upper-body movement. This can easily result in a forward tip or push from their toes when trying to prevent the backward push from their heels. So, when you feel unsteady on your feet, if possible, use a hallway when you practice. You will be very thankful to have another protective wall in front of you when you need it.

Stand with your back toward one wall. Position the heels of your shoes approximately one of your foot lengths away from the wall that's behind you, and then stand upright with relatively straight knees. Now **very slowly** move your shoulders back. Feel the pressure quickly increasing in your heels. Slowly and carefully repeat this, from flat-feeling feet to slightly increased pressure in your heels, and then back to flat feet. You need to understand this changing-pressure feeling very well, because this is how you unknowingly create it in your stance and movements. You are also learning how to correct the heel-heavy pushing problem: Moving your shoulders slightly forward in a controlled manner to avoid it.

Now, doing this again, pay attention to how quickly you begin to feel unstable as you move your shoulders backward just a little bit more. GO SLOWLY! Also note that the pressure in the ball areas of your feet becomes very light at the same time the heel pressure increases. Just as happened when you did this on the outside of the foot going sideways, you will very quickly move to the point of no return in the heel area as your shoulders move backward.

With the wall behind you, carefully experiment with that point of no return. With slow and controlled backward shoulder movements, feel how easy it is for your shoulders to suddenly be pushed to the wall. Learn to very quickly recognize the good pressure, the not-so-good pressure, and the point of no return that pushes you into a tip. This is vitally important.

Remember what else you are learning:

1. The movement of your upper body determines, adjusts, and controls the location of the pressure in your feet.

2. The location and distribution of the pressure in your feet determines your stability.

3. Your body is moved (pushed) by the increased pressure in an area of your feet, or foot.

INDUCED STIFFNESS

Some people with balance and movement problems also have a tense (guarded) posture. When their upper body is tense so is the lower body. When their arms and shoulders are tense, it is likely their knee movements are restricted.

Stand upright, knees straight, stay on flat feet, and focus your "feeling" attention on the *sides* of your knees. (Note: What you are intending to feel is relatively subtle and may take added time for some to notice.)

1. Act as if you are out-of-control angry. Tense your entire body and make hard fists with both hands. What happens in your knees?

Then relax your hands and arms without changing your posture. What happens to your knees? If you don't feel anything change, do it again with more vigor, exaggerate all of it, and pay closer attention to the outside parts of your knees. Feel it, then let your hands relax to feel the tension in your knees fade.

2. Standing upright with straightened knees, shrug your shoulders high and feel what happens in your knees. The forced **high** shrug of your shoulders adds slight tension to your knees. Now relax your shoulders while keeping your knees straight. The slight tension in your knees is released.

    The mild tensing and relaxing of your knees is very subtle as you do this, so pay very close attention.

3. Stand very upright on flat-feeling feet, and stay on them. With both arms down at your sides, straighten and stiffen your arms, and shrug your shoulders up. What happens to your knees? Stiffness increases in them.

4. Do this straight-armed shoulder shrug again while redirecting your attention to the pressure on the entire surface area of your feet on the floor. What happens?

    With stiffened arms at your sides and shoulders stiffly moved upward, the total pressure in your feet *slightly* decreases. Then, when you relax your shoulders and arms, the pressure in your feet is restored.

    Again, this change is quite subtle and requires very close attention.

If you cannot feel the pressure changes in your feet as described, but you are stable when standing, practicing the second stance will help wake you up to them.

Hint: it is easier to feel pressure in your feet when you mind is relaxed and quiet.

■ ■ ■

CHAPTER 7

SECOND STANCE: THE READY STANCE

Beware of missing the obvious.

To be successful in any movement, our body must be properly prepared for what we want it to do. Otherwise, the result of the then "forced" movement will not be what was expected. A forced movement too often results in poorly controlled, erratic, and reactive body movements that lead to instability and falls. This is the unfortunate dilemma many people with balance and movement problems deal with every day. With a tensed (guarded) posture interfering with natural preparation, the outcomes of many of their movements register on a scale from unsteady and unpleasant, to frightening and disastrous.

The "ready stance" is the foundation stance we use to begin the vast majority of our movements and activities. Walking, jogging, moving around the house or office, playing sports, or shopping in stores, the ready stance posture is our natural preparation.

The ready stance always involves some degree of flexing of multiple joints of the body. This is required to provide the necessary coordinated and cooperative bodily movements. In picture 1 of Figure 7.1, Ant is in an upright posture, standing in the first stance. Then in picture 2, he moves into a ready stance. Test question: Where is the increased pressure located in his feet? It is toward his heels in both pictures. Why and how? Look at his postural alignment. He is holding his shoulders back.

The ready stance is variable in how low or high it needs to be. However, it is always very specific to the movement we are preparing to do, are doing, or have just completed. In natural movements, the required posture *is not a conscious decision* we make. It is quite the opposite.

Naturally, *the required posture is set to create the pressure in the feet that is required for the task of the movement.* Thus, the posture is set according to that person's correct feeling for their movement. And what creates the correct feeling? The stability and comfort of the pressure in our feet, or foot, and the relaxed body.

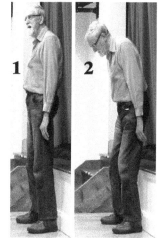

FIGURE 7.1: From the first stance to a high second stance.

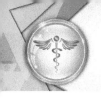

In this context, we reflexively adjust our posture in a coordinated and cooperative manner. Naturally, our posture is determined by what our relaxed body is required to do to keep us stable on our feet. In the example seen in Figure 7.2, Ant lowers his body with flexing knees, ankles, and hips. As the relaxed joints move, body parts are moved equally and opposite to counterbalance one another (per weight). For example, the head, shoulders, and knees moving forward counterbalance the hip area moving backward.

This is a very important point. Our natural movements are "thoughtless" movements when our relaxed body can adjust itself to the correct posture, and the correct posture sets and controls the required pressure in our feet for the stance and movement. Without thought we immediately recognize the feelings of the correct posture as comfortable and stable, and this is what we trustfully use in our movements and activities.

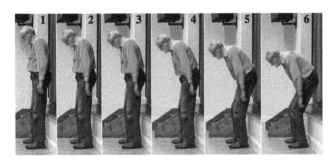

FIGURE 7.2: Ant is in the first stance in picture 1. In the remaining pictures, he's in the second stance and moving into a squat.

The intent and purpose of the movement is a creation of the mind. However, the movement itself is a reflexive counterbalancing creation of the body, to satisfy the desires of the mind. And importantly, the mind does not consciously control the body's movements—unless something doesn't go as expected.

PREPARATION

As we proceed through the six stances (postures), you will frequently be reminded to first move into a ready stance, relax, and focus on the correct feeling of the pressure in your feet. This reminder is necessary to bring your attention back to what many of you will forget to apply.

There is much to understand and remember about your posture and movements as we proceed. Therefore, until this information makes sense to you and is easier to use, *you may have difficulty applying it*. BUT please do not try to memorize any of it. Why? This information, this practical intellectual understanding of your movement ability that you are learning, is **not** meant to be memorized. Rather, you must learn how to use it, and recognize it without thought, just as you have done all of your life before you had any movement issues.

POSTURAL CONTROL

If you can't control your posture, you won't have control of your movements.

In the first stance, we use *static* postural control. Static postural control means having the ability to stand comfortably *in place* without bodily movement, with a firm and stable foundation. The second stance (the ready stance) is an introduction to *dynamic* postural control. Dynamic postural control refers to the coordinated independent and dependent movements of parts of the body. It refers to the stabilized

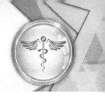

reflexive and coordinated, equal and opposite movements of the body's different parts. For those with a restrictive posture, this is challenging because the movements of the upper and the lower parts of the body are limited, and less coordinated with one another.

MOVING INTO A READY STANCE

The ready stance is critical to natural movement ability, because we rely on it for the preparation and completion of most of our movements. Therefore, the unsteady movement-impaired person should begin every movement from a ready stance posture (a prepared posture) with flattened feet on the floor, and return to it after the movement when possible. This helps ensure a more stable and balanced movement.

For those of you with guarding or stiffening (tension) in your posture, you should do the following to better prepare your body for movement. Before you move from an upright posture to a ready stance, remind yourself to relax your hands and arms, to relax your shoulders. Practice doing this in front of a mirror to see what you are feeling and doing. This relaxing movement of the shoulders is not slouching them forward, stooping the upper body forward, or pulling the shoulders backward. Simply allow them to relax downward on their own accord.

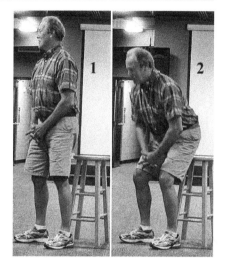

FIGURE 7.3: "Bottom down, sit" to begin the squat with a relaxed posture. Start the movement with your hips moving back and down, as you allow your shoulders to move forward and knees to flex forward and down.

Then with shoulders more relaxed, focus on your knees. When tensed shoulders relax, the knees will also begin to feel and become more relaxed. When they do, you will begin to feel the effects of slightly improved stability, because your body will be more relaxed and functioning better; because the guarding and stiffening has been reduced. It is this small bit of improved stability that will allow you to relax and lower more comfortably into a ready stance.

To help you transition from standing upright to a ready stance, try this next exercise. Use a stool that's only a few inches lower than your bottom, as shown in Figure 7.3. Now relax and simply sit down on the stool.

As Richie is practicing sitting on the stool, he is moving from an upright posture into a ready stance. As he is flexing his knees forward and down, his shoulders move forward to match the movement of his knees. The other movement you see is his hips moving backward to counter the movement of his knees and the forward movement of his upper body. This is an example of coordinated counterbalancing postural adjustments.

You do not need a stool to practice this movement. All you need is a relaxed body and stabilized feet on the floor, and then simply imagine you are *starting* to sit down. Some can do this movement easily by just relaxing and then bending their knees. Others need to imagine they are pushing their *bottom out and down* to sit, to do the very same thing. It doesn't matter which focus you use. What matters is the movement itself, and getting relaxed so your body can do it in a coordinated manner.

Allowing the knees and shoulders to flex forward as the hips move slightly backward and down is frequently problematic for people with a tensed posture. The typical problems are:

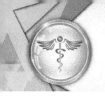

1. They cannot relax their posture enough to allow it to happen.

2. They overfocus on moving one part. Then the movement of another part is restricted.

3. Living with a tensed posture, they learn to overuse their upper body in their movements while underusing their knees.

4. Because of this, they begin by stooping forward from their hips rather than beginning to squat down with their knees and hips.

Lowering into a Ready Stance, Increasing Heel Pressure

When you bend your knees to move into a ready stance, do you feel increased pressure moving into your heels? When you do, the most common reason is that you are unintentionally holding your shoulders back. Be careful with this. During the movement, the pressure can increase in the heel area quicker than expected, causing a tip backward. This uncoordinated movement happens most when the posture is tensed. It also happens when you think too much about how to do the movement. Pay attention. When you first feel pressure moving into your heels, stop and correct it by moving your shoulders forward.

Standing Up Again

When you're in a ready stance, to return to an upright posture, simply reverse the squatting (sitting) movement. However, people with a tensed (guarded) posture frequently have issues with this movement as well. Common problems are straightening the knees too much and too quickly when standing, moving their upper bodies up and back too far and pushing their pelvis forward. Any combination of these mistakes can lead to instability, and typically a backward tip due to increased heel pressure.

Adding and Holding Pressure

As you move downward into a ready stance, feel for the small change that happens to the pressure in your feet. As your body descends, the pressure in your feet increases. The squatting movement forces muscles in your legs to do more work, and the increasing pressure is coming from this extra work. This pressure increase can be difficult to feel when still in a high ready stance. So, continue to lower down in a stable squatting movement until you begin to feel it.

Naturally, the muscles in our legs are always working to provide added pressure to the feet, because that is what is required to keep us stable in everything we do on our feet. We never stop applying this added stabilizing pressure, but we do fluctuate the amount.

But many people with balance and movement problems return to standing and release this added foot pressure. This is due to instability and a tensed posture, because their tensed leg muscles are doing less productive work.

They release it for two reasons. First, the location of the pressure in their feet changes during the movement. And secondly, they frequently straighten their knees too quickly.

To keep the muscles working, do the following. As you begin to lower yourself into a ready stance, imagine you're trying to flatten something under your feet. Or imagine you're trying to push the floor down a few inches as you lower into the ready stance. Keeping your feet flat, after you've lowered your body about six inches, feel the extra pressure you've created. This will feel like a heaviness in your feet. This is the feeling you want to keep as you return to standing more upright. But how?

To move back into the upright stance while keeping the increased pressure, use and feel the same push down into the floor as you did to lower into the ready stance. Push down into the floor and allow your knees to move, while keeping the location of the pressure in your feet stable. Do this by maintaining the proper shoulder position, and by allowing your shoulders to also slowly move upward. To more easily coordinate this knee and shoulder movement, practice it using only your eyes to guide the movement.

When you are relaxed, your head will gently tilt up as your eyes move upward to look up and lead the standing up movement. So, stand up using only your eyes, to look up to the level of a light switch on the wall, or a door knob/handle for example. Relaxing into the movement, your knees and shoulders will follow in the more natural movement, provided you do not try to control them.

Do not stop pushing down into the floor. Hold that pressure as you stand up. Now answer the same questions about how you feel. Are you more stable? If you've done this correctly, yes, you are.

Very importantly, every movement begins, continues, and ends with a stabilizing push down into your feet. Without it, our movements are hampered by limitations and inabilities.

Hinged in the Middle

When our ability to control and coordinate the connection between our upper and lower body is challenging, each and every posture, stance, and movement will be a problem. The upper and lower halves of the body function properly only when they serve as the structural support for the other half. So, functionally they are strictly dependent on each other.

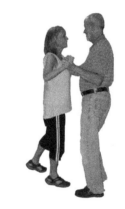

FIGURE 7.4: Tango lessons. Vicky and Jay enjoying the fun while learning to move into and stay in a ready stance.

Ready, Set, Go

In Figure 7.4, one person has a mild-to-moderate movement impairment. Compare their postures for the clues. See the difference. One is more relaxed than the other. This small difference in posture and flexibility makes a big difference in our natural movement ability. Vicki and Jay: One of them very much wanted to learn tango steps, but a "disabling condition" took that dream away.

Many people with balance and movement problems, especially those with a neurodegenerative movement impairment, cast themselves deeper into inability, even though they still have a great deal of normal function. They do this because *they don't know how not to*. Because of the movement problems they're experiencing, and those they suspect they will have, many people stop doing or trying things they would love to be doing.

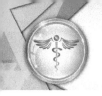

The first part of reversing this trend is knowing how to stabilize your body on your feet in a ready stance. The next part is learning how to remain stabilized during movement.

Working harder is not the answer.
Working smarter is.

PROBLEMS WITH THE STANCE

Standing up "too straight." When we do something long enough, it becomes the way we will always do it. The conscious and subconscious mind accepts that this is what we are required to do, because this is what we always do.

With the knees flexed, muscles in the legs support most of the body's weight. Standing with knees straight, the bones of the legs are supporting the body's weight. It is common to see people with natural ability standing with shoulders held back and hips pushed forward. This is a "lazy" way of standing because it requires less work. The knees are held straight and give the leg muscles a break from work. Is it wrong to stand with knees held straight? No. It only becomes a problem when the person cannot *easily and quickly* move off of straight knees and flex their knees.

Beverly's movements are mildly impaired. In picture 1 of Figure 7.5, she is standing as she normally does. Importantly, she doesn't stand this way because of leg weakness. Her knees work just fine.

So, why does she stand with her hips forward, knees straight, and shoulders held back? She adapted to it because she has been experiencing mild imbalance and clumsiness when standing and walking. Mild issues frequently cause reactions that lead to dramatic postural changes, and then additional movement problems develop. Initially this posture worked for her, but then her imbalance and clumsiness returned, with an added ingredient. She has been tipping and falling backward. In picture 5, do you see why?

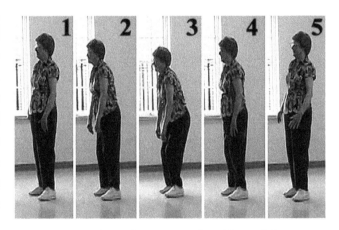

FIGURE 7.5: In the early stages with mild instability, many people develop the habit of standing on straightened knees while moving their hips forward and shoulders backward. This creates additional problems.

Many movement-impaired people dealing with clumsiness become accustomed to standing with straightened knees. To avoid bending their knees, they learn to push their hips forward and pull their shoulders back. This flattens their feet on the floor, or more commonly puts only a small amount of increased pressure in their heels, as shown in picture 1. Standing is easier and they feel more stable, because they've removed the need to control their knees and have reduced the work they must do. This allows them to relax while still achieving standing stability. For those with otherwise natural ability, this is an adaptive behavior for standing. However, it is a *maladaptive behavior when used for function and movement*, as many people with a movement impairment do.

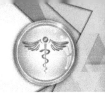

In this example, Beverly was asked to make her feet flat in picture 1, then move into a ready stance, and then return to standing upright while staying on flat feet the entire time.

In picture 1, she is stable. In picture 2, she corrects her posture for the movement by moving her hips back and shoulders forward, and flexing her knees. In picture 3, she lowers herself with flexing knees and hips, and then, in picture 4, she returns to a natural upright posture on flat feet. Consciously, she stopped in picture 4, but subconsciously she then continued moving into a straightened-knee posture. What does this mean? At the time, she was **un**aware that she had changed her posture from picture 4 to that seen in 5. What was the result?

In picture 4, she was very stable. Then, as soon as her knees straightened (picture 5), she said, "I'm feeling a little unstable."

Look at her left hand. It was relaxed, and now it isn't. Now compare her postural alignment to the vertical edge of the window in the picture. Her upper body is tilted farther back than it was in picture 1. This is typical for many people with a restrictive-posture movement impairment. They return to the wrong posture because that is where they subconsciously think they should be.

They create their own instability with uncontrolled and overcontrolled postural straightening and exaggerated upper-body movements. Much of this is because the correct feeling does not feel right to them in their mind. But they will not stop to feel and compare the actual difference. Why? First, the thought never enters their mind. Second, they typically are moving too fast between the beginning and end of the movement to notice. In the process, they're learning not to trust their ability as their fear of instability and falling increases, and they remain completely unaware that they are causing much of the problem they're desperately trying to avoid.

Because of this early maladaptive "reset" in her subconscious mind, Beverly could not recognize the naturally steadying posture she continued moving through. She had been very stable while consciously paying attention to keeping her feet flat in pictures 2 through 4. From evenly distributed pressure in picture 4, she moves increased pressure into her heels in picture 5, and that pressure is pushing her backward. This sudden change in posture also removes needed downward stabilizing pressure from her feet. How? In picture 4, the muscles in her thighs are naturally working and pushing added pressure into her feet. In picture 5, as her posture is stiffening in response to the backward tip, more of the work of her thigh muscles is directed to holding her knees straight.

She unnecessarily created the instability she hates to feel, and her response to it created more. This is common in people with balance problems, and *it is correctable*.

Weakness, Fear, and Instability

Individually, each person's reaction to their weakness, fear, and instability dictates how restrictive their posture will become through guarding and stiffness. Their reactions will place them in one of two categories.

1. Those with more guarding and stiffening are intimidated and very reluctant to flex their knees *and* hips. The result: They develop exaggerated stiffened and upright postures when standing and moving. These people seldom feel comfortable on their feet.

2. Those with less guarding and stiffness are also intimidated and very reluctant to flex their knees.

Thus, they often look more relaxed than they are when standing, and will then stiffen in varying amounts when moving. Consequently, many of them often develop stooping as their preferred alternative to squatting. The result: Depending on how stable or unstable they feel, this group will alternate between squatting and stooping.

Postural guarding, and especially stiffening, always limit the functioning of the knees, and to a lesser degree the hips. This forces the improper use and overuse of the upper body in an attempt to compensate for the underuse and dysfunction of the legs. This destroys coordinated and purposeful movement. The initiation and performance of the movement are reversed, and the cooperative nature of both the upper and lower body is very limited.

Inappropriately used leg muscles weaken. Instability worsens. Fear strengthens. The cause and effect that follows is a downward spiral into inability and dependency.

Susie's movement impairment is moderate. With *slightly* flexing stiffened knees, she is relatively stable in picture 1 of Figure 7.6. This is because her bottom is close to counterbalancing her stooping-forward upper body. But then in picture 3, her bottom has moved forward more than her upper body moved upward. Now she is unstable, tipping forward due to increased pressure in the ball areas and toes of her feet. In response to the instability and forward tip, she straightens her knees (indicated by the red arrows). To counteract and

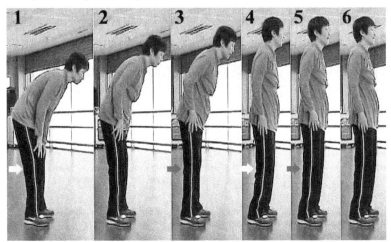

FIGURE 7.6: Resistant, stiff knees. The yellow arrows point to a small flex of the knee. The red arrows point to a straight knee.

stop the forward tipping, she uses the muscles in her calves to push added *downward* pressure into the ball areas of her feet.

The inserted yellow arrows point to slightly flexing knees. The red arrows point to straightened knees. Note how the straight knees coincide with postural instability.

Susie's legs are weakened from years of limited use with extended (straightened) knees, so now when asked to squat, she stoops forward from the hips with straightened knees (as shown in picture 1), rather than squatting with flexing knees. This forward stooping movement of the upper body often applies increased pressure in the ball areas and toes of the feet, and that causes her to tip forward. The tipping issue is the reason many of the movement-impaired people learn to overuse their calf muscles to stop the forward tip, and then chronically use them when it's not necessary.

Susie returns to an upright posture by raising her upper body (using core muscles) while also pushing into the ball areas of her feet to prevent a forward tip. In her movements, her upper body and hips move freely, but her knees move very little. This non-movement of the knees promotes instability.

When she feels unstable, her knees are straightened and stiffened (red arrows). When she's feeling more stable, her knees are slightly flexed (yellow arrows). In the fifth picture, she is mildly unstable with slightly increased pressure in her heels.

In Figure 7.5, Beverly has flexible knees. In Figure 7.6, Susie does not. When returning to standing, they both end up in the same function-restricting posture. To the casual observer, the issues with these two women appear to be different, but they are the same. Susie is merely farther along in living with her instability issues than Beverly is.

STOOPING

In Figure 7.7, Arpi's movement impairment is moderate to significant, and her knees resist flexing more than Susie's.

In picture 1, she has just moved into a ready stance from standing upright. Note that her shoulders are a little too far forward, which chronic stoopers do more than not. In this posture, she has increased

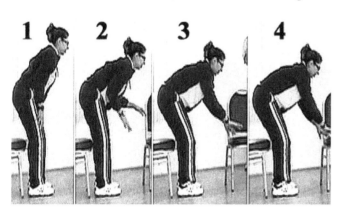

FIGURE 7.7: Stiffening of the posture is a reaction to instability and fear. It is an attempt to reduce instability and gain better control of the body and movement. But the increased stiffness, especially in the knees, restricts the functioning of the body, causing added instability.

pressure in the ball areas and toes. However, she does not use her calf muscles to compensate. Instead she continues the stoop, moves her bottom backward, and then flexes her knees slightly to stabilize on her feet.

Imagine how much improved standing stability, and ability, Susie and Arpi would have if they used a squatting movement instead of a stooping movement. Correcting a chronic stooping movement is challenging.

Arpi's legs and core muscles are just as strong as Susie's. Their instability and fear levels are also very much the same, and they both resist flexing their knees. But Susie has better use of her legs and pushes more pressure into her feet.

Yes, Arpi does flex her knees slightly more than Susie does, but then she stiffly holds them in this position. This reduces natural function of the involved muscles, lessens downward pressure in the feet, and creates instability.

Arpi increases her forward stooping rather than squatting. This increases her instability with quickly increasing pressure moving into the ball areas and toes of her feet. This also creates additional reactive stiffening of the slightly flexed knees. But the good thing about this is that she keeps them slightly flexed. This allows her to move her hips back, as seen in picture 3, and remain relatively stable on her feet. If she hadn't flexed her knees, she would have been applying a great deal of backward pressure to them and to her heels.

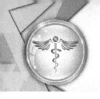

HYPEREXTENDING KNEES, NO READY STANCE

Stooping, instability, stiff *straightened* knees, and fear: This combination applies increased back pressure to the knees and, in time, pushes them farther back. Continually repeated over years, this excessive back pressure stretches the supporting ligaments of the knee joints. This allows the knees to move farther backward beyond their natural anatomical limit. Pushed into an unnatural hyperextended position, the function of the joint is compromised, and the stretching diminishes the integrity of the joint capsule.

When the supporting capsule and ligaments of the knee joint have been unnaturally stretched by the knee repeatedly moving into hyperextension, the *only* way these people can stand on their legs is with the knees "popped" backward. Why? With the weakness of the muscles and damage to the joint-capsule integrity, it becomes very difficult for them to control the position and movement of their knees. Through many years of excessive forward upper-body movements with straightened knees, the legs eventually weaken to the point where they essentially function as uncontrollable "stilts" with a free-moving joint in the middle.

Stooping causes it and stooping maintains it. The upper body must be forward to supply the back pressure on the knee to "pop" the knee backward in place and hold it there. This locks the person on their stilts. Now they support their body weight with the backward-angled bones of the legs, without the need to use their leg muscles. This is why people with hyperextended knees have a less-stiffened posture when standing, but they are forced to rely on something or someone for stability.

Standing on locked stilts in this manner, they can totally relax the muscles in their legs. The problem is, this escalates their problems. The leg muscles grow weaker and atrophy while the joint capsules of the knees are increasingly stretched and further destroyed. At the same time, their upper-body strength increases from the extra use, which further drives the overdependence on the upper body for support and movement.

This evolving situation quickly becomes a complicated ordeal with eventual full dependency on the upper body for movement and support. To transfer body weight and move one leg, they must lean their upper-body forward and to the side to relieve the pressure from the opposite knee, so that it can move forward. Reducing body weight on the leg and removing back pressure for the knee allows the knee to "pop" out hyperextension. Now they are able to move the knee and foot forward. However, they will most commonly do this by dragging the foot forward with added upper-body movement. Then, when they shift their upper body to transfer body weight back onto the leg, very suddenly the knee pops backward into hyperextension.

The use of the knees is uncontrolled, reacting only to pressure—or the lack of pressure. However, this situation is not uncontrollable. It began as a destructive maladaptive behavior, a compensation to their stooping movements. They didn't realize what they were doing and were unaware of the outcome. And, as the hyper-extension of their knees became evident, they were told there was nothing they could do to avoid it. Everyone believes it is merely a direct effect of the disorder. **But it is not.**

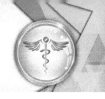

In Figure 7.8, Mandy is another unfortunate person with this condition. In this example, we were testing her ability to use her knees and *not* allow them to hyperextend when she transferred body weight onto the foot. Picture 1 shows that both knees are significantly hyperextended. Note the red lines marking the direction of the leg bones above and below the knee. The V where the lines cross shows the degree to which the knees are hyperextended. For external support, Mandy is holding and leaning onto the person beside her with her left hand and arm.

In pictures 1 through 3, she is transferring body weight to her right foot. Then, in pictures 4 through 6, she is moving her left foot forward with a flexing left knee. The green arrows in pictures 5 and 6 indicate the flexed, forward-moving left knee. Also note that in those two pictures, Mandy's right knee remains straight.

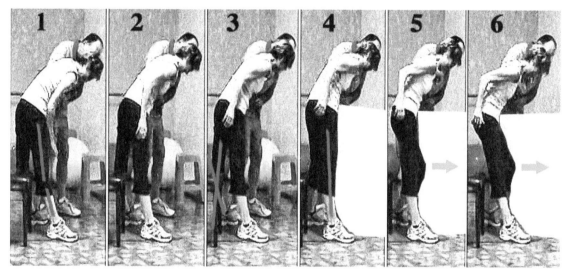

FIGURE 7.8: Mandy's knees very quickly hyperextend (backward) when she stands, making it extremely difficult for her to stand with flexed knees pointing forward. In pictures 2 and 3, she moves her right knee forward, and holds it straight in 4, as she then flexes her left knee forward. It's important to note that she is only partially bearing weight on her right leg as she flexes her left knee forward. She is leaning heavily on the person beside her. (Background in pictures 4-6 removed for clarity of left knee forward movement.)

In this example, she showed herself that her knees still work. Unfortunately, controlling the over-stretched supporting joint capsules is extremely challenging, and without the strong support of the leg muscles, it is next to impossible. Therefore, hyperextending knees are always a direct indicator of very unstable and very weak legs.

Can this condition be undone? Due to the chronic stretching damage of the joint capsule, a hyper-extending knee *is* a permanent condition. Realistically, about the only thing these people can do is work to understand how to stop their knees from popping backward. But understanding and doing that are two very different things. Once the problem has been created, the slightest error they make and, *pop*, the knee is forced backward. Therefore, the best treatment is prevention of hyperextension. To eliminate the condition, it must not be allowed to happen. Therefore, the situation that's causing it must be recognized early. In the beginning it is preventable, so the person must work to maintain

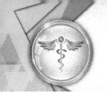

improved muscle strength and correct posture to eliminate or reduce the amount of back pressure being applied to the knee.

For those with the condition, preventing the knees from popping into hyperextension requires them to wear a very substantial and rigid brace around the joint. From experience, if it is not rigid and strong, the hyperextending knee will continue to be pushed back through the brace. The downside of bulky braces is that they are uncomfortable, especially in hot climates. Prevention is the best treatment.

As an interesting side note, Mandy and other people with this uncontrollable hyperextension problem can still drive a car, and do it well. Seated, they have near-natural control of their legs and knees. What does this mean? Again, they have more natural ability than they realize, and their knees and leg muscles still function naturally. Everything still works.

SITTING, STIFF KNEES, STIFF SHOULDERS, AND "NOT PAYING ATTENTION"

This may seem to be out of place, but it is very pertinent and something many of you need to know very early on.

With a stiffened posture, when you move from standing to sitting, you will frequently plop firmly onto your bottom. The underlying reason for this is actually obvious, and I am *not referring to your disorder or condition* as the excuse. The problem is that your bottom is moving unsupported and uncontrollably too quickly backward.

In Figure 7.9, Mary is plopping hard as she sits on the chair. More correctly stated, she is *pushing* herself into a plopping thud onto the chair. In picture 1, with a very tight grip on the back of the chair in front of her, and with her shoulders locked stiffly in place, she pushes her hips backward. She pushes her hips back because her knees are stiffly resistant to flexing more than they already are. But as you look at the sequence of pictures, it appears that her knees are flexing more than just slightly. Don't be misled. *They are not.*

In picture 2, her bottom moves closer to the chair as she continues to push her hips backward, and her shoulders also move farther back. Her shoulders are just behind her knees in picture 1, and then in picture 2, they are

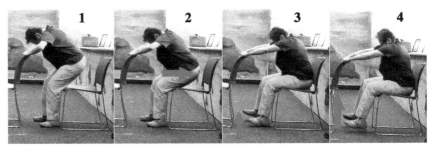

FIGURE 7.9: "Reaching for the chair with your bottom" will quickly put you on your heels. The increasing pressure in your heels pushes you backward and down into the chair, and also pulls the pressure from your feet. This is another avoidable pushing fall.

over the middle of her thighs. This upper-body movement quickly transfers increased pressure into her heels, which increases the backward push.

As pressure increases in her heels in picture 2, pressure is removed from the forward areas of her feet. Now the movement is without any control as she forcefully plops into the chair.

Again, and very importantly, Mary *did not fall into the chair*. The increasing pressure in her heels forcefully **pushed** her body quickly backward and pulled her feet from the floor, as seen in picture 4. For those wondering, yes, this is the way some people break toilet seats and toilets.

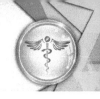

To improve your movement abilities, you must have the ability to control your posture. This is how you control the pressure in your feet and control your movements. Without this ability, you will always be without adequate control of your movements. You will always be unstable on your feet. You will always be pushing yourself into falls in every direction, thanks to the erratic and unstable pressure you create in your feet.

■ ■ ■

CHAPTER 8

RELAX THE HANDS TO RELAX THE KNEES; USE THE ELBOW TO GUIDE THE HAND

To relax tension in knees and feet,
relax tension in the arms and shoulders first.

Before they will gain the ability to improve their movement problems, people with a restrictive (tensed, guarded, stiffened) posture must first learn to release much of the tension in their body. Without the ability to relax tightened muscles, they will not improve their ability to stabilize and control the pressure in their feet, and their movements will remain a problem. This is because natural movements require a cooperative and flexible posture that their tensed muscles don't allow.

To *begin* relaxing the posture, the process must start with improved stability in their feet. For many, this means keeping the feet flattened on the floor. Then, as they begin to relax into stabilized feet, restrictive postural control is gradually replaced with a more relaxed postural control, and the body begins to work more naturally.

With a restrictive-posture movement impairment, the amount of postural guarding and stiffening often varies greatly from moment to moment. When standing and moving, the muscles of their body and feet frequently shift between extremes, from mildly stiff and mildly flexible to very stiffened and inflexible. There are many reasons this happens. For example,

1. Changes in the surface the person is standing on: soft, hard, loose, uneven, or sloping, or there are rocks, sticks, or other clutter on the ground. Another factor that complicates these things, and often dramatically, is the wind.

2. Variations in their wellness and body temperature: When rested, they typically are better. When tired, they're worse. When feeling healthy, they're better. When feeling ill, they're worse. They are often better when they're warm, and many are much worse when they're chilled.

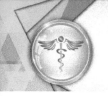

3. The presence of perceived physical obstacles or challenging characteristics of the path they would like to use. The path is narrow, or the sidewalk is uneven. There are items on the floor, or people and furniture within the space they must walk through.

The reasons people with a restrictive-posture guard, stiffen, and become fearful are endless. Sometimes the reasons make sense, but much of the time they don't. However, to the individual person, all their reasons and fears are vividly true. But to be honest, the individual reasons don't matter when considering the outcome. Why? It is because fear is fear, and to their movement-related fears, the physical reaction is always the same. Fear within the posture or movement for any reason, or from any source, leads to the same increasing postural guarding and stiffening reactions.

This part requires a great deal of emphasis. Fear is the trigger. To stop the guarding and stiffening reactions, that person's fear must first be tamed and resolved. Then the causes of the fear they believe to be true will also fade away.

Fear is psychological. The reaction to it is physical. Importantly, removing fear can only be done by the person who has it. With respect to movement, the physical response to fear can only be removed through their personal actions of creating and easily reproducing independent stability. Only then will they find the comfort and trust that will allow them to relax. Therefore, to release the psychological component, they must first resolve the physical component.

TIGHTLY HELD HANDS AND FINGERS

Consider this question: How much is a bird in the hand worth? That depends on many factors, but for our purposes it comes down to only one thing. The worth of the bird depends on how tightly you're holding it. If you gently hold the bird, it remains healthy and active, and it is worth a great deal. If you tightly hold and squeeze the bird, you will eventually kill it without realizing what you're doing. Well, hello! Many people with a restrictive posture need to stop squeezing the life out of imaginary innocent birds. More importantly, they need to see and feel the negative effects of what they're doing. With tightly held fingers and squeezing hands, they are squeezing the life out of their movement abilities.

When Eileen is standing (Figure 8.1), her feet and knees are very stiffened. This causes instability. She reacts with total-body postural stiffening. She holds her right hand and fingers tightly flexed, clawlike, while her left hand and fingers are held stiffly straight. Like most people with a reactionary and restrictive posture, she is unaware that she's doing this.

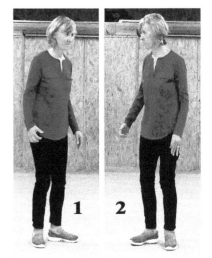

FIGURE 8.1: Stiffened hands, stiffened posture.

THE FOREARM

This abbreviated discussion is directed toward only the *rudimentary basics* of our anatomy.

On both sides of the forearm, there are multiple muscles. One end of some of the muscles is attached to a bone in the forearm, and some attach to the bone just above the elbow joint. At the other end of the muscles that control the wrist, hand, and fingers, the muscles have one or more long tendons that attach to a bone in the wrist, the hand, or a finger. When the muscle contracts (shortens), it pulls on and moves the wrist, parts of the hand, or a bone in a finger.

Muscles mainly do work by pulling. This is the reason there are at least two muscles that control any joint. For example, to move the hand and fingers, muscles on both sides of our forearms are required. When the muscles on the back of the side of the forearm pull, (palm down image on the right in Figure 8.2) they open the hand and extend the fingers. When the muscles on the "palm up" side of the forearm pull, they close the hand and flex the fingers (on the left in Figure 8.2).

Muscles have two basic functions. First, when they contract (shorten, pull), they move the smaller of the two bones they're attached to. Second, they help to stabilize the joint they cross over.

What is the difference between a naturally contracted and an unnaturally stiffened contracted muscle?

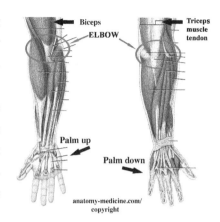

FIGURE 8.2: Muscles and tendons of the forearm.
copyright https://anatomy-medicine.com

1. The naturally contracted muscle is toned for productive work. It functions in a controlled and smooth manner and can be easily relaxed.

2. The unnaturally stiffened muscle is not toned for productive work and has limited function. The movement it does is either under-controlled or over-controlled, and is characteristically done in an interrupted manner. Stiffened muscles also do not easily relax in these people.

3. The unnaturally stiffened muscle is *not* toned for productive work and has limited function. The movement it does is either undercontrolled or overcontrolled, and is characteristically done in an interrupted manner. Stiffened muscles also do *not* easily relax.

4. A naturally functioning muscle is cooperative with the other muscles that are involved in the movement. The outcome is the intended coordinated movement.

5. An unnaturally functioning muscle is **not** cooperative with the other muscles involved in the movement. The outcome is most often *not* what was intended and *not* a coordinated movement.

    The purpose of postural stiffening is to maximize the stability of joints and *minimize* the movement of those joints.

    What does this mean? The purpose of any tightening or stiffening is not to produce purposeful movement. It is the opposite.

The purpose of postural stiffening is to restrict or stop movement.

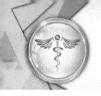

THE MUSCLES

See the muscles contracting and relaxing under the skin of your forearm when you move your fingers. Lightly place the fingertips of your other hand on the skin over the working muscles you see moving, to feel and follow them up your arm while you slowly move the fingers. How far up do they go? Where is the elbow in relation to the upper end of the muscles? The muscles begin and attach in the area surrounding the elbow.

With your fingertips on your forearm where you feel the muscles moving, make a fist, hold it, and then relax and open the hand. Slowly repeat this. Pay close attention to what you feel happening to the muscles with your fingertips, and to what you feel happening to the entire arm. When you make a fist, the muscles in your forearm tighten. This also causes your elbow to begin to tighten.

Now make a *very tight* fist. What happened in your arm? It tightened more than before. What else tightened? Feel for it as you slowly repeat making and releasing the fist. The shoulder is also tightening. Now, hold the *very* tight fist and move your arm. Take note that the arm does not move as easily and smoothly as it does with the hand relaxed. The tightened muscles are restricting the movement of the wrist and elbow. This is an example of postural stiffening causing all the muscles in an area of the body to contract at the same time, with the purpose of restricting movement of the involved joints.

PSYCHOLOGICAL VERSUS PHYSIOLOGICAL TIGHTENING

The *psycho*logical component is a response to anxiety and fear. It is a manifestation of the person's perception of what they expect will happen. It is based on their mental interpretation of what they see, think they see, or think might be. In general, as we become more anxious or fearful of our movements and falling, in a self-protective reaction the overwhelming tendency is to increase the psychological tightening or stiffening of muscles.

For people with natural ability, this type of psychologically driven physical reaction happens quickly, and then quickly is relaxed away. For those with troublesome movements, the relaxing process takes longer. For those with a restrictive-posture movement impairment, the reaction of overcontracting (stiffening) of the muscles comes *very* rapidly and remains for a prolonged period. They slowly return to their less-tightened (less-guarded) restrictive posture.

Why does this happen faster, stay longer, and take longer to resolve? Their background anxiety and fear are always present. This means when these people think they are relaxed, they physically are not. Their muscles remain contracted more than the naturally toned, relaxed posture people with natural ability have. With this primed level of *precautionary muscle contraction*, when people with restrictive-posture movement impairment have another "frightening" episode, their reaction very quickly becomes an exaggerated stiffening response. When the frightening moment is over, the stiffening response is very slow to release because they are not sure it's over. This is a learned precautionary reaction to another *expected* encounter.

The *physio*logical component of tightening happens on its own. In the context of degenerative neurological disorders, the tightening/stiffening is from the direct effects of the disorder. For example, many people stiffen as they become chilled, and the remedy is to warm themselves. As their body warms, the muscle tightness decreases. This is much more pronounced in many people with these disorders. These

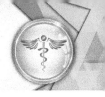

affected people are more sensitive to being chilled, and their stiffening comes faster and is more intense. Another common thing causing muscle tightening for them is prolonged sitting or standing.

In cooler temperatures, we must dress warmer to prevent our bodies from becoming chilled. When we're dressed appropriately, being out in the cold is less of a problem. For the standing- or sitting-too-long issue, when possible we must limit the time we stand still or remain sitting. When we are in the same position for too long, before walking, it's helpful to loosen up, do some range of motion movements to lightly exercise the legs, and flex and extend the knees.

Here's an easy way to do this. Move into a ready stance (a high squat) on stable feet. Staying on both feet, repeatedly, slowly shift your body weight toward one foot and then back toward the other foot. To loosen up further, vary how much your knees are flexed, while shifting from foot to foot or standing in place. How much of this you'll need to do will vary, and only you will know by feeling how much is enough. This gentle warm-up helps to prepare the muscles for walking. Then, when you decide it is time to walk, you also need to get in the habit of starting with very small steps until your body is relaxed enough for bigger steps. How will you know? You'll feel it. This topic is covered in more depth in later chapters.

Another component of physiological stiffening is the background tightening of muscles that is not related to any of the above triggers or fear. For unknown reasons, some of these people have a generalized tightening of muscles throughout the body.

Releasing Guarding and Stiffening

As covered in previous chapters, creating postural stability begins by first slowly moving the upper body to adjust the pressure in the feet, to make them flat on the floor.

1. This is the *first* thing to do because it creates the required initial improvement in physical stability that the rest of the process depends on.

2. The *second* part is to begin relaxing the body into the stabilizing feet. This process rightfully begins in the hands and arms, where the tensed muscles are easier to see, feel, and manage.

3. The *third* part is flexing slightly downward with the knees and hips to move into a ready stance. This provides additional stability in the feet that allows additional postural relaxation and stabilization.

4. Where does the pressure in the feet need to be to have them flat on the floor? The pressure must be equally distributed throughout both feet: equal pressure in the ball and heel areas.

Restrictive Posture: Relaxing the Arms to Begin Relaxing the Body

Sit on a chair. With your hands resting on top of your thighs, look at them and focus on what you see and feel. Are the fingers slightly curved inward toward the palm of the hand and loosely together, showing they are relaxed? Or are they straight, held apart, and feeling tense? What you see and feel in them

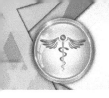

is showing you what is also happening with much more intensity in your legs and feet, and even more so when you are standing.

Now stand up. With your arms hanging down at your sides, do this feeling sequence again. If possible, do this in front of a large mirror to see what's happening. This will help you identify what you are and are not feeling and doing, exposing the things you haven't been aware of. Use a mirror!

Focus on and feel your arms. Look at them in the mirror. How far away are your hands from your thighs? Are they in front of, beside, or behind your thighs? Are your fingers relaxed? Are your shoulders held upward as if you're shrugging them, or are they drooping slightly down? Does your body look relaxed?

If your arms are not loosely lying at the sides of your body, you are not relaxed. When the arms are held away from the body, contracted (tightened/tensed) muscles are holding them there. The same is true for shoulders that are held up in a shrug. Many people with a movement impairment constantly hold their arms out and shoulders up without having a clue that they're doing it.

Slowly move the fingers of one hand and watch how they move. Are the fingers moving freely and easily, relaxed? Or are they being held straight or curled and moving slowly due to muscle tightness that serves no useful purpose?

Relax your hands. With *slow* and gentle movements of your fingers, allow them to loosen. The fingers begin to move more easily when the muscles in the forearms begin relaxing. The elbows also begin to relax. As the relaxation of the muscles in the forearms continues, the muscles in the upper arms begin to relax, followed by muscles around the shoulders. Feel this happening and also watch it happening in the mirror. Look for slight position changes of your fingers, hands, elbows, and shoulders. Typically, as the shoulders begin to relax, they will move slightly downward—but don't force them down. A note to those with a relaxed posture: You won't see or feel a change with this when you are not holding the same guarding or stiffening as the people you are intending to imitate.

When standing, another important feeling to be aware of is the one happening in your knees. As the hands, elbows, and shoulders relax, the knees begin to release a small amount of tightness as well. This small change is difficult for some to feel. Practice and play with it. Feel the change. Learn the feeling. Repeat it constantly throughout the day in everything you do and take note of the small improvements happening in your posture and movements.

SIMPLIFIED ANATOMY

Again, this abbreviated discussion is directed toward only the *rudimentary basics* of our anatomy.

Even though there are many functional differences of purpose between them, the structure of the bones in the arm and leg are very similar. Therefore, there are muscles and joints in the arms and legs that function in much the same ways, doing the same basic jobs. How can that be?

The bones and joints of the legs and arms are similar in basic design. The elbow is in the middle of the arm and has one big bone above it, jointed to two smaller bones below it. The knee is in the middle of the leg, also with one big bone above it, jointed to two smaller bones below it.

Muscles in our forearm control the hand and fingers, and the hand connects to the arm by the bones of the wrist. Likewise, muscles in our lower leg control the foot and extend the toes, and the foot connects to the leg by the bones of the ankle. Additionally, muscles on the bottom of our feet flex our toes.

Joints connect bones. One end of a muscle usually attaches to a larger bone on one side of the joint. The other end of the muscle usually attaches to a smaller bone on the other side of the joint. These muscles (or the tendons on the ends of the muscles) crossing over the joint control the movement of and stabilize that joint. This is the same as saying they stabilize and control the movement of the bones.

At precisely the same time and with precisely the same amount of opposite movement, when the muscles on one side of the joint contract (shorten), the muscles on the opposite side of the joint relax (lengthen).

When the muscles are strong and relaxed, with natural tone, the joint functions well within its natural range of motion and is very stable. When the muscles are weak, control of the movement of the joint and bones is compromised, and the joint is unstable. This often allows the joint to go beyond the natural range of movement.

Natural movements require relaxed, toned muscles with the strength to stabilize the joints and control the movement of the bones. For people with only muscle weakness, their remedy is muscle strengthening and conditioning. For those who have muscle weakness as well as postural guarding and stiffening, their remedy to improve their movement ability is threefold.

1. They must learn how to stabilize while standing on their feet.

2. They must learn to relax muscle guarding and stiffening, which they will not be able to do until they feel stable.

3. They must strengthen and condition their muscles in the same way anyone else must do.

USE YOUR ELBOW TO POINT YOUR FINGER

"Norm, there is a glint of a reflection from the duct coming through the slits of the vent near the top of the far wall in front of us. Do you see that?" I asked.

"Yes, I see it," Norm replied.

"Good. Point your finger toward that spot and hold it there." As Norm held his pointing finger (Figure 8.3), I asked, "Norm, why is your fingertip moving around so much?"

"I don't know," he responded as he watched his fingertip moving erratically.

"Do you feel the tightness in your arm right here?" I asked, pointing to his forearm.

"Yes, I do, now that you mention it. But I didn't realize it was like that. Now that I know it's there, it really feels tight," he added.

I replied, "It's tight because you're making it that way, but you don't have to keep it tight. Norm, look at what you're doing with your finger. Look at how you have it held so stiff and tight that it is actually bending backward. Look how the middle joint of

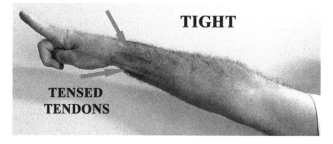

FIGURE 8.3: Norm's focus is on using his fingertip to point. His elbow is pulled straight. His hand is tightly clenched, and his forefinger is hyperextended.

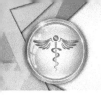

that finger is curving down. Feel the tightness in your finger, hand, and forearm. Your forearm is tight because that is where the muscles are that you're using to point that finger.

"The middle joint is down like that because a muscle in your forearm is aggressively pulling on the tendon that's connected to the tip of that finger. So, Norm, why are you trying so hard when all you want to do is gently point a finger? Well, you already gave the answer a minute ago. You weren't aware that you were doing it.

"As your movements became clumsy, gradually you began tensing muscles, trying to stop the clumsiness. It was a reaction without thought. Then you began tensing muscles as you were anticipating a movement, and gradually that led to the muscles stiffening during the movement. With time, this created another issue. After the movement, the tensing of the muscles didn't go away. That bad habit pattern is what you must learn to undo. You must relearn that only a gentle use of the muscle is needed most of the time. Additionally, you must learn how to relax your muscles when you're not using them, *and* when you are using them. That is what we'll begin working on now."

This overcontrolling, stiffening, and tightening habit is common in many people with restrictive and ataxic movement issues. They learn to hold things tightly, hold them close, and stiffen up as much as they can to gain more control. But doing these things only makes our movements worse.

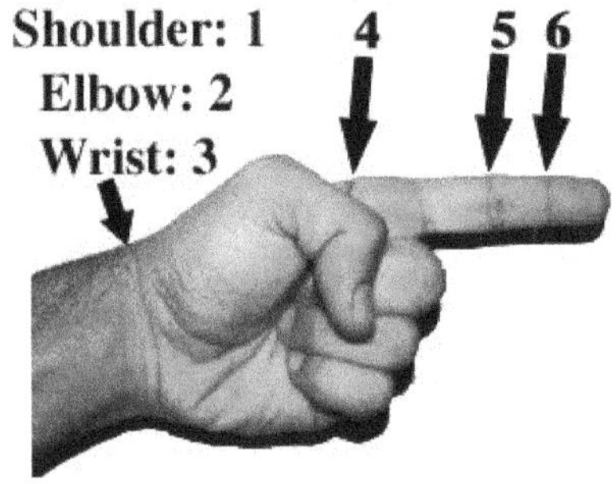

Shoulder: 1
Elbow: 2
Wrist: 3

FIGURE 8.4: From the shoulder to the fingertip, there are six joints. The two not shown in the picture are the elbow and shoulder.

For those with a restrictive posture, muscle tensing quickly turns simple movements into complicated and scary movements. The good news is, this can be minimized and often prevented.

From the shoulder to the tip of a finger, there are six main joints involved in this action. These include the shoulder, the elbow, and the four smaller joints marked with arrows in Figure 8.4. When the muscles in Norm's forearm tightened to hold his pointing fingertip still, all six of these joints became involved in an attempt to control the fine movement of the fingertip. But that is the problem. Tightened muscles destroy fine movements and restrict gross movement. As a result, the only options become very limited movements or coarse, overcontrolled, exaggerated movements. This is why Norm was unable to keep his fingertip still as he pointed.

The natural function of the hands and fingers requires fine motor control. Using tightened muscles as Norm was, fine motor control is substantially limited and very often eliminated. This is a common reason people with a restrictive-posture movement impairment tip and push things over when reaching for them, and shake food off their spoons and forks when eating.

"Okay, Norm, now we'll work on making this problem go away. You will be pointing a finger by focusing on just one joint, and using only the big muscles in your arm to control the movement. Yes, you'll still be using all the muscles and joints in the finger and arm, but this time nothing will be tensed, tight, or stiffened. This time you will be pointing and holding your fingertip using relaxed control of your entire arm. That will allow your hand and fingers to remain relaxed, and you will have fine motor control in them when you need it.

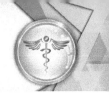

"By the way, you will *not* be pointing *with* your fingertip this next time, but you will be pointing it. This is an important concept to understand. When you pointed a few minutes ago, you were leading and directing your entire arm with a focus on the tip of that pointing finger.

"Now, consider what happened: Before you began the movement, you stiffened your finger into a pointing position, and then moved your arm to point it. What does that mean? Before you began the movement of using your arm to point with your finger, the muscles in your forearm stiffened, and that caused your elbow to tense. Then, to a lesser extent, the bigger muscles in your upper arm said "me too." Without realizing it, in the very first second of the movement, you tensed and stiffened your entire arm.

"Norm, all of that happened while you are relaxed and sitting in a chair. There you are, stable and comfortable sitting on your bottom, but you still stiffened your arm just to point a finger. Think about the bigger problem. What happens when you're standing on your feet, especially when you're feeling unstable? This same stiffening process is more intense, and it involves your entire body. What you're feeling in your arm, hand, and fingers while sitting in the chair is happening much, much more in your legs and feet when you're standing.

"There is a simple way to learn how to stop this bad habit. Instead of tightening muscles and essentially *pulling* your arm out into a pointing position, you will be pushing your hand and finger into that same pointing position while keeping the arm, hand, and finger relaxed. Because you'll be using relaxed postural control, all six joints will be functioning more naturally. The focus of this movement will be on using your elbow. The movement will be easier, and the results will be better.

"An important starting point is to relax your hand *BEFORE* you begin to move your arm. And keep it relaxed. Do that now. Relax your hand, and then focus on lifting your elbow to lift your arm. Next, push your elbow forward to make your arm

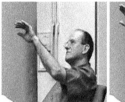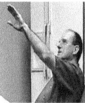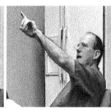

FIGURE 8.5: To move your hand and fingers where you want them to be, lift your arm and extend your elbow. Relaxed control. Natural movements.

straight. [I'm demonstrating this in Figure 8.5.] Now hold your relaxed finger, or fingers, *using your elbow* to control where the **arm** is pointing. Importantly, do not focus on moving your finger to put the fingertip where you want it. Only use your elbow to move and hold the pointing finger or fingers.

"Now, let's consider what's happening. The big muscles in the upper arm are moving the arm and extending the elbow to push the hand outward and straighten the arm. These bigger muscles are now pointing relaxed fingers and directing their movement with one joint, and that is the shoulder. The shoulder moves the entire arm, from side to side and up and down, to move and hold the finger on the spot. The muscles in the forearm are then used to extend the finger into a pointing gesture, or move the finger or fingers for a different purpose.

"Okay, Norm, forget about your fingers. Use your elbow and allow your shoulder to move your finger to that same spot. Good. How does your finger feel doing it this way?"

"It's not as shaky," Norm replied.

"Compare how the pointing finger feels now with how it was before," I said. "Move it around while pointing it with your arm. It moves better, but it is still a bit stiff because you're still holding

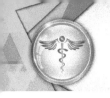

it too straight. So, drop your arm, again relax your hand and fingers, and this time point with all of your fingers.

"Great! Norm, look at the middle joint in all of your fingers. Instead of slightly curving down, now they curve up. This shows they are relaxed and flexible. Now feel for the tightness and stiffness in your arm, hand, and fingers. It's gone. Gentle, relaxed control always works better than tightened and stiffened overcontrol. Now gently move your fingers to feel how easily they move."

Focusing on controlling the elbow to move the hand provides improved abilities in the use of the hand and fingers. Now use your imagination. If you did this same thing when eating, less food would be spilling off your fork and spoon. Putting food in your mouth, drinking from a glass or bottle, touching your nose, all are simply other examples of finger pointing. The only difference is that with a spoon or fork in your hand, you are directing the utensil instead of your fingertip.

When you're holding a spoon tightly, your tightened arm causes the jerky movements that throw things off the spoon. Shorten the time it takes to eat, and do it without the "toddler mess" around your place at the table. Relax and use your elbow to improve your odds of keeping the food on your spoon all the way to your mouth. "How do I do that?" some still ask.

Question: What is the easiest and simplest way to direct the spoon in your hand into your mouth? Simply raise your arm (using a relaxed shoulder), and then bend the elbow.

How far away from your mouth are your fingers when your arm is straight, or when your elbow is partially flexed? *Functionally*, the distance is always only a simple bending of the elbow. To touch your nose with a steady finger, no matter where your relaxed arm is, simply bend your elbow. Try it. Play with it. Let your relaxed arm move from the shoulder joint as your elbow directs the movement of your hand, and the entire motion will happen naturally. Many will be pleasantly surprised to find that their shaking is less, so continue practicing to reduce it even more.

Prove all this for yourself. Straighten your arm out wherever you want, and then bring your fingers back to your mouth by *only bending your elbow*. Repeat it with your arm extended in different locations and with differing amounts of elbow flexion. Feel the difference.

Stop the foolish chasing games between your head and your hand. Stop making the mess around your plate. Stop feeling foolish and more "disabled" than you actually are. Relax your fingers to gently grip and hold the spoon. Then easily move the spoon between your plate and your mouth using only your elbow. Is this any different from what every person with natural ability does? *No!* It's exactly the same.

Where else should you use this elbow technique in your daily life? Hint: Every time you use your hands. Why? It's what we naturally do.

Relax your hand and fingers first, and then push your relaxed fingers out with your elbow to reach for a glass, the saltshaker, the phone, or anything else. As your hand moves toward the object, keep your fingers relaxed. Do not open your fingers until you need them to open, and then pick up the object with relaxed fingers. Next, remind yourself to grip the object *just* enough to hold it securely. Then use your elbow and shoulder to move the object where you want it to go. Simplify your thoughts, movements, and life by doing things more efficiently. Feel better about yourself. Stop the embarrassment at restaurants.

Do the same for the finger-pointing exercises you're asked to do when you go for checkups with your doctor (Figure 8.6). Use your elbow. Relax your hand and push your finger out with your elbow to their

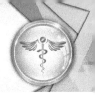

moving finger, and then bring your finger back to your nose by only bending your elbow. When you use this natural way of relaxation, you will perform better in many areas, and your doctor will be amazed at the improvement in your condition.

BUT stop right there. Your condition **did not** improve. You only improved how you are using your body. And, surprise! Many of you are discovering that your body still works much the same as it did before your disorder or condition became the problem.

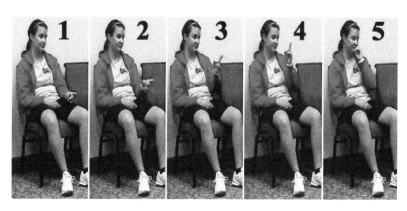

FIGURE 8.6: Keep your hand and fingers relaxed. For the finger-to-nose test, point your relaxed finger. To touch your nose with that finger, bend your elbow to move the finger to your nose.

Picking up and holding a bar of soap, or catching, throwing, and holding a ball is often challenging for those with a restrictive posture. We fumble the ball because our fingers and hands are stiffened. The bar of soap squirts out of our hands because we hold it too tightly. To improve these activities, use the same technique. Relax your hands, use your elbows to position your hands, and remind yourself to stay relaxed during the movement and activity.

USE THE KNEE TO CONTROL THE FOOT

Here is another way to make things better. Use your knee to control your foot, exactly as you are using your elbow to move and control your hand. When you're asked to rub your heel against your shin, *STOP* focusing on moving the heel of your foot. Practice using a relaxed knee to move your heel to the other leg, to stabilize and control the foot. Also, do not focus on holding your heel against the front of the leg. Instead, focus on the movements of the knee. This will help stop the erratic movement of your heel, and it will stay in line with the bone in your lower leg much better. Once again, you are proving that *you are more normal than you are not!*

Relax your elbows to relax your arms, hands, and fingers
and they will work better.

Relax your knees to relax your legs, feet, and toes
and they will work better.

■   ■   ■

CHAPTER 9

THIRD STANCE: SQUATTING

You must learn to help yourself
before any of the help you receive from others will make a difference.

Squatting begins with standing on stable flat feet in the ready stance, with your hands, elbows, and knees relaxed. This will allow your relaxed arms to dangle at your sides. During the squatting movement, the goal is to stay on flat feet as your knees and hips flex, and your body moves downward. When you do this correctly, your shoulders, knees, and toes will move into vertical alignment, as shown by the red reference line in picture 3 of Figure 9.1. This alignment will happen when you relax your posture and the movement is coordinated, and when you keep equal pressure in all areas of your feet (flat feet).

Your relaxed arms dangling loosely at your sides can be used for two purposes. First, this tells and shows you they're relaxed. And second, they will serve as a guide in the squatting movement. When you stay on flat feet in the squatting movement, your relaxed and dangling arms will gently brush against the fronts of your knees. Then, as you continue downward, your dangling fingertips will touch the floor in front of your toes, as illustrated in picture 5.

Study the sequence of pictures in Figure 9.1. The knees flex. The upper body moves forward as the hips flex and the bottom moves backward. When we're relaxed, this is a perfectly coordinated counterbalancing movement that keeps us centered on the starting pressure in the feet. Everything moves where it needs to move, and when it needs to move. It happens this way because it is directed by the stabilized pressure in our feet, and allowed through relaxed postural control.

This is not as difficult as some with impaired movements think. So, what happens that makes it difficult for them? Most commonly, the difficulty stems from one, and often both, of the following two reasons. These two reasons lead directly to a third.

1. Fear and stiffness. The fear of falling makes their postural tensing stronger. As it increases, their body's ability to flex and squat decreases.

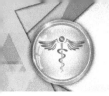
2. Diminishing strength. As fear in their mind increases, so does the tensing in their posture. This restricts natural movements and forces the use of modified and/or unnatural movements. Another consequence of living with chronic postural tensing is the muscles involved are poorly exercised. The outcome is muscle weakness.

3. Self-doubt, fear, uncontrolled postural tensing, and weakness cause instability, awkwardness, and the development of additional maladaptive behaviors. Living daily with these issues, many people with balance and movement issues quickly learn not to jeopardize their safety by trying anything that seems scary.

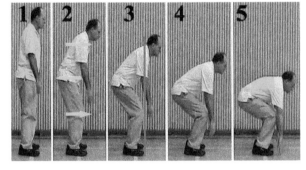

FIGURE 9.1: Use your relaxed arms as a natural guide to know where the pressure is located in your feet. When your feet remain flat during the squat, your arms will gently brush against the fronts of your knees.

SQUATTING, ARMS HANGING OUT IN FRONT OF THE KNEES

There are two common reasons for the arms to be dangling in front of the knees, but not *touching* the knees (Figure 9.2). First, the shoulders have moved too far forward. Second, the knees are not flexing enough. This indicates the person is stooping forward at the waist more than squatting with the knees.

The "stooping squatter" typically begins the movement by moving the shoulders forward and down, and then adds very little movement in the knees, as shown in pictures 1 and 2. With this excessive movement of the upper body and hips, they are showing the greater stiffness in their legs compared with that of their upper body. What else are they showing? Weakness. The longer they use stiffened knees, the weaker their legs become.

These people can surprise the casual observer. They perfect the "butt out" and shoulders down on straightened legs so well that they usually don't show fear when doing it. However, when it comes to other simple movements, the opposite is quickly obvious.

Another problem occurs when the stooping upper body causes back pressure to be pushed on the knees. When the knees are straight, the back pressure on them is high. With the knees slightly flexed, there is less back pressure, but enough that it hinders flexing the knees more than they are. This issue is fairly common in people who are accustomed to walking stooped over a walker.

Also, always remember: When a person is beginning a movement and their knees do not easily flex, their upper body is much more likely to move first, and its movement is very often excessive. This is the opposite sequence of most natural movements.

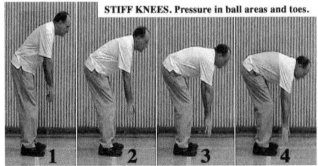

FIGURE 9.2: This is a stooping squatter posture. Stiffened knees force stooping forward from the hips. During the stoop, to make up for the non-movement of the knees, the upper body moves too far forward and downward, and this moves pressure forward in the feet.

For walking and other movements done while standing on our feet, we naturally begin these movements using our legs. The upper body is responsible for setting and controlling the location of the pressure in the feet, *but does not include starting the movement*. The lower body, the legs and the feet, start and do the movement. This is our natural order.

Now, to be clear. There is nothing wrong with stooping if that is what you intend to do, and you are stable and comfortable while doing it. The issue we're working on here is to keep your feet stable on the floor while improving the use of your knees and hips in a squatting movement, to then be better prepared to improve on other movements.

SQUATTING, HANDS RESTING ON OR BESIDE THE THIGHS, ARMS BEHIND THE KNEES

What does it mean when you're moving down into a squat while keeping your feet flat on the floor, and your arms and hands are resting on your thighs? Or when your relaxed arms are hanging down alongside your thighs, behind your knees? In both cases, your shoulders are not moving forward enough. Unless you compensate for this with your knees, there is increased pressure in your heels. Then, as you continue to move lower in the squat with shoulders held back, *the pressure in your heels increases*.

Consider the following two ways to move the extra pressure out of the heel area. One, move your shoulders forward. Two, push your knees farther forward to counterbalance the back position of the shoulders. An example of pushing the knees forward is shown in picture 2 of Figure 9.3. In comparison, John's postural alignment in picture 1 is good.

Looking at Joan's posture, with the green zone-of-stability overlay it's easier to see that she is slightly overcompensating in her counterbalancing adjustment. There is a small part of her bottom out of the back of the zone, but her knees and head are both out of the front side of the zone. This shows there is slightly more body weight forward on the ball areas of her feet, mainly due to the forward position of her knees, than there is toward the heel.

This zone of stability is described in more detail in chapter 15. But briefly, it is defined by the outline of the parts of the feet that are in contact with the floor, with an imaginary projection to the top of the head. This graphical representation helps to define the relationship of posture to the location of pressure in the feet.

When you are in the same sort of posture as Joan, you will say one of three things about the pressure in your feet:

1. My feet feel flat.

2. I feel increased pressure toward the ball areas of my feet.

3. I feel increased pressure in my heels.

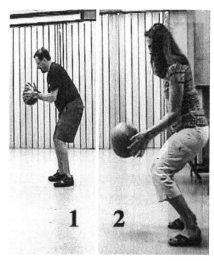

FIGURE 9.3: Counterbalancing. Picture 1: John's shoulders are slightly forward. This moves increased pressure into the ball areas of his feet. Picture 2: Are Joan's feet flat? No. There is increased pressure in the ball areas and toes. Her knees are forward and shoulders slightly back. She is also pushing increased downward pressure into her feet, which adds to the ball-area pressure.

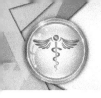

All of these are possible. This is due to the use of additional muscles to compensate for the postural alignment, and/or how the individual has learned to interpret what they feel in their feet. There is another issue that can be a factor for some, and that is wearing shoes with a prominent heel that alters the angle of the foot relative to the floor. For example, when the heel of the shoe is higher, added pressure is often shifted into the ball areas of the feet. Therefore, wearing footwear with a low heel to keep the feet closer to parallel with the floor is preferable in order to initially feel and work with these pressures.

When your posture is relaxed enough to allow your knees to move forward beyond your toes like this, you will move the increased pressure forward and out of your heels, unless you compensate with shoulder movement. Joan did not feel the extra pressure in the ball areas of her feet because she was holding her shoulders back and adding pressure to her heels. With her thoughtful intent to do a simple squat while focusing on the exercise with the ball, she overthought how to do the movement.

Most people with natural ability will say their feet feel flat on the floor and they feel comfortable when they are in a squat with knees or shoulders slightly forward. In contrast, those with a movement impairment will NOT feel comfortable in this same posture, and both will have increased pressure in the ball areas of their feet. What is the reason for this difference? The posture of the person with a movement impairment is not as relaxed. And remember, when standing, they typically have increased pressure in their heels. So, when they're in a knee- or shoulder-forward posture, the additional pressure going forward in the ball areas registers as much, much more than it is.

As Joan was bouncing and then catching the ball, she said that her feet felt flat. Why does she not feel the increased pressure in the ball areas of her feet that her posture shows she has? With her natural ability, her posture is very relaxed, and the working muscles in her legs are strongly *pushing stabilizing pressure into the entire surface* of her feet. This diminishes the effect of the increased pressure in the ball areas while increasing the total pressure in the feet. Yes, the pressure in the ball areas is mildly more than in the other parts of her feet, but she is also pushing that pressure straight down into the floor. This negates the forward tipping that the movement-impaired person routinely feels, because they are not directing that pressure straight down into the floor. The counterbalancing and compensating Joan is doing with her natural ability shift the effective pressure in her feet.

This highlights another important message about the so-called right and wrong ways of how we choose to do our movements. While there is a right and wrong way in our use of the natural basics, there is *not* an absolute right or wrong way to do all our movements. We see this everywhere we look. People are doing the same things, but some people's posture looks a bit different in the same movement and activity.

So, our natural movements are based on the same foundation fundamentals. But our natural ability also allows us to modify the style or character of our movements while using these same fundamentals.

Joan was very stable in this posture as she bounced and caught the ball. *But*, because this posture applies added strain into the legs, she was somewhat restricted in going farther down into the squat. This doesn't normally create much of a problem for people with natural movement abilities and relaxed postural control, because these issues are easily corrected or overcome. However, people with balance and movement problems, especially those with a tensed posture, do have additional problems with it. Their muscles are tense, which means the muscles controlling the knees are being used more to hold the

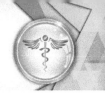

knee in position, rather than allowing them to move. This also means these muscles are not being used as much as they normally would be for adding pressure into the feet for stabilization.

With her natural ability, when the ball does not bounce straight back up, Joan can easily adjust her posture to remain on stable feet to catch the ball. People with a restrictive (tensed) posture often struggle doing the same thing when in this same posture. When they reach for the ball as it bounces slightly away from them, they often do not stay on stable feet. Why? As their tensed posture changes position to catch the ball, the location of pressure in their feet also changes. The common result is induced instability.

When people with these issues squat with their hands resting on their thighs (arms behind the knees), they typically are holding their shoulders back. This means they are very likely beginning the squatting movement with increased pressure in their heels, and creating difficulty for themselves in the very beginning of the movement.

In panels A and B of Figure 9.4, I begin the squat with shoulders held back, with increased pressure in my heels. In both panels, the intended movement is a squat while staying on flattened feet.

In panel A, I'm holding my knees in place as if they are stiffened. That's why the position of my knees doesn't change in pictures 2 and 3. Starting the squat in picture 1, I move my upper body (shoulders) forward. But look at what happens to my feet. This adds more pressure to my heels, and then the fronts of my shoes come up off the floor in picture 2. In picture 3, I continue to move my shoulders farther forward to move pressure off my heels, but the toes of my shoes are up higher than they were in picture 2 (red arrow).

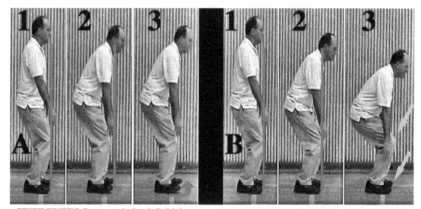

STIFF KNEES:Pressure in heels is high, and PUSH into feet from legs is weak.

RELAXED KNEES: Pressure in heels is low, and PUSH into feet from legs is strong.

FIGURE 9.4: A small amount of stiffness negatively affects our posture, the pressure in our feet, our stability, and our movement ability.

Why is this happening? It is because of stiff knees. When I move my shoulders forward, my knees move backward. Compare the red vertical line in pictures 1 and 2 and note the small space between my knee and the line in picture 2 that was not there in picture 1. The amount of backward movement of my knees is small, but the effect is significant. This is a very common reason why many movement-impaired people with restrictive postures tip and fall backward when attempting this and similar movements.

Now, another question. Why am I holding my arms forward in all the pictures, except the third picture in panel B, where they are relaxed and hanging straight down? If I had relaxed them in the other pictures, they would have moved backward and added the weight of my arms to the pressure in my heels. So, I'm holding my arms forward to move pressure forward in my feet, to keep me from tipping backward.

FEET VERSUS MIND

In the two panels of Figure 9.5, Nigel's posture and movement look very different. In both, his intent was to do the exact same squatting movement to touch his fingers to the floor while keeping his feet flat.

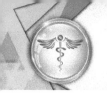

In panel A, I had instructed Nigel to focus only on controlling the positioning of his shoulders during the squatting movement. Then immediately after, in panel B, I instructed him to focus only on keeping his feet flat.

The difference between the two movements is striking. In panel A, he is controlling the movement with the thought of how he should be doing it, while controlling the position of his shoulders. This focus causes him to overcontrol his shoulders and greatly limit the movement of his knees. Using thought control, he destroys his natural movement ability.

A few moments later, in panel B, Nigel's focus is back to where it had always naturally been, with the only additional consideration of making and keeping his feet heavy (pressurized) and flat. This *is* an additional thought part to the natural movement. However, *it is **not** distracting to* the movement. Naturally, we always, always, always begin and continue our movements with additional stabilizing pressure pushing into our feet. So, with Nigel's mild instability issues, I was only reminding him to do what he was beginning to not use as much. Then, as he was using it again, his squatting movement was naturally perfect.

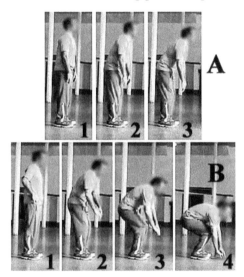

The previous problem vanished. This time he easily and naturally moved into a very low squat on flat feet. Every part of his body moved exactly where it needed to be, because he was totally and naturally relaxed. His balance was perfect as his body counterbalanced and "collapsed" down with relaxed, flexing joints—just as it is designed to do.

Panel A shows guarded dynamic postural control.
Panel B shows relaxed dynamic postural control.

FIGURE 9.5: Panel A: Focusing on controlling shoulder movement, Nigel restricts other parts of his body in the squatting movement. Panel B: Focusing on keeping his feet flat, he moves freely into the squat.

This is the difference those with problematic movements are working to achieve. They are striving to get out of their overthinking and overcontrolling minds, to get back into their bodies' truly natural guiding focus: the stability of their feet.

NATURAL SQUATTING

Standing in an upright, relaxed posture with straight knees on flat feet, how do you begin the squatting movement? Or, the same question asked in a different way: When standing upright and then moving into a ready stance and squat, to remain balanced and coordinated and not change the location of the pressure in your feet, which part of your body moves first? The answer: Your hips are the first part to move.

So, when standing upright on flat feet, simply push your bottom out and down to begin the squat. Think of it as beginning to sit down onto a bar stool. This will easily move you into a ready stance. The rest of the squat is like sitting on a low chair with flexing knees lowering you down. This helps take some of the thought out of what you might think you should be doing. *But* there is one thing that needs to be added. What must you do before pushing your bottom out and down? Relax your hands to relax your knees.

How does this work? This initial backward movement of the hips actually results in a tilting movement of the pelvis. This combined movement of the pelvis and hips alters the pressure on and positioning of the bones of the knees, which allows the knees to flex.

This third stance, the squat, requires improving control of the upper and lower body in both an independent and codependent functioning manner. To control the location of the pressure in the feet, the upper body is dependent on the stabilization and support of the lower body. To start and complete the movement, the lower body is dependent on the proper functioning of the upper body. Each half must have the ability to do its job without assistance from the other, but neither can do that job properly without the other.

CORNERS: USE THEM FOR SUPPORT

Lean into a smooth corner for support to practice relaxing and using your knees, as Megan is demonstrating in Figure 9.6. Her bottom and back are against and sliding on the walls, which isolates work to using only the knees. This is very helpful for people who are unstable and have weak legs and knee issues.

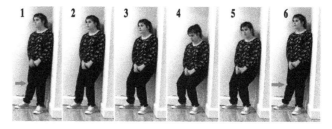

FIGURE 9.6: With weak legs and uncontrolled knees, Megan's mind is preoccupied with instability and a fear of falling. These things prevent her from doing movements she would like to be doing, and learning how to feel pressure in her feet. Working in the corner stabilizes her posture and allows isolated work on knee function and leg strengthening, and also allows her mind to quiet so the feelings can be known.

Using a corner, foot placement is key. The feet need to be forward enough out of the corner so there is increased pressure in the heels when the person is standing with their bottom and back against the corner walls. This heel pressure pushes them safely into the corner so they can relax and then focus on using their knees to do the movement. Importantly, though, the feet must not be too far forward out of the corner. If they are, they're less supportive and are liable to slip forward on the floor, causing the person to fall.

When they are coming up out of a squat or rising from a chair, many people with weak legs and knees push their knees together to gain added stability. When they do this, each leg is bracing the other. Megan has learned to depend on doing this, as is seen in most of the pictures. Because they have allowed their legs to substantially weaken, typically out of habit, these people do not like to hold them apart.

WHERE IT BEGINS

Realize that what you are reading and practicing is not new to you. Realize that you are simply learning how to renew the same very natural and comforting feelings you grew up using. This means you are only searching to rediscover yourself in everything you'll be doing. You will be finding your way of stabilizing your movements according to the natural workings of your body, guided and controlled by the stabilized pressures in your feet. None of this is new to your body. It is only new to your mind.

Naturally, we trust the ability, not the thought of the ability.

We balance on our feet, not on our head. We stand and walk on our feet, not on our head. We control our natural movements with our feet, not with our head. Our natural movements require no thought,

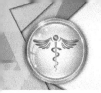

because we learned to totally trust how we use our body and feet long before we knew what thinking was. We learned to trust how we use our body and feet long before we developed the capacity to understand intellectually what we were learning to do physically.

Keep reminding yourself of this. Why? Because you will consistently search in your mind for an answer to your movement problems. But the answer will not be in your mind until you learn it and put it there. Relax.

■ ■ ■

CHAPTER 10

KNEES AND SHOULDERS

Your best teaching and learning examples, improvements in ability,
and personal discoveries will mostly come to you while you're doing simple things.
Especially when you're having fun.

Staying in good physical condition is frequently ignored, and is often a problem for many people with balance and movement problems. Why?

People with these issues view doing things that seem to make their condition worse as very impractical. For example, often when they begin exercising they initially become clumsier with added instability. Too often this leads them to believe that their condition will not allow them to exercise. So, they don't. Then, neglecting exercise, these people drift deeper into their disability and become weaker. Collectively, by regressing into a relatively inactive lifestyle to minimize their clumsiness, they gradually slide into increasing inability, instability, and clumsiness.

Being less active allows their physical conditioning to decline more quickly, even more so than that of a person with natural abilities who leads the same sedentary lifestyle. Due to their instability, clumsiness, restrictive movements and fear, people with problematic movement issues don't use their muscles as efficiently as people with natural ability do. Then, with this sedentary pattern, the interpretation is that their increasing movement problems are the result of their age, condition, or advancement of their underlying neurological condition, when much of the trouble is due to the deconditioning and weakening of their muscles. This tunneled focus on age, condition, or disorder is convenient, but frequently is a very poor rationale to explain their weakened physical condition.

My message is this: Most of you (us) with balance issues and problem movements, or a movement impairment, have the ability to improve. But first you need to have *your proof* to accept this as true, so you can then go about doing it. For most, this will not be easy, and it will not be a quick fix. Instead, it will be a very personal, lifelong therapy process of learning, improving, and living the benefits. But let's be honest. This is the way it is for everyone, with or without natural ability.

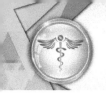
PROBLEM KNEES

When the leg muscles are not strong enough to adequately support the body weight, using the knees in any movement will always be a problem.

When your legs *are* strong enough, but staying balanced and stable while squatting is still challenging, look to the position of your knees and shoulders for a probable reason:

1. Your knees don't flex, or they don't continue flexing during the squatting movement.

2. Your shoulders don't come forward enough to begin the squat, and/or they don't stay forward during the movement.

3. Both result in increased heel pressure.

4. The restricted-knee-movement problem aggravates the restricted-shoulder-movement problem.

When the leg muscles are weak, a person doesn't have much control of the movement of their knees. Thus, flexing the knees with weakened muscles often creates immediate instability. The result: Weak leg muscles encourage standing with straight knees. To do this, the person forces their knees backward and then holds them relatively locked in place, forcing the bones of the legs to support the body weight. This allows the person some stability while standing, but it also creates a great restriction of all movements.

Strengthening the muscles of the legs and the rest of the body is the remedy that restores much of the knees' stability and functioning. Posture control will also improve, and the dependency on assistive devices for external support will slowly diminish. The exception to this is injured or deformed knee joints, especially when they're painful.

POOR POSTURE CONTROL and WALKER ISSUES

In Figure 10.1, William's legs have become very weakened because he has spent so much time in his wheelchair (picture 1). Thus, his postural control is very poor, and he is totally dependent on the walker to stabilize himself when standing. In this example, William's body weight is centered over the ball areas of his feet. This is shown by the centered red line within the green zone of stability.

Note how he stands with aggressively stiffened and straight legs. His upper body is leaning forward onto the walker. This applies the back pressure on his knees that effectively locks them in place. In this posture, his arms are pushing additional pressure onto the walker and causing another issue. His hands are located on the rear areas of the upper bars. Combine that with the distance he's standing away from the walker, and notice that the pressure he is pushing into the walker is angled (red arrows). Therefore, instead of helping to stabilize him, the way he's using the walker is causing added instability.

In this example, his body is tipping forward from the pressure in the ball areas of his feet. Also note that his feet are spread slightly farther apart than the legs of the walker. What problems does this create?

To make any movements, this forces him to stand farther away from the walker so he can move his feet without kicking its legs. Now he must lean farther forward, and that pushes more pressure into his hands and the walker.

The distance he is standing away from the walker determines the angle of his forward-leaning body. This lean causes the increased pressure he's placing on the walker to be at an angle, which causes a tipping action of the walker. By itself, this applied pressure causes the top of the walker without wheels to more easily tip backward. To counteract the tip, the person pushes forward on the walker with stiffened arms. (With a four-wheeled walker, the pressure pushes the walker forward, and then the person constantly pulls the walker back while applying the brakes.)

Now let's consider another factor that often goes unnoticed. Note that William's hands are toward the back of the walker's handgrips. Also note that the walker's back legs are perpendicular to the floor rather than slightly angled back-

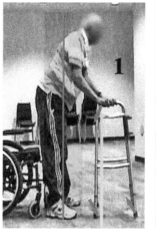
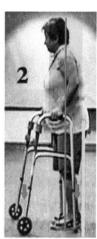

FIGURE 10.1: Two factors determine the stability of the walker. The first is your stability on your feet. The second is the pressure you are pushing onto the walker.

This means, by controlling your posture, you control the walker.

The purpose of the walker is NOT to control you.

ward, as they are on Betty Lou's walker (picture 2 of Figure 10.1). The back legs of William's walker are straight upright because the front legs have been incorrectly adjusted (lengthened) to keep him from tipping the walker forward. How would he tip it forward? When the walker is pushed forward the legs skid on the floor. But when he pushes it forward in this posture, he is also pushing down on it, and that pressure often causes the front legs to stick on the floor. The result is a forward tipping tendency of the walker, and William.

Now compare William's posture with Betty Lou's. Her body weight is centered just behind the ball areas of her feet, and her posture is upright. Look where her feet are positioned. They are inside the legs of the walker, and her knees are slightly flexed. She is stable on her feet and using her legs more than the walker for support. She is using the walker appropriately and pushing less pressure into her hands than William is. Her hands are on the centers of the handgrip areas and pushing pressure straight down equally into all the walker's legs. She is using the walker for limited secondary support, while William is forced to depend on his for primary support. This gives Betty Lou the stability, movement abilities, and postural control that William does not have.

Interestingly, they share similar disorders, but Betty Lou's disorder is much more aggressive and involved than William's. Still, Betty Lou's legs are slightly stronger than William's, although they've both spent most of each day sitting in a wheelchair for the same number of years. This implies that their relative leg strength is not the only determining factor in the differences shown in this comparison. Two other determining factors are the placement of their hands on the walker, which is determined by where they are standing relative to the device, and the width of their stance.

The truth: *In this comparison, they both physically have the same relative level of functioning. Thus, the differences and discussed points in this example highlight how they are both using, or not using, the ability they*

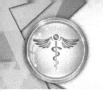
have. William's setup posture is poor. Betty Lou's setup posture is good, and that gives her better ability while using the walker. See and understand it. Our posture is a huge determining factor in everything we do. To have better standing and movement ability, we must pay closer attention to using the correct posture that enables that ability to be realized. Unfortunately, too many people with movement impairments pay little attention to this and then complain about how bad their "condition" is. It is up to each person to change their poor posture and maladaptive behaviors, and the first step is to become aware of their mistakes. We can all do better!

These basic errors are very common in people with weak legs using walkers. They push themselves forward onto the walker with an upper-body lean and expect the walker to support and keep them safe. Here is a news flash, my friends. The walker is a piece of aluminum and plastic and has no ability or responsibility to save you from yourself. *When you do something foolish, the walker will only do something foolish along with you.*

BACK TO THE WALL

At the end of the previous chapter, I suggested that those with very weak legs use a corner for practice. For those with better ability, a good tool to use is a flat and smooth wall. The wall provides *partial* support for isolating and working on flexing the knees and strengthening the legs while doing squats.

Be careful, because this can also be a very scary thing for many. Why? The wall is smooth and is not supporting you at either side, unless you are standing very near a corner or large piece of furniture. Doing this against an open wall will be tough for many, as it was for me when I first began doing this in 2005. During the down and up, I would slide to the side across the wall. Why? I wasn't pushing enough pressure down into my feet. I was using too much upper-body movement, and because of that excessive movement, I was pushing different pressure into each foot. I temporarily corrected this lateral instability issue by using a wall where there was a filled four-drawer filing cabinet (very heavy) on each side of me, with each cabinet approximately one foot away from each shoulder. This was a small enough distance to stop me from falling when my side slip happened. But the cabinets were far enough away that they didn't hinder my efforts to relearn my responsibility to use my legs and feet properly. Within a short time of dedicated practice, I didn't need the side support any longer.

Using the wall, begin with the heels of your shoes approximately one of your shoe lengths away from the wall. Then allow your shoulders and bottom to rest against the wall, as shown in picture 1 of Figure 10.2. This setup creates a small amount of increased heel pressure that will lightly push and hold your bottom to the wall. Next, focusing only on your knees, while keeping your back against the wall, slowly lower yourself into a squat as far as you can comfortably go. In the beginning, it doesn't matter how low you go. But it does matter that you keep your upper body centered over your feet with equal pressure in both feet. Keep your posture relaxed and comfortable while working to remain stable. As you do these things, the movement will become easier, and you'll be able to go lower with flexing knees.

To stand back up from a squat, you need to do only one thing: Push down with as much force as you can into your feet. Your knees will straighten (extend) as your body moves upward while your legs and feet keep you stabilized.

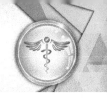

What is the very first thing every person with natural movement ability does *for every movement* they do? We push down into our feet for strength and stabilization. So, as you practice lowering your body

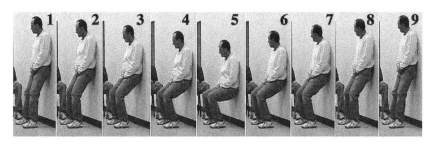

with flexing knees, begin and continue this movement while pushing down into your feet. Then, when you want to come back up out of the squat, continue pushing down into your feet to push your body up with extending knees.

FIGURE 10.2: With better balance and ability, use a flat wall instead of a corner to work on knee movements and leg strengthening. This isolates the movement to only the knees.

Every movement begins and ends with a push down into the feet, or the foot that is doing the movement.

Many people with a movement impairment are functionally more impaired than they should be because they are not applying and holding this downward pressure when standing and in movement.

When standing, every person with natural ability holds stabilizing pressure in their feet to support their body.

Therefore, there are two things you need to do to make moving into and out of a squat easier:

1. Keep your knees slightly flexed when you're standing, as shown in pictures 1 and 9.

2. Push down into your feet as if you're trying to push them through the floor.
   Learn to hold the same feeling of pressure when you begin the squat, during the squat, and when you stand back up. Learn to hold it in all stances and movements.

Doing squats with your back against a wall eliminates having to coordinate the movement of your shoulders with the movement of your knees. This allows you to isolate work to strengthening your legs, stabilizing your body by pushing and holding equal pressure into your feet, and using your knees independently.

As the strength in your leg muscles increases, your balance will also improve. As you feel that happening, allow the squat to go deeper toward the floor to strengthen the muscles and function of your knees.

Correct a leaning body by correcting the pressures in your feet. When the same amount of pressure is pushed equally into both feet, your relaxed body will naturally center between them. What is the point here? The pressure in your feet also directs the movement of your relaxed body.

When your body leans, push it back to the center by increasing **and holding** pressure in the weak and/or lazy foot. The weak and/or lazy leg/foot is the one your body is leaning toward. To keep your body centered between your feet, you must learn to continue **holding** this pressure in that foot, even though it will often seem like it is too much.

Also remember that having a mirror directly in front of you lets you see what's actually happening. What you see in the mirror is your physical truth. The reflection of your postural alignment also shows you exactly what you're feeling. This is highly beneficial and necessary before many of you will believe me, yourself, and the other people telling you what they see you doing.

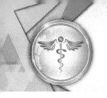

Be skeptical of what you or others think might be. Instead, always stop, see, and feel the truth. Then apply the necessary corrections to make things more natural in your posture and stance.

Now, another news flash: Everything you are learning to do on two feet, you must also learn to do on one foot. Natural movement requires it. Therefore, when you have the stability and strength to squat on two legs, you need to begin practicing squatting centered on just one leg, and then the other. This doesn't necessarily mean that you must lift one foot off the floor each time. Many of you can't do this and stay balanced while leaning on the flat wall.

So, if you need both feet on the floor while using a wall, practice having both feet in contact with the floor but shifting more body weight onto one leg. The challenge then is to continue holding your body over that one leg as you do the entire movement. Be careful. Many of you will find this very challenging, and the risk of sliding across the wall and hitting the floor is much higher.

For those of you who *slide on the wall* when trying to use one leg, **stop** and use a corner. The double-bracing corner will hold you stable, making it possible to lift one foot off the floor to work entirely with only one leg, knee, and foot.

BACK AGAINST THE CORNER

Sang Dong has extremely weakened legs (Figure 10.3). Thus, standing is challenging for him, and walking is extremely difficult because he can't control his knees. The remedy for this situation at a minimum is twofold. The first is strengthening his legs. The second is learning how to relax the stiffness in his legs to use the strength he does have, but this is much easier said than done. With the leg weakness and stiffening, he is very unstable when standing. This instability will not allow him to experiment with relaxing his knees enough to use them. So, to provide him with standing stability, we moved him into a corner. With his back against the two walls and the increased pressure in his heels pushing and keeping his back in the corner, he now has the support and stability he requires to isolate and exercise his knees and legs.

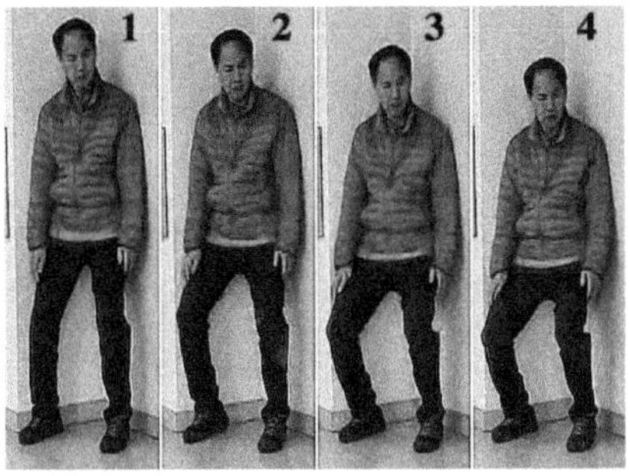

Now consider this question: What is he showing himself in this example? *Very importantly*, he is showing himself "*my legs still work.*"

Far too many people begin using wheelchairs because they tire of struggling and/or others advise them that it would be easier if they were using a wheelchair. Far too many people resort to wheelchairs because they don't know how not to, or they simply stop trying. Most commonly, this happens because they and others don't realize how it can safely be avoided.

Those who are caught in this wheelchair trap of convenience would give anything to change their predicament. But they have two big issues to contend with:

FIGURE 10.3: A corner is more supportive for people with very weak legs. It is also a good place to work on one-leg squats for those with stronger legs.

1. They must find the self-motivation and determination to do what it takes to get out of the chair and off their bottoms to exercise, to begin creating their very-much-wanted improved strength and ability.

2. Their path to recover lost strength and ability is a long and frustrating ordeal, and many of them don't have a good support system to help them stay with their recovery program.

SHOULDERS OFF THE WALL

As you improve in squatting with your shoulders against the wall, then you need to advance and begin practicing the squatting movement with only your bottom against the wall. To do this, the placement of your feet on the floor stays the same, but the pressure you feel in them during the movement is different.

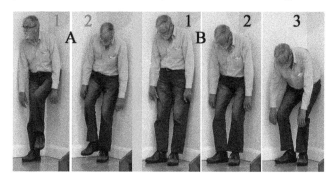

FIGURE 10.4: Panel A: One-leg corner squat. Panel B: Bottom in the corner. Shoulders off the walls.

Why? When the upper body (shoulders) move forward, the pressure in the feet also moves forward. Therefore, as you lower into the squat and your shoulders move forward, the pressure in your feet will become nearly evenly distributed throughout. Your feet will feel flat on the floor with only your bottom staying on the wall.

While keeping your bottom against the wall, or in the corner as Ant is doing in Figure 10.4, begin the squat with your knees and allow your shoulders to move forward off the wall as shown. While doing this, some of you will note that there is still increased pressure in your heels, but not quite as much as before. The reason is that your shoulders are not coming far enough forward.

How far should you allow your shoulders to move forward? Let them come forward so your hands are just in front of your knees, as shown in picture 3 in panel B. In this posture, you'll feel the same pressure throughout all areas of your feet. This may seem impossible for some people to do, for three reasons:

1. Weak leg muscles or painful joints will not support the body to allow moving into a lower squat.

2. Stiffened, injured, or painful knees won't flex enough to allow the body to move into a lower squat.

3. The feet are too far away from the corner. This puts too much increased pressure in the heels, and that pressure pushes the body into the wall. Also, with the feet too far forward, they are not able to provide enough support and independent stabilization to continue the movement.

   Be careful. When your feet are too far away from the wall or corner, they may slip out from under you during the stance or movement.

When using the corner or the open wall, keep your bottom *lightly* against it until you're stable enough on your feet that you don't need the wall for support. This will happen when you feel and trust the stability you create with flattened feet on the floor, when your legs are strong enough to support your body and the movement. Learn and understand how you create this feeling, what it actually is, and how you relax and move your body into the proper posture to get it. These things are required to build your confidence and wean yourself from needing the corner or a wall for support, so that eventually you can

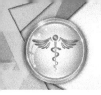

do squats on the open floor with no support. More importantly, this is your gateway to more advanced movement ability.

While practicing moving your shoulders forward, many of you will feel that the pressure in the front of your feet becomes too much, even when your bottom is still staying against the wall. This happens for these basic reasons:

1. Your mind is registering the small amount of increasing pressure in the ball areas and toes as a great deal of pressure. This happens when you have been unknowingly keeping the pressure light in these areas of your feet. Now a little extra pressure seems like a large amount.

2. Your feet are too close to the wall or corner. When they're too close, you'll be feeling that you are about to tip or fall forward as you begin the squat and/or as you move your shoulders forward.

3. Some people will feel that they're tipping forward, even with their bottoms pressing on the wall. A common reason is that their shoulders are moving too far forward and/or their feet are too close to the corner. Be careful.

    When your feet are too close to the wall and you squat with your bottom firmly on the wall, you are creating two pressure points that will act to push you forward. One, the increasing pressure in your bottom can push you out of the corner and/or away from the wall. Two, increasing pressure in the toes and ball areas can tip and push you forward.

    So, when you feel yourself tipping forward, stop, stand up, and recheck the position of your feet.

4. If the backs of your feet are at least one of your foot lengths away from the wall, the problem is almost always that your knees are not flexing enough and your shoulders are moving forward too much.

    This is much more common in those who habitually stoop forward at the waist rather than squat with the knees. If this applies to you, have something solid and very supportive in front of you to stop a forward fall as you practice correcting this problem. Of note, in pictures 2 and 3 of panel B in Figure 10.4, Ant is moving his upper body forward more than he is flexing his knees.

    For those who are prone to tipping forward, a good place to practice is a hallway that's approximately four to five feet wide, so that you have a wall in front of you.

UPPER- AND LOWER-BODY CONTROL

In natural movement, your body adjusts to the situation of the movement to keep you stable on your feet. The movements of the upper half of your body are highly coordinated with, cooperative with, and responsive to what's happening in the lower half of your body (your hips, legs, and feet). And the movements of your hips, legs, and feet are highly coordinated with, cooperative with, and responsive to what's happening in the upper half of your body.

Our relaxed body is superbly coordinated with, cooperative with, and responsive to creating and holding the correct pressure in our feet. This keeps the body stable and ensures that the movement will

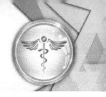

be purposeful and will continue as intended. So, from a movement perspective, while we're on our feet, everything the body does is for one purpose: Keep the feet comfortable, stable, and properly functioning. This is the *"keep Mama happy"* purpose.

When the entire body is relaxed and working cooperatively, the pressure in the feet is where it needs to be for *the feet to produce the movement.* Relaxed, stable, and purposeful movements are the result. When the body does not work cooperatively, restrictive movements and instability in the feet are the results. Keeping the feet comfortable and stable is the ultimate goal. Without it, not much else matters.

The body functions best when the mind is *not* trying to control it. When the feet are stable, so is the body. When the feet are stable, the mind and body can relax. When the mind is relaxed, it is focused on other things, and not the details of the movements. This is exactly how our natural movements work. Our natural, thoughtless movement abilities are created with relaxed dynamic postural control—with the mind focused on other things and not trying to control the body.

In the movement of squatting and standing back up, you are reminding yourself how to allow the upper and lower halves of your body to work in a coordinated and cooperative manner. You are practicing how to relax multiple parts of your body to let them move independently and cooperatively together at the same time. This is what the dynamic part of relaxed posture control means. The naturally smooth, flowing, and unrestricted movement of the entire body requires a relaxed posture. Every part is codependent on all the other parts, and each part is moving independently as required to complete the movement.

Coordinated Squatting: Knees and Shoulders

Some will find it challenging to keep their feet stable when practicing squatting low without support. The common reason for this is twofold. One, the movement of the shoulders and knees is uncoordinated. Two, the movement of the shoulders and knees is restricted.

Is it okay if the pressure moves a little in your feet during the movement? Yes, provided you remain stable and in control the entire time. When you're doing basic movements and you become unstable because the pressure moved, this is telling you that you need to work on coordinating your body movements to stabilize the pressure in your feet. Check how relaxed your body is, and check to make sure you're in the correct setup posture for the movement you are about to do.

Naturally, we adjust our posture according to what "feels right" in our feet. When our feet are flat and our body is relaxed and comfortable, our posture will be exactly where we want and need it to be. When it "feels right" in our feet and our body is relaxed, our shoulders, knees, and toes will be lined up where they need to be. This is the simple, straightforward, and natural concept everyone with natural ability uses in every posture and movement.

In review, we use three main counterbalancing body parts in a squatting movement. These are knees moving forward and down, hips moving backward and down, and shoulders moving forward and down. The centering point for their movement is our feet. Using the hinge points of our hips and knees, and movement of the ankles, our body "folds" as shown in Figure 10.5, just like a trifold door that many homes have for closet doors.

This is illustrated by the inserted green zones of stability in pictures 1 and 5 in Figure 10.5. Note how there are close-to-equal parts of the body (per weight) on each side of the zone in both pictures,

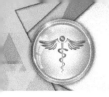

showing that the body is centered over flattened feet throughout the movement. (See Chapter 15 for further explanation of green "Zone of Stability.")

Holding the pressure in your feet constant, you control the natural squatting movement *by not controlling it.* Your body controls it by doing what it must do to cooperate with itself, by counterbalancing all its parts while being guided by the stabilized pressure in the feet. This is why the matter of relaxing the hands and knees to begin relaxing all of the body is so vitally important. When the body is not relaxed, this natural mechanism does not work very well.

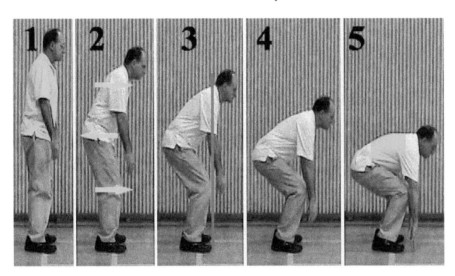

FIGURE 10.5: The feet are flat when the body is relaxed and the shoulders, knees, and toes are in vertical alignment, as shown by the red line in picture 3. The green areas show that the body remains centered over the feet.

The two most common issues causing restricted movements are knees and shoulders:

1. *Knees.* They won't flex or won't flex enough, and/or don't remain flexed during the movement.

This is by far the most common movement problem people with balance and movement issues experience. It is especially so for those with a neurodegenerative cause for their movement impairment.

Whenever you're having difficulties with any of your postures and movements, the first place you should look for the source of the problem is your knees. When your knees are not flexing as freely as they should be, your postures and movements will always be negatively affected.

2. *Shoulders.* They won't move forward or won't move forward enough, and/or won't stay forward during the movement.

The shoulders are the second place to look for the source of the problems you're having with your posture and movements. This is why you need to get in the habit of immediately checking the position of your shoulders while you're working on relaxing your knees.

USING SOMETHING STURDY

Standing and holding on to something that is very sturdy and supportive is another important tool. Unfortunately, many people are so weakened and unsteady that the object they use must be something sturdy enough to stop their fall when they lean or pull on it. When they tip back on their heels, they will often fall backward. Just as often, they will lean or move their shoulders too far forward and unexpectedly fall forward. Also remember that leg weakness and instability will often cause them to fall to the side. For all these reasons, they need to have a good hold on the object, but not a death grip that causes them to stiffen.

Many need to use their hands and arms for support while they relearn how to balance, strengthen, relax, and provide more of their support with their feet and legs. This means they must also become very aware of their tendency to overuse their hands and arms. The goal is to transition into learning to relax their grip so they have better use of their body and legs. This is a challenge for many people with a restrictive-posture movement impairment.

For those with instability: Without realizing it, your hands will be tightly gripping what you're using. Especially for those with a neurodegenerative movement impairment, this frequently will stiffen your arms, and then the rest of you and your knees will stiffen too. For this reason, you must constantly remind yourself to relax your fingers, to help relax your posture and flex your knees, in order to remain stable on your feet. Remember, *only* the stability in your feet produced by your legs and posture alignment will allow you to relax your fingers and arms.

Use a handrail, the countertop in front of the kitchen sink, the back of a couch, or any other similar household surface that is very stable, secure, and easy to grasp. With your hands and arms ready, stand with your toes pointing forward and the toes of your shoes about one of your shoe lengths away from what you are standing in front of.

Please, *be very careful if you're using something with a smooth surface, such as a table or countertop.* This offers you very little support for unexpected excessive forward, backward, or sideward movements. When you're falling forward or sideways, your hands will slide across the top. Moving back onto your heels will pull your hands away from the surface, and there will likely be nothing for you to grab onto as you fall backward.

I suggest you do at least these three things to help keep yourself safe:

1. If you are using the kitchen countertop, use it at the middle of the sink and wrap your fingers down on the inside of the sink. This provides a more secure handhold.

2. If you must use a table, it's better to use one that is lower than your waist so your hands are pushing down onto it as you lean slightly forward. But stay alert! When you're pushing down into your hands, you must pay closer attention to keeping your elbows flexed and relaxed. Weak legs will very quickly cause you to stiffen and straighten your elbows, and then use your arms to help your legs support your body.
   Stiffened elbows cause stiffening knees.

3. Keep the increased pressure in your feet *SLIGHTLY* forward toward the ball areas. This pressure will help to keep you in contact with what you're using for support, but not so much that you are leaning into it. It also helps to keep you from moving onto your heels as easily when you make small mistakes. Having the pressure slightly forward in your feet will help you relax your elbows and hands, and allow you to place some downward pressure into your hands on the surface without trying.
   To set this slightly forward pressure, simply move your feet a *little* farther away from what you're using. Be careful. When the pressure is too far forward in your feet, your body will be pushed into a forward lean. This will cause you to overuse your hands and arms.

In Figure 10.6, Mandy and Jon both have the correct pressure in their feet, as shown by the centered red line in their zone of stability. This provides them with a small amount of pressure pushing into their hands. Keeping this postural alignment, they will both remain stable and able to practice flexing their hips and knees in the squatting movement.

Mistakes happen. When Mandy tips slightly back on her heels, the heavy frame she's holding on to will keep her from falling backward. When Jon tips slightly back, he won't have anything to hold or grab as his hands are pulled off the table. Because of this, he must be very aware of keeping his shoulders slightly forward.

Another important point: When your weak legs become tired, a slightly forward posture will give you the ability to easily, safely, and quickly push more pressure into your hands. This allows you to use your arms for support and prevent falling, so you can then sit.

What else is happening here? Do you remember Mandy from Figure 7.8 in Chapter 7? In that example, her knees were hyperextended, and she was having difficulty transferring body weight while attempting to keep them forward. In Figure 10.6, Picture 2, Jon has the same neurological disorder and the same hyperextending knee issues as Mandy. But in this example, their knees are functioning normally as they move from a high ready stance to a squat, and then return to a high ready stance (seen also in Figure 10.7). Thus, knees that hyperextend are capable of normal function when they are not hyperextended, provided the involved muscles are strong enough to support them.

FACING THE WALL

When you stand against a wall, your bottom and back sliding against the wall or in the corner helps to keep you stabilized as you work on using your knees and leg muscles and feeling the pressure in your feet.

Holding on to something in front of you with your hands allows you to transition into increasing your support and balance using only your legs and feet.

As shown in Figure 10.7, facing the wall and placing only your fingertips lightly on the wall forces less dependency on your hands and arms. This setup demands improved use of your legs and feet for your stability and ability to do the movement.

The movement is the same as in the previous exercise: focusing on doing squats while keeping increased pressure *SLIGHTLY* forward toward the balls of your feet. The setup begins with positioning the toes of your shoes approximately one of your shoe lengths away from the wall, but not more than one-and-a-half shoe lengths. With your elbows flexed and only your fingertips on the wall, you will be standing comfortably in a high ready stance (picture 1).

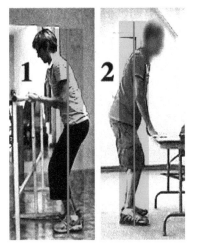

FIGURE 10.6: Use something that is very stable and won't move, because you will push and pull on it.

Your fingers should be *very LIGHTLY* on the wall at approximately eye level. This is also the position you want them to stay in throughout the down-and-up movement using your knees. Do not put the palms of your hands on the wall, because they won't slide easily, especially if they have any moisture on them. Also, when your palms are on the wall, typically it's too easy to push added pressure into them.

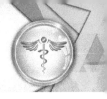

In this example, note that the toes of Jon's shoes are too far back from the wall. This is because his legs are very weak and unstable. They are strong enough to stand on and practice squatting for a short while. With this limited strength and ability, if he should make a mistake and unexpectedly move back on his heels, he would quickly lose his balance. This is why his feet are farther away from the wall. This added distance moves the increased pressure into the ball areas and toes of his feet, and that pushes him forward toward the wall. Yes, this adds extra pressure to his fingertips, but that is easier to manage than being unstable on one's feet.

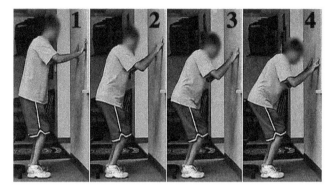

FIGURE 10.7: Flat feet with flexing elbows, knees, and hips, and with fingers lightly touching the wall. This brings the wall up close in your personal space, which many of you will not like.

The fingertips on the wall serve as a guide to how well you're doing. As you lower yourself into a squat with flexing knees and hips, your fingers should remain at eye level, sliding lightly on the wall *as your nose moves closer to it*. If your fingers don't remain in this position, it means you're moving them with your upper body or arms. When your fingers slide very easily with your body movement and stay on the wall at eye level, this shows that you're doing the squat correctly. This is important because it shows that only your legs and feet are supplying your support and balance in the movement.

Hips and knees only. Bottom down. Sit.

Seeing their nose coming closer to the wall reminds me of another problem many movement-impaired people deal with. Many of them do not like anything or anyone coming near them when they are on their feet, especially when their close personal space is invaded. This is because they have difficulty controlling their posture and movements. In a wide-open space, their poorly controlled movements don't matter as much. However, when they get close to things or people, they are forced to have more control. But they can't, because they don't know how. So, their response is standing in place while fearfully guarding and stiffening their posture—and waiting. What are they waiting for? They have learned to be reactionary to everything around them. This means they don't move until they're forced to move. Instead of changing anything about their standing posture or movement to avoid a conflicting situation, they freeze where they are and hope that the thing or person in their space moves away before they're compelled to move. They do this because they don't trust their movements, especially starting and stopping a movement. More on this later.

Jon and Mandy were *very* unstable when standing without external support, so controlling their knee and shoulder movements was a big problem. And they have another issue that makes them unstable. When standing, they quickly hyperextend their knees in an uncontrollable, snapping-backward knee movement. Then, for any posture change or movement, to flex their knees forward, they must first unlock them. This results in another uncontrollable knee movement when the knees suddenly pop forward. With both knees doing this, it has become next to impossible for them to support themselves on one leg to allow the other knee to flex forward.

The only functional remedy for them is to prevent their knees from popping backward into hyperextension, and keep them flexed slightly forward. This means when standing, *they must not allow them to*

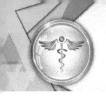
straighten. However, this is extremely difficult to do because the weakened leg muscles and the damaged joint capsules make it nearly impossible to control the knees when they're extending. Thus, strengthening the leg muscles to gain partial control seems to be the best they can hope for.

But can that alone provide a solution to the popping-knee problem? Yes and no. Consider this example as a good contrast. There are some people who are said to be "double jointed." Actually, these people appear to be very normal in their anatomy, with the exception that their joints are hypermobile. This means their joints move beyond the range that's natural for our anatomy. In these select people, their hypermobility may allow their knees to bend backward (hyperextend), but they also have the ability not to let them hyperextend. How? Strong and naturally functioning muscles control the position of the joint.

Therefore, if people who are "double jointed" have the ability to control their hyperextendable joints, so should the people with hyperextending knees due to a different condition or disorder. When this hyperextension movement stems from *muscle weakness and poor postural control or misuse,* these weakness and posture issues can be corrected. However, when the hyperextension is a result of damaged or deteriorated nerves, or other uncorrectable anatomical conditions leading to muscle weakness and poor postural control, the person has very limited ability to correct the situation or cannot do so at all.

The bottom line for these people is to correct as much as they are able to, and most have the ability to correct much more than they realize. The first place to begin is with improving their strength and postural control. Therefore, all of them should work to improve their total-body fitness level, to seek better control of every part of their body. The leg muscles must be strong to support the body's weight. The core muscles must be strong to control the movement of the upper body, in order to control the posture and the location of pressure in the feet. However, the best remedy is not allowing the condition to occur. Prevention!

Your Body Provides the Feedback

In this facing-the-wall exercise, understanding the feeling of the pressure in your feet and fingertips will tell you exactly what your posture is:

1. When the increased pressure moves forward in your feet, your fingers will be pushed harder onto the wall and will not slide easily up or down.

2. When the increased pressure in your feet moves toward your heels, your fingers will be pulled away from the wall, and your elbows will straighten to keep your fingers on the wall.

3. *Control the pressure on your fingertips by controlling the pressure in your feet,* because the pressure in your feet is controlling your posture.

RESTORING STABILITY

Easily moving down into a squat is your self-made recalibration and restabilization "go-to" posture. Learn this squatting movement very well. Become very comfortable with it. You must know that you can trust it. Importantly, you will be using it often to correct many of the mistakes you make in your posture and movements.

Now for your stubborn mind-set of "I don't want to look funny." *Get over it!* Don't be shy to use a squat, *even in public with other people around*, to correct a movement problem.

Remember, it's much better to do a squat in front of other people than to clumsily fall in front of them.

This brings up a very common question. "When I become unstable, how far down into a squat do I need to go to correct it?" This is variable. It depends on how unstable you are and the posture mistakes you need to correct. However, there is always **only one** *absolutely correct answer.*

The correct answer is always, you continue moving down into a squat until your "mama" says, "This is how much." When the increasing pressure in your feet is enough to stabilize your body to stop the nonsense you've created, this is exactly how far down you need to go. Anything less won't fully correct the instability situation. Anything more is unnecessary.

The important point is this. When you begin to feel a mistake happening and/or you're beginning to feel unstable, immediately begin to correct it. Immediately move into a ready stance and continue into a squat until the pressure in your flattening feet completely stabilizes your body, and you feel balanced and secure. This is **always** *the only correct answer!*

PROBLEMS STANDING, AND RETURNING TO STANDING

The following sections discuss common postural mistakes people with a restrictive-posture frequently make, for the same common reason. That reason is instability, and the maladaptive habits the instability creates.

The instability is in the feet, but a big part of their reaction to it is directed to the knees. People with movement difficulties commonly have weaker leg muscles than those with natural movement ability, and are weakest in those with a restrictive posture.

For people with a restrictive-posture movement impairment, as the muscles weaken, the first response is to stiffen the muscles to limit the movement of the knee joints in an effort to provide better support for the body. But this response creates four additional problems:

1. Movement ability decreases.

2. Involuntary shaking occurs within the affected muscles.

3. Increasing instability ensues.

4. The muscles weaken further.

The person's response to these problems is to hold their knees straight. This eliminates the need for the leg muscles to control the knees' movement, and now the muscles are not directly responsible for

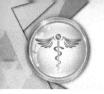

supporting the body. Instead, when standing, these muscles are now used primarily to help hold the knees straight. This further weakens the muscles, increases instability, and destroys movement ability.

Because of their weakening leg muscles and lack of control of their knees, people with this difficulty learn to move quickly from one rather straight knee posture to another. They do this to decrease the amount of time their knees are flexed.

Shoulders Come Up Too Fast and Move Too Far Back

This quickened and excessive backward movement of the shoulders most often moves the location of the pressure in a person's feet to the heels. Suddenly the person tips backward, and they typically react with a fear response and increased postural stiffness. This response then causes another exaggerated and quickened upward and backward movement of the shoulders that pulls the knees straight and moves the pressure farther back in the heels. This overreactive response forces them into a greater likelihood of continuing to fall backward. But, more correctly stated, the increasing pressure in their heels is forcefully and abruptly pushing their body backward.

Correcting this habit of quickened upper-body movement is challenging, but can be done. The transition begins by deliberately slowing the movement and paying attention to what is physically happening in their feet and body. But how do they slow down when they're prone to being unstable? They do this by keeping their feet flattened and stable with downward pressure, as previously described. Without this, they will not be able to slow down. When their feet are stabilized, only then will they develop the ability to relax enough to control changes to their posture.

Another remedy to add is *using the eyes to raise the shoulders*. When standing up from a squat, many people whose shoulders too rapidly lurch up and back are in effect "pulling" themselves up with their shoulders. This is the exact opposite of what they should be doing.

Pushing the body up using the feet and legs with extending knees is the natural way. However, until these people strengthen their legs, gain better control of their knees, and can stay relaxed during the movement, this natural way will remain challenging. Using the eyes to control the rate of shoulder movement helps this transition and is effective even while their legs are relatively weak. This is done by simply *looking up to the horizon with **only** the eyes* when beginning to move up out of the squat.

Be gentle. **Don't use your head to move your eyes.** Tilting the head upward to look up with the eyes is the most common problem, and doing so complicates the movement. *Only* look upward with your eyes. With a relaxing posture, your shoulders will follow in a controlled fashion.

When the neck is relaxed, the head and shoulders will naturally rise with the lifting eyes. So, to those with a restrictive-posture: Practice this eye motion and relaxed non-movement of your neck when you're seated, in order to understand it when you're standing. Feel for the difference between the two. Some of you even need to relax the muscles in your face to relax your neck.

News flash: A stiff neck forces you to turn your shoulders to turn your head. Bigger news flash: This is why many of you tip, stumble, and fall when you "turn your head." The problem is, instead of using your neck, you are using your shoulders to move your eyes to look in another direction. This stiffened upper-body movement moves the pressure in your feet to a new location. That is what causes the tip, stumble, and fall. Even a small amount of restricted movement of the neck due to guarding or stiffness of the neck

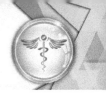

muscles leads to exaggerated upper-body movements and pressure changes in the feet. Experiment with this. Hold your neck stiff and play with different shoulder movements to turn your head. You must *feel* it to understand the effect. Having a stiff neck frequently causes awkward movements, even for those without a movement impairment.

Slow down. Relax your hands. Play with slow mouth and jaw movements to help relax and get some freedom of movement in your neck. Learn to stop moving your head to move your eyes. Practice moving your eyes first, and then follow them with a turning head. Next, allow your head to move with the movement of your eyes.

How high do you need to raise your eyes while rising to standing when you're indoors? Use door handles or light switches on the wall as the limit. Look at these things without straining anything. Do not lift your chin. Do not point your nose up to the ceiling.

When you're stable and following these two suggestions, your head and shoulders will slowly and naturally come up. Their movement will be much better coordinated with the movement of your knees, and you'll be more likely to stop coming up while you are still in a high ready stance. You'll be better stabilized on flattened feet. The overall movement will be better controlled and more comfortable, and your body will be more relaxed.

Quickly Straightening Knees

Knees straightening too fast is a problem that is more commonly seen in people who have stiffened knees caused by leg-muscle weakness and instability, and in those with a higher level of fear. Therefore, many people with adequate strength in their legs have this problem because they've forgotten how to use that strength, or simply don't trust using it.

Why do they do it? Again, this quick straightening movement of the knees is done to avoid the need to control flexed knees. Flexed knees require more work. So, when standing, these people have become dependent on using their leg bones to support their body weight. Therefore, when forced to flex their knees, they are habitually very anxious to straighten them again.

Many of the people who straighten their knees too quickly will stay on flattened feet when their knees are straightened. This is good, but it encourages another problem. It is also very easy for them to move their shoulders back a bit too far as well, and they often do. See it in their posture. They are very high in an upright, straight-knee stance, so it takes only a very small amount of shoulder movement to quickly cause a heel-heavy problem. Also remember, these people frequently have a good deal of body sway while standing, and they easily become unstable while swaying.

Why do they sway? It is the direct result of the decreased downward pressure in their feet in combination with their straight, stiffened knees. As their knees straighten too quickly and essentially lock into the straightened position, the pressure the muscles had been pushing into their feet is lost. It's lost because the muscles are now being used to keep the knee straight.

The person reacts to this self-induced instability by increasing postural stiffening. The result is very tenuous stability that is extremely restrictive to any movement. For all practical purposes, this makes them a living standing statue.

Decreased pressure in the feet combined with stiffened knees causes the body to become top heavy and more susceptible to body sway. In this overly upright stance, people are very sensitive to the quickly

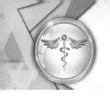

changing pressure in their feet. As the upper body moves very little, the pressure in the feet moves a great deal.

When the pressure shifts to a new location in the feet, it pushes the body in a new direction. This forces the person to react to stop the unexpected movement. However, too often their reaction is an overreaction that forces additional corrections and overcorrections. This is *always* followed by increasing instability and postural stiffening. Because this happens so frequently, they quickly learn that their only recourse is to grab onto something or someone to stop the escalating instability and uncontrolled movements. What they are creating fuels their fears, subconscious negative thoughts, and dependency on external support. It forces them further into their impairment and disorder.

There is an alternative to this downward spiral of circumstances. In large part, it is correctable. How? Consider this question. When the person is rising from a squatting position and this destabilizing situation begins, *what should their reaction be to keep all or most of this from happening*?

They should stop moving up and go back down! They must go back down to restabilize to correct the mistakes they've just made. They then need to remind themselves to hold the pressure in their feet with purposeful working muscles as they move upward again. They need to remind themselves that they can control this situation by keeping their feet stable, leg muscles working, and knees slightly flexed. Then they need to remind themselves to begin to relax, and that all or most of their body *still works*. Fact: Most of them are not as disabled as they have been led to believe.

Yes, there are people with deteriorated physical conditions who can't avoid moving onto straightened knees. But how did many of them get that way? Too many of them allowed it to happen because they did not know how to prevent it. Another yes: There are those with quickly advancing degenerative disorders that do not allow them the opportunity to prevent it. However, many of them can learn how to keep it from happening so quickly.

Quickly Straightening Knees While the Shoulders Move Too Slowly

This mistake puts the person on their toes with straightened and locked knees in an upright, forward-leaning posture. This is very common in those with a habit of stooping. The reasons are twofold. One, they are not bringing their shoulders up to match the movement of their knees. Two, they are bringing their knees up too quickly for the same reasons just described.

As previously discussed, the easier way to learn how to control the upward head and shoulder movement is with the eyes. Yes, previously the discussion was about using the eyes to slow the movement of the shoulders, while this discussion is about quickening the same movement. But also understand, we are discussing the same underlying topic of converting *stiffened* postural control to *relaxed* postural control.

While the *observed* movement of the shoulders in these two examples is the opposite, the *functional* correction and control for them is identical. Additionally, the correction to dysfunctional overly fast or overly slow movement of the knees is also identical.

We've talked about how people moving their shoulders too fast must remember to begin the rising movement with their knees and then use their eyes. But when the problem is moving the upper body too slowly, these people need to *begin* the movement of rising from the squat with the movement of their eyes to gently start to bring their head and shoulders up, and then use slower movement of their knees to continue the standing-up movement.

But please be careful. Some of you "stoopers" will very easily overreact and mistakenly use your shoulders to move your eyes. This frequently causes excessive shoulder movement. Then, as you continue standing up, this mistake will quickly move the pressure in your feet toward your heels. This leads to a very unexpected backward fall.

The purpose of using the eyes to begin the upward movement of the head and shoulders is to move the person into the proper alignment while they are in the squat. Then they use their knees, while continuing to use their eyes, for the rest of the movement, just like everyone else. First correcting the upper-body lagging problem, the remainder of the shoulder movement will more easily coordinate with the movement of the hips and knees during the upward movement of the body.

Pushing the Hips Forward and Moving the Shoulders Back

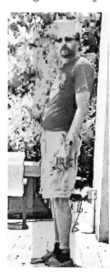

FIGURE 10.8: Hips forward, shoulders back: not a good posture for movement purposes.

This is a "lazier" supportive posture. People with natural ability using this posture stand on stable feet with *flexed* knees and feel comfortable. For this reason, they have a difficult time understanding what is wrong with their posture until they see themselves in a photograph or video.

However, when people with a restrictive-posture movement impairment use this posture, commonly their knees are held straight, and their hips are pushed farther forward to counterbalance the back-leaning shoulders. Still, even with the straightened knees, many of them feel stable while standing. However, when they initiate a movement, their instability quickly begins.

What causes this? As shown in Figure 10.8, this is a heel-heavy posture. Note how his shoulder and arm are well outside of his personal zone of stability. (See Chapter 15). To begin a movement, people with natural ability easily transition out of this posture. But those with a restrictive-posture movement impairment very often cannot easily transition out of it. The primary reason is that their body is not as relaxed and cooperative. Another factor: The movement-impaired person is depending more on their body weight and straight knees to keep them standing stable. Thus, they're not using the muscles in their legs to push pressure down into their feet as much as a person with natural ability continues to do.

Even when a person with natural ability is standing with straightened knees and not using their leg muscles as much as they normally do, they always immediately activate these muscles before changing anything about their posture.

Many movement-impaired people have difficulty doing this, or they do not do it. Transitioning out of the standing movement, they either don't use their leg muscles enough, or they begin to move before putting their leg muscles back to work. Because of this, they create instability before the movement begins.

Holding the Shoulders Slightly Forward, Straightening the Knees

This is not stooping, and it is not a quickly straightening knee issue. This is the opposite of the hips-forward and shoulders-back issue. In this posture they are leaning slightly forward, but with slightly increased *pressure toward the heels* and feel relatively stable on their feet. But they do *not* feel comfortable. The uncomfortable feeling comes from the back pressure they're applying to their knees, which is forcing increased pressure to move toward their heels. This posture typically develops from an inappropriate correction to a mild tipping-forward problem, where there is increased pressure in the toes and ball areas of the feet. To correct this, instead of moving their shoulders back slightly, they push their knees back.

Try this to feel and understand it. Stand with your shoulders held slightly forward and then push your knees back as far as you can. Feel the pressure pushing into your heels. Now, keeping your knees where they are, move your shoulders forward just a little bit more. The pressure is still on your heels. *Hyperextended knees push pressure* **toward** *the heels.*

When the person is in a weakened condition, moving out of this posture is problematic for the same reasons as for those who have their hips forward and shoulders back with straight knees. The only difference between the two is the direction the body has moved into due to the instability.

Unless they correct this posture first, people with locked knees and shoulders slightly forward typically will become unstable in a forward tipping/falling movement when they release their locked knees. Think it through. They are standing with increased pressure in their heels, so:

1. If they first move their shoulders back, the pressure in their heels increases more, and they tip or fall backward.

2. If they first move their knees forward, that removes heel pressure while the forward-positioned shoulders are holding pressure in the ball areas and toes. Suddenly the increased pressure is forward in their feet, and they are tipping or falling forward.

SIMPLIFYING THE MOVEMENT

Actually, our movements are only as complicated as we make them.

- The more we think about how to do the movement, the more we overcontrol our body.

- The more we try to control the movement according to how we think it's supposed to be, the more problems we create.

■ ■ ■

CHAPTER 11

Sitting and Standing

If you are NOT willing to do all you can to help yourself,
why should others be expected to do it for you?

Whether you have a big bottom or a small one, many of you let your bottoms plummet down with a crashing boom onto the porcelain throne and break the toilet seat. You may be small framed, "big boned," thin, skinny, or supersize—none of this size stuff matters very much in this discussion. What does matter is the delivery, or the force you create with your moving bottom. With bottoms essentially in free fall onto the toilet, normal-size people crack toilet seats too.

Now consider this. Some people almost never plop down onto the toilet. But they are very guilty of plopping into chairs and couches and onto the bed. They plop when sitting down, and they often plop back down when trying to stand up. Why do these people plop into furniture but not onto the toilet?

What is this man doing in Figure 11.1? Is Blair standing up from sitting or is he sitting down onto the chair? But first ponder this question. What is the difference between sitting down on a toilet, sitting down on a chair, or squatting to touch your fingertips to the floor?

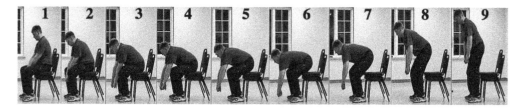

FIGURE 11.1: For people with movement difficulties, rising from a chair is best described as two functional movements: 1. Moving into a flat-footed squat. 2. Standing up from the squat.

The one-word answer is NOTHING. We use a squatting movement to do all of them.

What does this mean for those of you having difficulties sitting down and standing up, yet your squatting ability seems to be okay? It means your sitting and standing problems are not as real as you think they are.

As stated at the end of Chapter 5, every movement we make is based on one or a combination of our six basic stances. The larger meaning is that all our movements are simply repetitive movements using the same muscles and body parts. The changing activity, or purpose of a movement, *does not* change the mechanics of our body. The only difference in the quality of the movement is in how well our body functions—*doing the same repetitive movements* in varying order for the different activities.

SITTING

We actually covered this in the previous two chapters. Squatting down is sitting. Sitting down is squatting. Prove it to yourself. Stand with your back to a chair. Now, with flexing hips and knees, lower yourself into a flat-footed squat to touch your fingertips to the floor just in front of your feet. When you squat *and do not stoop*, your bottom will touch the chair before your fingertips touch the floor. And your bottom will not plop onto it.

There are grand benefits to keeping your feet flat when sitting down and standing up. It keeps you stable and gives you options. It allows you to stop the movement when you want or need to. Ladies, when sitting on a toilet, it allows you to stop when you notice the seat is up.

STANDING FROM SITTING

For people with balance and movement difficulties, standing up from a chair is best separated into two movements. Referring to Figure 11.1, the first movement is transitioning into a flat-footed squat, as shown in pictures 1 through 5. The second movement is standing up from a flat-footed squat, as discussed in Chapter 9.

Getting Your Bottom off the Chair

From a seated position, the first movement of transitioning into a flat-footed squat has four important parts. Jia demonstrates these in Figure 11.2.

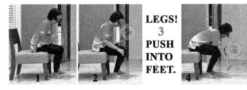

FIGURE 11.2: When getting out of a chair, the four basic parts of moving into a flat-footed squat before standing up are: 1. Set your feet. 2. Align toes and knees. 3. Push into feet with strong legs. 4. Move shoulders forward.

1. Move your feet close to the chair. Push pressure into them, and then *do not move them.*

2. Move your bottom forward. This pushes your knees forward to align them with your toes.

3. Using your legs, push a great deal of increased pressure down into your feet.

4. Move your shoulders forward and down as if you are picking something up off the floor.

ONE, Feet Flat on Floor

Place your feet close to the chair (picture 1). Jia's feet are physically flat on the floor because the soles of her feet are entirely on the floor.

"How far should my feet be apart?" is a common question. Except for "put them where it feels comfortable to you," the answer is, there is no set distance that works for everyone. The general rule for those with a movement impairment is to begin with the feet about shoulder width apart. This wider distance offers some increased stability. But if you are stable and comfortable in the movement with your feet closer together, then position them that way.

TWO, Knees Forward

The second part of transitioning into a flat-footed squat is vertically aligning your knees over your toes. Do this by lifting your bottom off the chair enough to move it forward, to push your knees forward. With your knees aligned with your toes, you also will have moved a small amount of body weight forward and changed the angle of your lower legs relative to your feet. This will cause your feet to feel slightly flatter and heavier, and, the pressure in your feet will have moved slightly forward.

A common comment after moving the knees forward is, "This feels odd." In response, many of you will again move your feet forward away from the chair. What problem did you just create? This takes you back to part one, with your knees behind your toes, with more pressure back in your heels.

Another common mistake in response to this odd feeling is that some people release the small amount of downward pressure they just created in their feet. This allows their feet to easily move on the floor and destroys the foundation they're working to create.

Many people have problems moving their bottom forward in the chair. They try to scoot it forward, but it doesn't move. So, many of them push their shoulders against the back of the chair to push their bottom forward. Others very quickly rock their shoulders forward to slide their bottom forward, but often the chair rocks forward with them. Could the cause of this stuck-bottom difficulty be their disorder or condition? No!

This is a mechanical problem. The person creates this non-moving bottom with too much of their body weight holding their bottom down on the chair. The second issue: They are not using their legs to push their bottom up off the chair before trying to move it forward.

It's a simple concept. To move your body and not the chair, you must first remove the body weight that is pushing your bottom down onto the chair. More specifically, you must transfer your body weight from your bottom to your feet.

Can you use your arms? Yes, but the primary job of pushing your body upward belongs first and foremost to your legs and feet. Far too many people with balance and movement issues forget this and overuse their arms and under use their legs. This allows their legs to become weaker.

With your feet physically flat on the floor and close to the chair, the correct thing to do to move your bottom forward is to push down with your legs and hold that pressure in your feet, for three reasons:

1. So your feet don't move.

2. To remove pressure from your bottom so it can be moved forward.

3. To provide stability and control of the movement.

This is very important because:

1. The most common mistake people with balance and movement issues make when standing up from a chair is *not* moving their knees forward.

2. The second part of this knee mistake is moving the feet forward after moving the knees forward, and not correcting it before they try to stand.

3. Not aligning the knees with the toes is the most common reason they plop back into the chair in their failed attempt to stand. They plop back down because the increased pressure in their heels *pushes* them back on the chair.

When you're standing or squatting and your knees and shoulders are behind your toes, the increased pressure in your feet is in your heels. The exact same principle is true when you're sitting in a chair. When sitting, this pressure is often difficult to feel because most of your body weight is on your bottom. And when sitting back against the back of the chair, the only weight going into your feet is from the portion of your legs that is not supported by the chair, and that little bit of created pressure is in your heels. Moving your body forward to move your knees forward adds body weight (legs) and pressure to your feet, while also moving the pressure forward in your feet.

Thinking knees and toes are lined up

Are they lined up? Many of you will think your toes and knees are lined up when they are not. For this reason, in the beginning I strongly suggest you do a visual check to test what you think you feel. You must know the difference between lined up and not.

You can check your toe and knee alignment by bending forward to see if your knees are vertically aligned with your toes. But frequently there is a problem with this. Many will not bend far enough forward to properly see the vertical alignment. This is the situation with Blair in Figure 11.3. He is looking from an angle and is convinced his knees are in vertical alignment with his toes. Then I placed the stand in front of his feet so he could physically see how far his knees were behind his toes. This is a very common mistake. I suggest you use a reference object that can stand alone on the floor, because it leaves no doubt and can't be argued with. This is an easy and uncontroversial way to show true alignment. Another suggestion is to use a large mirror located to the side.

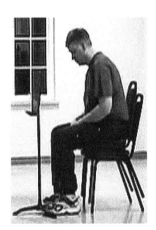

FIGURE 11.3: "I thought they were lined up."

To look out over the edges of your knees, lightly push pressure into your feet and then lean forward from your waist, as if you're about to pick something up from the floor.

"But I'll fall forward out of the chair!" is a common reaction. No, you won't, when you are using your legs and feet properly. Not supporting the movement with your legs and feet is the reason many of you

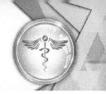

fall out of a chair when leaning forward or to the side. This is also the reason many of you tip the chair over with you in it, while hanging on to the chair with one hand and leaning to pick something up with the other. Support your body with your feet first, then do the movement.

THREE, *Stronger Legs Pushing Down*

To transition into a squat and then stand, you must have the strong support of your legs, a stable foundation, and a cooperative posture. The beginning of the stable foundation is the alignment of knees and toes. To improve the functional stability of your feet after moving your knees forward, increased pressure is then pushed into your feet using the strength of your legs.

The core muscles in your abdomen, lower back, and pelvic areas are also being used to stabilize and control your upper body on your legs. This strengthens your stance and allows the cooperative, coordinated, and counterbalancing movements of all parts of your body.

Knowing how to increase the pressure in the feet is confusing to many people with balance and movement issues, but there is an easy way to remind them:

- Women who have gone through childbirth should use the same strong labor push they used to deliver their baby.

- Men and women, imagine sitting on a toilet. Push as if you are very constipated and desperate to get things moving.

- Both use the same muscles to provide the same stabilizing push down into the feet.

Without this added pressure pushing into your stabilized feet and the strong support of your legs, getting your bottom off the chair will always be a struggle. Without this natural part of the movement, you must rely on your arms to pull or push you up.

The second-most-common mistake people with balance and movement issues make when standing up from a chair is *not* pushing enough increased pressure into their feet. They either forget to do it, don't continue it, or try to do it after doing part four.

FOUR, *Shoulders Forward*

There are two important points that first need to be clarified.

1. Moving into the squat, your legs **do not** move your bottom off the chair. This means your bottom is not coming off the chair in part three.

2. Moving into the squat as you come off the chair, your legs **do not** push your body off the chair.

Yes, your legs have a critical role in getting your bottom off the chair. However, they are merely supportive in this counterbalancing body movement. Remember, for the movement-impaired person's

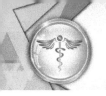
purposes, I am dividing "standing up from sitting" into two separate movements: One, moving into a flat-footed squat. Two, standing up from a squat.

This is not to say that we never use our legs to push our bottom and body up and off the chair in one movement, because many people with and without natural movement abilities often do. However, doing it this way demands more precision, immediate corrections, and additional work in the movement.

With natural ability and relaxed posture, regardless of how we choose to stand up from a chair, it is almost always very easily done. With natural ability, we easily combine and instantly adjust to the required movements. But people with balance and movement issues often can't make those quick adjustments and often have difficulty managing the increased work that's required.

With natural ability, we don't have to do our movements exactly right. We can get away with being a bit careless, because we have the ability and strength to correct the movement and the postural mistakes we make. This luxury is frequently not possible for those with balance and movement issues, and that is because their abilities and choices are too limited. This is the reason they need to learn to move into a flat-footed squat before they stand, and to keep their feet flat during the standing movement. They require this stable foundation to learn how to relax and control their posture and the movement. Then, after improving their ability to keep the pressure stable in their feet with a cooperative posture, they can take shortcuts in their movements.

When you've done parts one, two, and three correctly, there is still increased pressure in your heels. Then moving your shoulders forward moves the pressure forward and creates flat feet *and* lifts your bottom and body off the chair. This completes the transition of moving into a flat-footed squat, as shown in Figure 11.4.

Moving your shoulders forward moves the pressure out of your heels and into the centers of your feet (pictures 2 and 3). Moving your shoulders farther forward and down lifts your bottom off the chair (pictures 4 and 5). Of special note: This only works when your legs stay strong with increased pressure pushing into your feet. In part three, you must start and hold the push. If you don't, part four will not work.

With strong legs from part three, *your bottom will move up as your shoulders move down.* This is a natural counterbalancing body movement of relaxed dynamic postural control. As one body part moves one way, another part moves the opposite way to keep you balanced exactly where you need to be on your feet.

Practice these four parts of transitioning into a flat-footed squat until they become very easy and feel natural. While you're practicing, always pay close attention to what's happening in your feet. Learn to trust the feeling and stability of flat feet using strong legs.

Practice continuing to move your shoulders forward and down by imagining you're reaching

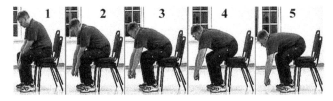

FIGURE 11.4: Moving your shoulders forward and down moves the pressure forward in your feet, and then lifts your bottom off the chair.

for something in front of you on the floor. Feel how easily your shoulders lift your bottom effortlessly from the chair as you move onto stable flat feet, without tipping forward as you feared would happen.

Feel how you don't strain or struggle to get off the chair. Take note that you are not plopping back down on the chair.

Four Parts = One Movement

One, set the feet. Two, push the knees forward. Three, grunt with a bigger push down to make the legs strong. Four, shoulders forward. This natural sequence makes the movement easier to do.

Missing or not completing any of the parts will make getting out of the chair much more difficult, so here's a reminder: The most common mistake is not lining up the knees with the toes. Forgetting to make the legs strong and push increased pressure into the feet, and hold that pressure, is the second most-common mistake. The third most-common mistake is not moving the shoulders far enough forward.

When everything goes well and you are in the squat with flat feet, the only thing left to do is stand up. That movement was covered in the previous two chapters.

HANDS: SITTING AND STANDING UP

When you can squat to the floor and then stand back up without support, you'll also discover that you can get up from and sit down on a chair without using your hands. But it is still perfectly fine to use your hands when you want to. If you want to touch the chair with your hands or hold on to something else to help, do it. Just keep the use of them to a minimum.

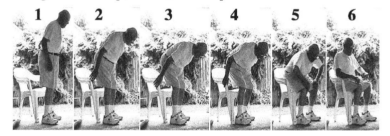

FIGURE 11.5: Instead of shuffling your feet backward to find the chair when sitting, squat and use your hands to move and adjust the chair's position. Then continue sitting only after you have moved the chair to where it needs to be.

In Figure 11.5, Charlie is sitting down onto the chair after adjusting its position with his hands. In Figure 11.6, Philip is standing up from the chair while using his hands. Both are in complete control, stable, and using their legs, hands, and arms appropriately.

Both men correctly move into a squat to transition into or out of the chair with relaxed fingers and elbows. Philip is using his hands and arms to steady his upper-body movement and provide only minimal assistance to his legs. He pushes a small amount with his arms to help his shoulders continue moving forward and down. This ensures that he moves onto flattened feet.

Natural movement depends on the proper use and function of the legs. Without the strength in your legs to provide stability and trust, your movements

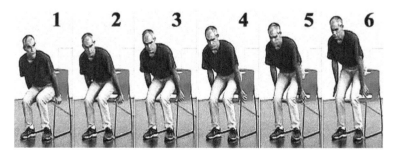

FIGURE 11.6: Proper use of hands and arms to assist the legs when getting up from a chair. Philip uses his arms to help guide his upper body forward and to help stabilize his body on his feet before standing up.

will never be anything close to what you would like them to be. So, pay close attention to the basics of each movement. Practice using your arms less, and your legs more. Rebuild the better ability to stop cheating yourself of your true potential.

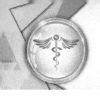

Common Mistakes and Problems

Struggling to Get Out of the Chair

When you are struggling to get up from sitting, most often it's because there is increased pressure in your heels and/or you're not using your legs enough. Both of these make your bottom seem heavier, because it is. Increased pressure in your heels is pushing your bottom backward and down.

When you're struggling to get up, the one thing you need to remember is to stop, sit, and reevaluate your setup. The very first place to look is the position of your knees relative to your toes. Remember, not moving your knees far enough forward is the most common mistake. The next thing is remembering how to count from one to four, to reveal the second most-common mistake.

This mistake is forgetting part three: making the legs strong with a strong push into the feet. Or, it is using the legs *after* moving the shoulders forward. Many people having trouble getting up move their shoulders *too far forward* **before** putting their legs to work. This is because the fulcrum effect provided by working muscles of the legs is not present to allow the bottom to move up as the shoulders move forward and down.

When the shoulders move forward and the legs are not doing their work properly, now the required work you must do to get off the chair is significantly increased with your shoulders this far forward. Count and do part three before you start part four.

Knees and Shoulders Held Back

When your knees and/or shoulders remain behind your toes, increased pressure stays in your heels. This always pushes your body backward as you try to get up. In picture 1 of Figure 11.7, Jack's knees and shoulders are behind his toes and causing increased pressure in his heels. Still, his bottom is coming off the bench. In this example, he is forcefully using his legs to counteract the heel pressure. He then quickly corrects the posture mistake in picture 2, moving his shoulders and knees forward. The red dots on his shoulder and knee graphically show this change.

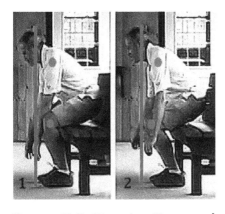

FIGURE 11.7: Picture 1: Knees and shoulders behind toes, pressure toward heels. Picture 2: Equally distributed pressure in feet. Knees slightly forward of toes, and shoulders slightly back.

Those with natural ability frequently do this, and then make the necessary postural adjustments as they continue the standing movement. So, what does this say about Jack with his mildly moderate impairment? He had more natural ability than he realized. This is the case for many people. Too many think they are more impaired than they actually are.

Weak Legs

In pictures 1 through 3 of Figure 11.8, Sangwon's posture for standing up from the chair appears to be good. But then in picture 4, the good has changed to bad. Why did this happen? Look at the position

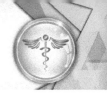

of his upper body and arms in pictures 1 through 6 and note that the forward angle of his upper body and his outstretched arms do not change. This shows postural stiffening. This is the reason he did not complete the forward-and-down shoulder movement to lift his bottom off the chair, to move onto flat feet. As Jack had done, Sangwon was attempting to forcefully push himself up with his legs with increased pressure in his heels.

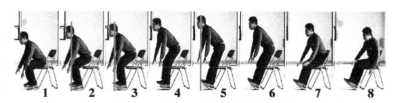

FIGURE 11.8: Sangwon comes off the chair with his knees and shoulders slightly behind the toes of his shoes, which means there is still increased pressure in his heels. He then tries to overcome the backward push from the heel pressure with more push down into his legs, but that only increases the backward push from his heels.

Sangwon's movement impairment is significant, and he is very unstable when standing independently on his feet. His legs are weak. He stands with straight knees. His posture is always stiffened, and his feet are very stiff. When he is standing and pressure moves to the forward part of his feet, he tips forward into an out-of-control, stiffened, shuffling fall. When the pressure moves toward his heels, he tips backward into an out-of-control, stiffened fall.

In pictures 1 and 2, he has a small amount of increased pressure in his heels. In picture 3, he begins straightening his knees. This pushes additional pressure into his heels. Look closely at his feet in picture 3 to see the proof of this. The toes of his shoes are moving upward. In pictures 4 through 6, note the changing angle of his feet. As he continues straightening his knees, the heel pressure continues to increase as it becomes concentrated into a smaller area. In picture 1, he is in control. In picture 3, that control is quickly lost.

Does he fall onto the chair? No, he *does not* fall onto the chair in picture 7. With the increasing pressure in his heels, Sangwon pushes himself backward onto the chair. In picture 1, there is an inserted green dot in the picture over his head next to the window, and the same dot is in the same location in picture 8. Note the distance his head moves away from it. This shows how strong the push from his heels is, to push him and the chair that far backward.

Because of their stiffening reaction, it is very, very difficult for people with a moderate or significant movement impairment to correct this heel-heavy posture mistake. Therefore, their only viable solution is to prevent it. So, do that!

Stop and check your toe and knee alignment before you begin to move your shoulders forward. Feel for the proper pressure in your feet. Also, before you move your shoulders forward, make sure your legs are working strong.

Jerking Upper Body Forward

In picture 10 of Figure 11.9, Amy is one second away from plopping back down onto the chair. Note, in all the pictures she has increased pressure in her heels and reactive stiffness in her arms. In pictures 6, 9, and 10, the fronts of her shoes are up off the floor. Now the question. Why did she stay on her heels the entire time?

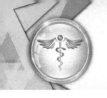

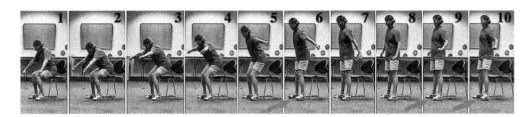

FIGURE 11.9: Stiffened arms ensure that the rest of your body will have stiffness, especially in your knees and feet. Amy doesn't move the increased pressure forward off her heels to begin the movement, and her stiffening posture holds the pressure in her heels during the movement.

She did not move her shoulders forward enough. Why is she stretching her arms out in front of her? This is to help move some body weight forward—the weight of her arms—so she doesn't need to move her shoulders as far forward. Amy's failed attempt here is, in large part, due to the way she tries to get out of the chair. She jerks her upper body forward, but not enough to move the pressure forward out of her heels. All of this is due to postural stiffness, and the heel pressure is constantly pushing her backward.

In picture 6 the forward part of her shoes lifted off the floor (red arrow) because her arms moved behind her. She regains her balance in pictures 7 and 8 but then her shoulders move backward in picture 9, causing the front of her shoes to lift again as increased pressure is applied to the heel areas.

Overusing or Misusing Arms

Pushing into the Chair with Hands

Using our hands and arms is a natural part of everything we do. However, when you are overly dependent on them rather than using your functioning legs, you are creating additional problems. Assistive arms are toned, relaxed, and flexible, and the joints easily moved. Overused arms are much more likely to be inflexible, meaning the joints cannot be easily moved.

- Relaxed and flexible arms and hands are useful during the entire movement.

- Stiffened and/or "stuck in place" arms and hands will help during the beginning of the movement, but they often become a resistant nuisance during the remainder of the movement.

In Figure 11.10, Jim's arms are restricting his movement, but they are not stiffened. In picture 5, his elbows are fully extended with the palms of his hands supporting too much upper-body weight. This stops the remainder of the getting-off-the-chair movement.

In this example, Jim has no problem with his legs. He simply forgets to use them. He forgets part three, and then attempts part four using his arms.

This example of overdependency on arm use has three visual clues in the pictures.

1. His hand is open and relaxed in picture 1. But in the remainder of the pictures, his fingers are clutching the seat of the chair as he pushes into it with the palm of his hand.

2. In picture 2, he moves his upper body forward to apply added pressure into the palms of his hands, to push his bottom up off the chair.

3. In picture 3, he then moves his knees forward over his toes, but his shoulders can't continue moving forward to align with his knees and toes because his arms won't allow it. They are supporting too much body weight.

This example was taken from one of Jim's not-so-good days, which are the days our movements and balance frequently do not feel good. These are the days we tend to use our arms more, and these are the days we make "lazy" mistakes. Our not-so-good days bring out our bad habits, which we must learn to be aware of in order to catch and correct them. These are the days we need

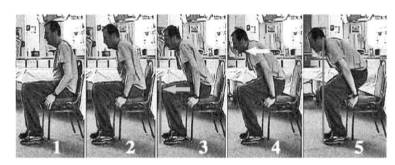

FIGURE 11.10: Jim is overusing his arms to push himself up from the chair. When his elbows straighten, the standing movement stops. This shows how little he is using his legs in this instance.

to slow down, to be more tuned in to the basics of what we're doing. This will help turn not-so-good days into better days.

Amy's and Jim's shoulders were held back behind their knees, keeping increased pressure on their heels. However, the results for them were different. Amy stood and then plopped uncontrollably back onto the chair. Jim corrected his mistake. He paused while in picture 3's position and then began using his legs. In the process he removed much of the pressure in his hands by transferring it to his feet, and continued moving his shoulders forward to move onto flat feet. He then stood and remained standing.

What was the most obvious difference between them? Amy's posture was very stiffened, while Jim's was not. Amy's stiffness was enough that she had no actual control of the movement. Her movement was nonfunctional. Jim had guarding in his arms from overusing them while pushing himself off the chair. This was functionally restrictive but still controllable. When he made the correction and transferred body weight from his hands to his feet, he restored stability in his feet and continued the movement.

Pushing Hands into Thighs

When getting up from a chair, many people push their hands into their thighs to help stabilize their posture and push added pressure into their feet. Provided their elbows remain flexible during the movement and they continue to use their legs appropriately, there really is no problem with doing this.

However, when your arms stiffen with straight elbows pushing down into your thighs, this often does create a problem.

The benefit of this stiffened setup is that it creates a very supportive and rigid A-frame to stabilize your posture. But that rigid frame also locks your upper body in place and will not allow your shoulders to move forward independently to line up with your toes and knees. In addition, the pushing force from your upper body into your thighs is not just pushing pressure into your feet. It is also pushing additional pressure into your bottom. As you attempt to move out of the chair, frequently this setup ensures that the increased pressure in your feet stays in your heels.

This is not saying that pushing into your thighs is something you should never do. What it is saying is that when you use your arms, they need to remain functionally useful and not hinder the movement. This means your elbows need to stay flexible and must allow your upper body to move to where it needs to move for the movement.

1. Using stiffened arms to push hands into your thighs frequently locks your elbows, elevates your shoulders, and stiffens your posture. This commonly results in decreased use of your legs, with less pressure moving down into your feet from your legs.

2. Some of you will say that pushing into your thighs actually increases the pressure in your feet. Yes, you're correct. When you push your hands into your thighs with your upper body, some of that pressure goes into your feet. However, the remainder of the truth is, stiffened arms with locked elbows do not "help" the legs. They do the exact opposite.

   To overcome the restricted movement of the upper body from stiffened arms pushing into thighs, many people with weakened legs will abruptly jerk or rock their stiffened upper body forward. Too often this only creates another instability problem, which is number 3, below.

3. Immediately after the person moves from sitting to up on their feet, the pressure pushed through their arms and into their feet from their upper body is released. When this pressure from their upper body is not immediately replaced with transitioning pressure coming from their legs, the pressure in their feet suddenly decreases. The result is instability. Why? The supporting foundation in their feet is quickly reduced as the added pressure retreats. Suddenly their upper body's abrupt forward movement is relatively uncontrolled.

   Consider the starting posture sitting in the chair. Better yet, put yourself in this posture to feel two things. One, leaning your upper body forward into your hands with straight elbows rigidly holds and blocks the forward movement of your upper body. Two, in this stiffened setup, what happens as your bottom comes off the chair? (Note: People with natural ability often do not add postural stiffening when trying to mimic those with restrictive postures.)

   With a stiffened posture, when a person rocks their bottom off a chair, they do one of two things: They hold the pressure in their hands, or they release it.

   With a mild impairment, most commonly the pressure in their hands is released *as* they transition into using their legs.

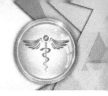

With more of an impairment, typically they *will not* transition enough into using their legs, and the pressure from the upper body on the thighs is not immediately released. People with this degree of impairment frequently have tensed knees and feet. Then, due to their inability to control the quick change in the amount and location of the pressure in their feet, the sudden upper-body-initiated movement is very uncontrolled. When they rock their bottom off the chair onto stiffened feet, the movement commonly ends in one of two ways:

One, the upper body rocks too far forward, which quickly moves increased pressure into the forward part of their feet. This causes them to tip or fall forward.

Two, the increased pressure from the stiffened arms pushing into the thighs limits the upper body from moving forward, keeping increased pressure in the heels. This pushes them back onto the chair before they can move up onto their feet. Then, what do they typically do? The failed effort is most commonly the setup for a more forceful upper-body, jerking-forward attempt.

4. The pressure being pushed into the bottom increases as the hands are positioned higher on the thighs, toward the hips.

The pressure pushing into the bottom decreases the closer the hands are positioned toward the knees. When the hands are on the knees, all the pressure from the upper body is pushed into the feet.

Therefore, rather than putting your hands on your thighs to get up from a chair, a better place to put them is on your knees, as Joanne is doing in Figure 11.11. The picture at the left shows her hands on her knees, but her elbows are straight. Try your best to avoid straightened elbows, because they tend to complicate the movement, as described above.

Pictures 1 and 2 show her elbows flexed. This allows her upper body to move freely and her legs to be used more appropriately.

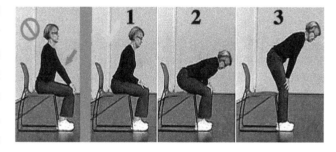

FIGURE 11.11: Straight, locked elbows restrict upper-body movement. Relaxed, flexing elbows allow movement.

Folding Arms across Your Lap, Hugging Your Tummy

For many people, this restricts forward upper-body movement.

1. With a relaxed posture, when you can compensate for it during the movement, getting up while hugging your tummy with your arms is not a big deal.

With a restrictive posture, many people do not have the ability to compensate for it.

2. If you are thin in the belly, folded arms don't block the forward movement of your shoulders. But when your belly is big, the added bulk of your arms against your thighs blocks much of the movement.

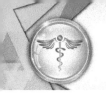

If you have a big belly, you need to free up space for it to move into, otherwise you will be in a grunting struggle with your belly every time you get up. Those with this issue already know that the extra space is made by spreading the knees and feet.

3. With the weight of the arms held against the body, the shoulders must move farther forward to compensate for the weight of the arms *not being held out to the front* of the body.

Allowing the Muscle Tone and Strength of Your Legs and Core to Evaporate

Many people with balance and movement issues experience this problem. They start with strong legs, but then forget to hold them strong as they begin to move their shoulders forward. This happens for four reasons:

1. They fear falling forward out of the chair. As they begin to feel pressure moving into the ball areas of their feet, their mind shouts, "This is scary!"

2. Their legs are relatively weak and tire easily, and they don't trust standing on them without using their hands and external support.

3. They don't know how to continue pushing pressure into their feet. Through years of instability, they have learned to stop doing it.

4. They forget while thinking of other things, are lazy in the movement, or are physically tired.

Falling Forward When Standing Up from a Chair

1. Straightening the knees too quickly while holding the shoulders forward is the most common reason people with balance and movement issues, and a restrictive-posture, tip forward.

   This was discussed in a previous chapter, on the topic of standing up from a squat. Do you remember what to do to help correct this problem? Use your eyes to guide the coordinated movement of your head, shoulders, and knees, and then stop the standing movement when you are in a high ready stance.

2. When standing from sitting, people with a tendency to stoop forward rather than squat have a habit of using excessive upper-body movement. They very frequently tip forward coming off the chair. Then, while they are standing while tipping forward, they're typically slow to bring their shoulders up, or simply don't bring them up at all.

   A contributing factor to the delay in moving their shoulders upward is their reaction to tipping forward. Using their calf muscles, they are actively pushing into the ball areas of their feet to stop the tip, their knees are straight, and their other leg muscles are also tensed. This makes it difficult for them to correct the forward-leaning posture. They are so locked up they're unable to do anything else.

3. Falling forward out of the chair also happens when a person with moderately weak legs uses a repeated rocking motion to "help" them get their bottom off the chair. Far too often, this quickly moves pressure into their toes as their upper body lurches forward in a relatively uncontrolled movement.

4. Having your feet *too far back* toward the chair puts increased pressure on the toes and balls of your feet, and lifts your heels. Uncorrected, this will cause you to immediately tip forward when attempting to stand. Hint: It only takes one or two seconds of paying attention to your setup to avoid this mistake.

Tipping or Falling to the Side When Sitting or Standing

1. A common reason people with balance and movement issues fall to the side is the lean of the upper body to that side. This applies increased pressure to the outside half of the foot, on the side the body is leaning toward, and that pressure pushes the body. This occurs much more frequently with stiffened postures.

2. Another cause is unequal distribution of pressure between the feet, meaning there is much more pressure on one foot than the other. This is more common in people who have painful knee or hip problems and is often combined with one leg being weaker than the other.

   The painful and/or weak leg is not used as much as the other leg, so the person subconsciously learns to overcompensate with the "good leg" in all movements. Thus, the good leg gets relatively overexercised while the bad leg gets less work. When this is combined with a movement impairment from another condition or disorder, their movement abilities degrade more rapidly.

   Therefore, for those people with correctable hip or knee problems who have a condition or disorder that leads to movement impairment, *I strongly advise that the joint problem be corrected as early as possible.* Many unnecessary disabling effects and much increasing disability can be avoided when the successful joint correction and recovery period are done early.

Blind Sitting

And now a pet peeve. When I hear of a person being taught to find the chair with the backs of their legs before they sit, I cringe and want to yell, "*Stop spreading this nonsense!*" This is synonymous with the blind teaching the blind to drive a car. I understand, those advocating this disaster waiting to happen think they're doing the right thing. But finding the chair with the backs of

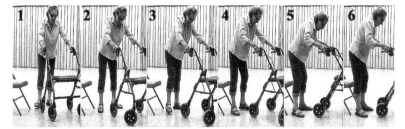

FIGURE 11.12: Alayne walks in front of the chair, then backs up to it and sits down on it without looking to ensure that it is where she needs it to be.

their legs often causes additional problems for those with a restrictive posture, balance and movement issues. (See Figure 11.12.)

1. As people shuffle backward, they often bump into the chair before they're expecting it, and many are mildly startled. What happens when movement-impaired people with a stiffened posture startle? They frequently react with added postural stiffening, causing a shift of the pressure in their feet that creates added instability.

2. When the chair is easily movable, that bump from their leg often pushes the chair farther back or rotates it. It is common for the person not to realize the chair has moved, especially when they've learned not to look for it.

   How far did the chair move? It depends on the chair's weight, how forceful the bump was, whether the chair is on wheels, and what the surface of the floor is.

   By not looking for where the chair is after they've bumped into it, they are assuming the chair is still in the same place. So, what happens when they sit down but the chair has moved? Too often there are mishaps, falls, and accidents.

   This is more of a problem than many people without the problem realize.

■ ■ ■

CHAPTER 12

GETTING UP FROM THE FLOOR

I was asked to teach movement-impaired people how to "fall properly."
*I responded, "NO. I would rather teach them how **not** to fall."*

People with balance and movement issues experience increased instability during the transition from standing to kneeling, to then sitting on the floor. In a squat, when their knees don't flex enough to lower their hands to the floor, they will tip forward the rest of the way and catch themselves with outstretched hands. Typically, they will then plop down onto the side of one hip and thigh instead of transitioning through their knees; and those with more restrictive postures will often uncontrollably roll onto their side.

The remedy for this movement issue begins with remaining stable while squatting and touching fingertips to the floor. The next part is transitioning out of the squat with fingertips remaining in contact with the floor, and lowering the body onto hands and knees. This requires added flexing of the ankles, knees, and hips with coordination of the arms, legs, hands, and feet. And what else does it require? Strength.

Consider the following movement as an example of why working on total body strengthening is required. Many weakened people either cannot turn over in bed, or have a very difficult time doing so. Many of them say it's because the mattress is too soft. Well, if it is due to the softness of the mattress, what is the excuse when the same problem happens on a hard floor? Oh, now I remember. The floor is too hard, and it hurts their knees. Face the truth and repeat the following in a loud voice: "*It is not the fault of the mattress or floor! The fault is mine.*"

To get safely down onto the floor, squat and follow Blair's example in Figure 12.1. But, now that you are "on all fours" in a crawling position on the floor (picture 11), how will you get back up to

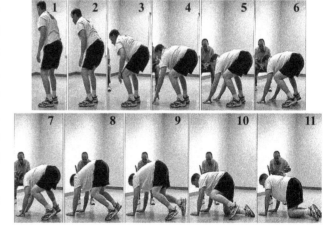

FIGURE 12.1: From standing to hands and knees on the floor, the transition posture is a flat-footed squat. Squat to touch the floor with the fingers, transfer body weight to the hands, and then walk the hands forward to gently lower the knees to the floor.

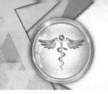
standing upright without scary things happening? For that answer, closely study Figure 12.2, and then compare it in detail with Figure 12.1. Look for the similarities in the movements of getting down on the floor and getting up from the floor.

What are you *actually seeing* when comparing the series of pictures in both figures? Be careful. Stop imagining what you think you should or might be seeing.

There is absolutely no difference. One is simply the reverse order of the other, meaning the pictures in these two figures are the exact same pictures. The movement of getting down is the exact same movement as getting up, only done in reverse order. Naturally, the movement of getting up from the floor is moving into a squat and standing up. For those with balance and movement issues, the squat often needs to be done using flat feet.

Down. Squat and touch your fingers to the floor. Then *walk your hands* forward away from you to lower yourself down onto your knees.

Up. To get up from hands and knees, *walk your hands toward you* to move into a flat-footed squat. Referring to Figure 12.2, to do this, you must:

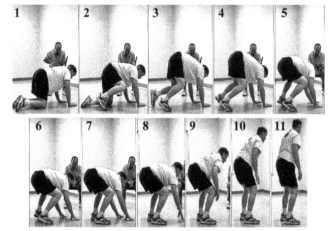

FIGURE 12.2: When moving from hands and knees on the floor to standing upright, the transition posture is a flat-footed squat.

1. Starting on hands and knees, push into your hands and then move your shoulders forward over your hands. This is to reduce the amount of body weight on your knees.

2. Shift your body weight to both hands and *one* knee.

3. Lift the other knee and move it forward. Then push pressure into the toes of that foot (picture 2). Now you must transfer body weight off the knee on the floor and into the toes of the forward foot.

4. Now move the other foot forward and push pressure into the toes of both feet (pictures 3 and 4).

5. Walk your hands back toward your feet to move into a flat-footed squat. This transfers all body weight to your feet (pictures 5 through 8).

6. Stand up from the squat (pictures 9 through 11).

GETTING UP FROM SITTING ON THE FLOOR

No, the movement is *not* pulling with the arms. Naturally, with a rotational movement of the body, we use the coordinated movement of our feet, knees, hands, and thigh to move from sitting to a hands-and-knees position, as shown in Figure 12.3.

1. Sitting on your bottom, lean over to one side (in this example, it's the right side) and put your right hand on the floor (pictures 1 through 3).

2. Lean to the right, onto your right hand. Allow your right elbow to flex as you push into the hand (picture 3).

3. Now rotate your body to move onto the right cheek of your bottom and your right thigh (picture 4).

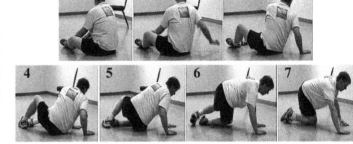

4. Continue pushing hard into your right hand as you also push hard into your right knee. This is to continue rotating your body to the right and move up onto your right knee (pictures 5 and 6).

5. Continuing to push strongly into your right hand, knee, *and foot*, keep your body moving onto both hands and knees (pictures 6 and 7).

FIGURE 12.3: Moving from sitting on the floor to hands and knees is a difficult chore for many people with a movement impairment. The difficulty stems from instability and muscle weakness. This restricts them from transferring body weight between hands, knees, legs, and feet to reposition their bodies.

6. Now complete the instructions for standing up from this position as explained above for Figure 12.2.

CRAWLING

When you can't adequately support your body and control your posture, weakness and instability make it very difficult to do most standing movements. Therefore, the weakened condition must be corrected before work on the other standing issues is possible. However, some stability and transfer-of-weight issues can be worked on while on all fours on the floor. Understanding how to improve these problems while crawling and exercising on the floor will help to clarify what needs to be done when you're standing on your feet.

On hands and knees, things aren't as scary. Thus, using this position the weak and frail group will have a better opportunity to focus on hand and knee pressure, and transfer-of-weight issues. For optimal stability, use a firm floor, with a thin mat or non-slip knee protection, if desired. Yes, most carpeted floors in the home are fine, provided the carpet is fixed to the floor and can't move. However, using a very soft surface will prove to be challenging and unproductive for many in the "*this is scary*" group.

Below are some things to work on.

1. We feel pressure changes more easily in our hands, so experiment with this. Understanding the pressure changes in our hands helps greatly in feeling and understanding the pressure changes happening in our feet during transfer-of-body-weight movements.

2. Learn how to relax your posture and balance, and stabilize on hands and knees.

3. While supporting your body with both hands and knees, as well as your toes, learn how to move your body to shift body weight between your hands and knees in varying amounts.

4. Practice adjusting your body weight to stay stabilized and balanced using only two hands and one knee, or two knees and one hand. When doing this, lift the free knee or hand off the floor.

5. This prepares you for crawling, which many of you need to relearn and practice. Learning how to transfer body weight using hands and knees in a crawling movement helps all restrictive-posture movement-impaired people, whether they have mild or advanced impairments.

When these simpler things become easier, kick it up another notch. Practice balancing *and relaxing* on two hands and one knee, or two knees and one hand, until it's easy. Then practice crawling on the floor like a baby until it feels natural again. With this, you are practicing body-weight transfers, creating and holding pressure and relaxing your posture in advancing movements. Also practice balancing on one hand and the opposite knee until that, too, becomes easy. Hint: Look up Pilates exercises and start doing them. Having an instructor showing and explaining the correct methods and positions is a very wise move.

Imagine watching a young child crawling on the floor toward a chair and using the chair to stand up. Now imagine what the difference would be between that child and an adult doing the same thing. What is the difference? Naturally, nothing in the movement would be different except in our minds. Young or old, we use the chair in the same way for the same purpose.

To use a chair to help you get off the floor, as shown in Figure 12.5, an important point is first moving close to the chair so your shoulders are directly above your hands throughout the movement (picture 1). This provides you with better stability as you push pressure into your hands and straight down into the floor equally through all four of the chair legs (pictures 1 through 7). This posture allows a great deal of body weight (pressure) to be transferred into your hands, and into the stabilized chair, to help you transition onto your feet. Then, when your legs are stronger, you won't need to depend on the chair to help you as much.

In Figure 12.4, John's movement abilities were significantly impaired, and he was in a very weakened condition. Slowly, over the years, he came to distrust his natural movement abilities as his fears increased. As a result, his level of physical activity drastically declined. His muscles weakened from lack of use, and his movement abilities progressively decreased to severely impaired. This caused him to fear his movements even more and to do less.

Living with the uncorrectable direct effects of their disorder, combined with the correctable *indirect* effects that are not realized as being correctable, many people become victims of this same perpetual cycle of decreasing ability due to lost strength. The combination of the direct and indirect effects ultimately put John in a wheelchair, substantially exacerbated his sedentary lifestyle, and accelerated the decline in his muscle strength and ability. Still, there is one very important aspect in John's presentation that cannot be denied, and is frequently overlooked by the people in this predicament and those looking at them. What is it?

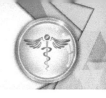

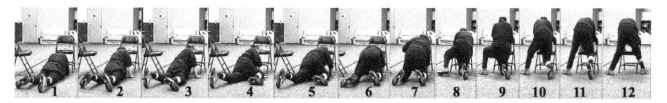

FIGURE 12.4: The chair John is using to get up from the floor is stable only when he is applying pressure straight down onto it. To produce a straight-down pushing pressure, to apply equal pressure into all four legs of the chair, your shoulders must be directly over your hands. This is to avoid tipping or pushing the chair away.

Look very carefully at what John is doing in the sequence of pictures. He is using and has control of every part of his body. His arms and legs, elbows and knees, hands and feet. They still function. For heaven's sake! What is this showing? Everything still works. This means, if he improves the conditioning and strength of his muscles, his level of function will be that much better. And *still*, there is something more to it. If **he**, and those treating and caring for him, had been more observant and practical many years ago, he likely would not have been in the very poor physical condition he was in on this day. These facts are loudly shouting that his level of functioning would be better *if he had not given up* on his need to remain in a more fit physical condition.

Why do so many people allow this to happen? Ultimately, they give up trying. They resign themselves to being what the disorder forces them to be. They stop trying because they don't know how to change the outcome. They're too tired of struggling with the frustrations. They are constantly warned against doing things. However, *do not* discount another factor that also applies to many of them.

It's easier to play it safe and sit in a wheelchair than it is to struggle with exercises and attempts to keep up with the overall effects of the disorder. I understand their dilemma and their very personal choices. Admittedly for some, *ultimately*, they don't have a choice about being confined to the chair, because the direct effects of their disorder are such that there is nothing they can do to alter the outcome.

But *ultimately* is a very relative term. Individually, our "ultimate" situation living with these disorders has many variables that we *do* have the ability to alter. The problem is that too many people are frequently blinded by others and themselves to what they could be doing to help themselves do better. Too many are prematurely convinced that it's useless to try. Too many are persuaded that it is not possible if they did try. Why? Too many believe we are at the mercy of our controlling condition or disorder, a belief that has not been helped by advice given by some professionals. Too many see

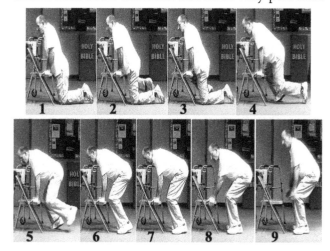

FIGURE 12.5: Shoulders over hands. Arms support the upper body and push pressure straight down to stabilize the chair equally in all four legs. The remainder of the body weight is transferred to one knee, then to the ball area and toes of one foot, and then to both flat feet. Then, the pressure in the hands is gradually transferred to the feet as you stand up from the squat.

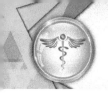

only the negatives so clearly that any potential positive has little to no chance of ever being recognized. This is a victim mentality.

Ultimately, everyone is responsible to themselves, for what they will or will not do to help themselves in their personal situation. Ultimately, it is each person's choice despite what anyone thinks or says. Ultimately, each person must decide on their own, because it is their life. But too many movement-impaired people give up their responsibility—because they do not know how to apply and use it. But now they have a positive resource to help them change this dilemma. This book fosters that change. It provides them with answers and methods to help them make an informed choice in how they can help themselves.

In many cases, much of the quickened decline can be prevented and the quality of life better maintained. Sadly, for others, not much can be done to alter the course of the aggressive nature of their disorder. Still, how much function can any of these unfortunate people maintain for a longer time? On an individual basis, none of them will know until they put forth the effort to allow the potential difference to become the possible.

Stop complaining and start doing something positive for yourself. Stop the self-degrading thoughts. Look at yourself with an *honest* and open mind. Are you afraid of succeeding, or are you afraid of looking silly working and practicing crawling on the floor? Play games with kids. Learn from watching and having fun with them.

You have everything to gain, and *nothing to lose*.

■　■　■

CHAPTER 13

Turning to Look
without Moving Your Feet

Wishful thinking only works when you put those wishful thoughts into action.

Turning our head without turning our shoulders requires a very relaxed neck. For many with balance and movement issues, especially when their posture is restrictive, turning to look in another direction is simply not a very good option. Why? Their tensed posture often includes the muscles in their neck. This makes turning their head challenging, and often they quickly become unsteady on their feet when doing so. So, turning their head to see what's behind them is something they learn not to do. Instead, to "turn" to look in another direction, they first stop. Then they shuffle their feet to "turn" their body in the direction they wish to look.

Not Turning

The movement of "turning" to look behind you is rightfully **not a turning movement**. It is a rotational movement. And that is the main reason many people with balance and movement issues have difficulty with it. This is also why my golf game is not as good as I would like it to be.

The problem. With a restricted posture, the upper body moves more easily than the lower body. As a result, the person twists from the top instead of naturally pushing their body into the rotational movement from the bottom.

Executed correctly, the rotational movement of "turning" the body in another direction is done with very relaxed knees and is powered by the feet. The movement of the knees and flexing foot rotates the hips *and* the upper body. The head rotates independently on the neck. Note: In this rotational movement, *the shoulders are not used to power any part of the movement.* Naturally, they merely go along for the ride.

To rotate your body as Paul is doing in Figure 13.1, you must be relaxed from your neck down to your toes. In the example, he begins in a ready stance with mildly increased pressure in the ball areas of his feet. Powered by his right foot, he then pushes and flexes his *right* knee forward. This forward-moving right knee pushes his hips and upper body into rotation to the left, and the slightly extending *left* knee allows the movement to go easier and farther.

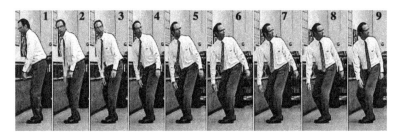

FIGURE 13.1: Turning in place to look behind you. Using only the knees, this is a rotational movement of the body. The hips and upper body cooperatively follow the movement of the knees.

As the knee pushes the hips and upper body into rotation, in a cooperative and coordinated movement, the relaxed body does four basic things. These are seen in the pictures.

1. The movement begins with increased pressure in the ball areas of both feet. Then, with a push from one foot, the knee above it moves forward.

2. Both knees are used. To rotate to the left, the right knee moves forward and slightly down as the left knee moves backward.

3. Pushed by the forward movement of the right knee, the hips and shoulders rotate. This rotational movement holds the pressure constant in the ball areas of the feet throughout the movement, exactly where the body requires it to be.

4. To rotate the body and hold it in the rotated position, the push from the ball area of the pushing foot must be continually applied.

The *rotational movement* of the body is powered by the pushing foot and controlled with the forward and downward movement of one knee. The right knee is used to rotate the body left, and the left knee is used to rotate it to the right.

The "balancing act" on the feet that allows the movement to happen is the responsibility of the upper body. The upper body must simply remain relaxed, to stay in position and hold the pressure constant in the feet, as the movement happens.

Paul makes this look very easy because his posture is totally relaxed. His relaxed, balanced rotational movement is what allows his golf game to be so much better than mine. In his game, his knees remain totally relaxed. In mine, my knees and posture tend to be intermittently slightly guarded. This relatively small difference in the comparison makes a *huge* difference in the quality of the movement.

TRY IT

With equal pressure in the ball areas of both feet, relax your posture. Hands and elbows first. Then push your relaxed right knee slightly forward to effortlessly begin to rotate your relaxed body to the left. When your

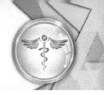

body remains relaxed, your shoulders will rotate and self-adjust to hold the location of the pressure in the ball areas of your feet constant. *Then and only then* will your posture—and especially your knees—stay relaxed.

When your posture is mildly guarded or stiffened, this rotational movement can quickly become complicated. You must focus on holding the pressure *toward* the ball areas of your feet and keeping your posture relaxed. For those with a restrictive posture, this means you must also remind yourself "shoulders forward" as you begin the movement. Why? Because your shoulders will have a very strong tendency to move backward and up. Also note that you must allow the forward-moving shoulder to come slightly down as it rotates forward, as shown in the pictures. This lowering of the forward-moving shoulder is the result of the lowering knee below it. Therefore, DO NOT focus on moving the shoulder. Forget about it. Simply relax and allow it to go where your body wants to move it.

As for the knees: What else must you be reminding yourself about them? *Stay down. Relax.* This is the biggest challenge in doing the movement when the body is *not* relaxed.

Relax your hands to help relax your body and knees. Shoulders forward to hold the pressure in the ball areas of your feet. Knees down to keep them flexed and more relaxed. Focus. Practice.

Always, always, always, in all *basic* movements we do standing on our feet, we naturally use our lower body to supply the power and to control the movement. Working on this rotational movement helps demonstrate this very important point.

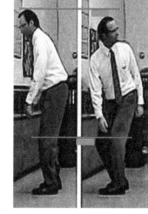

The pictures in Figure 13.2 show the start and completion of the movement and are the first and last pictures from Figure 13.1. This side-by-side comparison is to show the extent of the movement of the right knee, hips, and shoulders, and the change in height.

The red lines mark the top of Paul's head and the height of his right knee at the start of the movement. The blue blocks under the red lines are the distance his body lowered and his right knee flexed downward. Both blocks are the same dimensions. This graphically shows that the flexing knee lowered the body as it rotated the body. Also note that his head is centered over his feet when his body is rotated, in the picture on the right.

FIGURE 13.2: This is a rotational movement done with the knee. It is not a shoulder-turn movement.

This ability provides many people with good athletic skills in a wide variety of sporting activities, and it is also a necessary part of our everyday movements. Not having this completely relaxed ability is a primary reason many people struggle to keep their balance during movements.

GOING BACK

To return out of the rotation, to looking straight ahead in a ready stance, simply relax the pressure in the pushing foot and lightly pull the forward knee back into extension. Practice **not** using your shoulders to do or undo the rotation.

SHOULDERS LEADING THE MOVEMENT

Ann begins centered in the proper posture (picture 1 of Figure 13.3) but then quickly moves out of it. Note that in picture 2, her body has moved to the left. Do you see why this is happening? She's

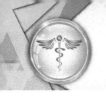

attempting to rotate her body by first turning her shoulders with very little movement of her left knee. In Ann's case, this was a result of three factors: One, learned behavior of using her upper body to begin movements. Two, mild postural stiffness, causing restricted knee movement and hip rotation. And three, overthinking how the movement was to be done. In picture 3, she flexed her left knee farther forward, but could not avoid additional lateral movement of her hips and shoulders that began in picture 2.

Now compare the obvious differences between Ann's movement and Paul's in the previous examples. Her movement begins with a turn of her shoulders, followed by a rotational movement of her body using her left knee. Paul's rotation is done with his knee. His body stays centered over his feet. Ann's body does not.

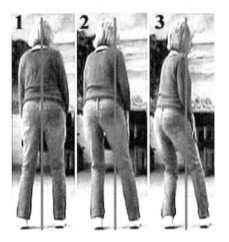

FIGURE 13.3: Example of a rotational movement begun using the shoulders and then followed with movement of the knee.

Mild knee stiffening or guarding encourages the use of the upper body to begin any movement. When the stiffening is more than mild, this forces the increased use of the upper body throughout the movement. When you forget to release the guarding stiffness in your hands and elbows in the setup posture, you are also forgetting to begin relaxing the guarding stiffness in your knees. This complicates the performance of the movement and often creates instability. This is also a large part of the big mystery of why you have so many problems with other movements. The slightest restriction in the flexibility of your knees makes a mountain of negative difference in the performance of any movement.

Stiffening and straightening knees restrict and destroy natural movement.

GUARDING STIFFNESS

Lenore's movement impairment is significant. When standing, she is very unstable, so any movement she attempts is highly problematic. In Figure 13.4, her intent is to look at the chair behind her. She is attempting to rotate her body to the left in the upper panel and then to the right in the lower panel. But her stiffened knees are not allowing it.

In pictures 1 through 8, she is practicing rotating to the left, but the movement of her right knee is slight. This is evidenced by the slight change in the space between her right knee and the corner of the chair. In these pictures, she moves her shoulders quite easily but *does not move her head*, and continues looking forward. But she remains stable. (Take note that her movement impairment is significant, yet she has increased function in her upper body. This is an atypical finding that will be explained later in this example.)

In the lower panel (pictures 10 through 17), Lenore becomes very unstable as she attempts to rotate to the right. This happened because before picture 10, I had just reminded her to use her knees for the movement. But when she tried to use her left knee more, her first response was to bend forward at the waist (picture 9). Next she added upper-body turning in order to help move her knee. When she moved the knee, it moved forward more than she expected, while her hips moved very little (pictures 10 through

14). With the changing pressure in her feet from the upper-body movement and the unexpected increased knee movement, she became more unstable. Ill-supported by weak legs and stiffened knees, she then tipped forward with a stooping movement of her upper body. In pictures 14 and 15, the forced stoop lifted the heel of her right foot off the floor (red arrow); it was then pushed back down in picture 16.

When Lenore is standing, her feet are rigidly stiff. This is best seen in pictures 14 and 15. Her right foot doesn't flex in the slightest when its heel is pulled off the floor. It functions more like a thick piece of wood that cannot bend.

In picture 17, note how she bends at the waist to put her hands on the floor. If she is as stiff in her legs and feet as I've described, how is she so relaxed in her waist? She enjoys a winter sporting activity in which she is seated with her legs strapped down. She then has relaxed use of her upper body for the activity of skiing on the snow. Make no mistake here. I applaud her efforts and determination in doing this, and it is a grand accomplishment. She is staying as active as she can be in spite of her disability. However, it is also a saddening predicament that she has worked herself into. The sporting activity that has enabled her to maintain the relatively relaxed use of her upper body comes with a huge price.

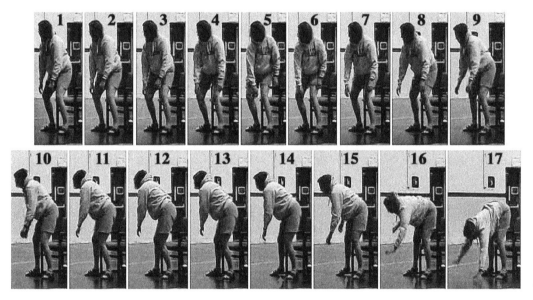

FIGURE 13.4: Weak legs with stiffened knees and feet make standing very challenging. When standing is challenging, any attempted movement is difficult. For movement ability to improve, weakened legs must first be strengthened.

In this activity, Lenore has taught herself how to better use her upper body to do things she enjoys. This is the *very* happy part. The sad part is, while having her legs strapped down, she essentially learned how to be a paraplegic. Why do I say this is a sad thing for her with this significant movement impairment? It is because this reinforced a dependency on the upper-body movements of a person whose legs are functionally useless.

Yes, her legs are problematic due to her disorder. *But* she still has functional legs, which we proved as we continued with the working sessions. So, imagine what the difference could have been if she had been exercising her legs as well as she had been exercising her upper body. Her legs would have more function and ability, *and* she may be doing even better in this sport she loves.

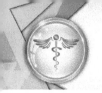

There is another important point that was only briefly mentioned in Lenore's example, and needs to be discussed. In picture 11, she slightly flexes her left knee forward. This knee movement creates a support problem that clearly illustrates the weakness of her legs.

When the left knee flexes forward, this releases too much of the muscle stiffness *that has been holding the knee in place* and supporting her body. When the stiffened muscle support is momentarily released, her upper body immediately stoops forward at the waist to stop her forward tip, so she can support her unstable body with her hands on the floor. In this same instability situation, most people with a movement impairment would have continued to tip forward and likely fallen to the floor—with straightened knees. Again, what does this say about Lenore with her flexed knees? She has more function and ability in her legs than she realized, and it would be much better if they were stronger.

People with weak legs have a very difficult time
transitioning from releasing stiffened muscles to using functionally working muscles.
The result. Poorly controlled knees.

Probe a little deeper into the issue of seemingly "nonfunctional" weakened legs. True, many people with a movement impairment have legs that by many standards are uncontrollable and useless for standing and in movements. But in reality, many of you prove every day that your legs still work better than you claim they do. For example, your legs DO work fairly well when you are *not* standing on your feet. And they DO work fairly well when you are leaning on something for support. And, with legs that you cannot stand or walk on very well, many of you **still drive a car**.

WAKE UP! If your legs work okay for driving a car, they also have the functional ability to do work when you stand on them. What is the big difference? Strength.

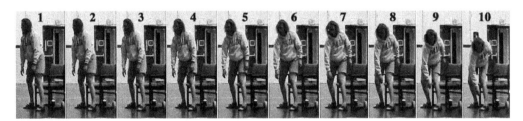

FIGURE 13.5: Improved postural relaxation allows increasing knee function and movement, which improves postural stability. Will you look at that? Rotational movement is now possible.

With practice, Lenore improved her ability during our two-hour working session (Figure 13.5). She began rotating her body with her knees as her ability to control the pressures on her feet improved. With better use of her leg muscles, she became more stable while allowing her knees to flex even more. This tells you her legs were not as weak as she considered them to be. So much realized in a short period of time. Imagine the possibilities, especially if this work had begun when her movements were only mildly impaired.

Stiffness hides strength and prevents it from being used.

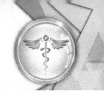

SEEING WHAT'S BEHIND YOU

As Ellen is doing in Figure 13.6, looking at it is the best way to ensure that the chair you are about to sit on is in the proper position.

Fear, stiffening, and induced instability—the same issues Carmen is dealing with in Figure 13.7—are the reasons some people don't look for the chair behind them anymore. Take note of his very tight right hand gripping the walker, and his elevated shoulders. His posture is stiffened, which means his knees and feet are very stiff, and he is also leaning on the walker for support. Because of this setup,

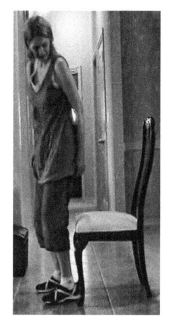

any postural adjustment or body movement he does moves the walker. This is the reason he is constantly squeezing the brake handle. He is overdependent on using it, so any movement of the walker increases his instability and reactive stiffening.

In Figure 13.7, Carmen is attempting to look at the chair behind him by rotating his body. But, with a moderate movement impairment his posture is too stiffened to allow it. There is no body rotation in his attempt because his knee will not flex to lead the movement. Instead, both knees remain straightened in all the pictures. Therefore, the only thing he can do is partially turn his shoulders and head.

In picture 2, take note of the location of his right hand, indicated by the blue arrow, and compare its location to the background in pictures 3 and 4. Beginning in picture 2, he pushes the walker slightly forward as he turns his shoulders to the right. This moves more pressure into the forward part of his feet, which adds forward tipping. This forces him to turn his shoulders back to the left to then correct the tipping instability. Picture 5 shows he has pulled the walker back toward him by moving his shoulders back. This flattens his feet,

FIGURE 13.6: "I know where it is, because I see it."

so he regains some stability, and this allows him to again turn his shoulders to the right and increase the turn of his head to the right in picture 7. In response to the instability he experiences, he adds more postural stiffening as he squeezes harder on the hand brake. The red arrow in picture 6 points to the left brake handle that he is tightly squeezing.

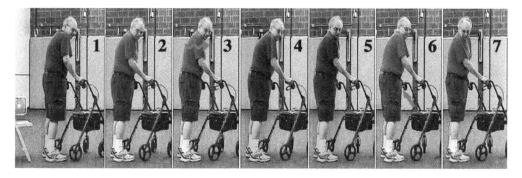

FIGURE 13.7: As Carmen attempts to look at the chair behind him, his increased level of instability and stiffness in the movement prevents him from adequately moving his body.

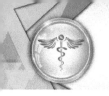

This example shows him in his first attempt, and it was toward the end of a two-hour work session. Because of this, he was growing tired, and his leg muscles were weakening. The importance of this example is to show the extent of the issues many movement-impaired people with restrictive postures deal with on a daily basis—the same issues that Alayne in Figure 11.12 (Chapter 11) intends to avoid by simply not trying to look for the chair. Importantly, what else is being shown here? These examples of Carmen and Alayne also highlight the overdependency on their walkers many people develop to control and correct their postural mistakes.

Sue's movement impairment is mild, but still her knees resist flexing as she attempts to rotate and look for the chair in Figure 13.8. In picture 1, she begins with flexed knees and then starts the body rotation using her left knee. However, the movement of the knee is slow, and then both knees begin to straighten while she continues to turn her shoulders (pictures 3 and 4). The reason: She had become unstable.

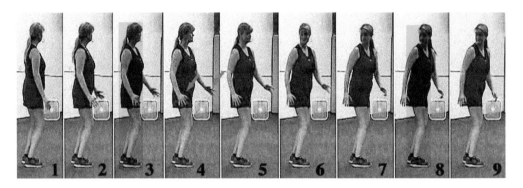

FIGURE 13.8: Sue begins with a stiffened and too-upright posture. The result is very restricted knee movement, leading to upper-body turning, straightening knees, and instability.

The carpeting on the floor is mildly spongy. This adds to the other reason Sue feels unstable, and contributes to postural stiffening, which her stiffly held fingers show. Her upper body is also too upright in picture 1 and stays in this position until picture 6. Because her posture is too upright, the increased pressure in her feet is slightly toward her heels. On the spongy carpet and with her postural stiffening, this is increasingly destabilizing and greatly limits the movement.

Standing on the spongy carpet, she has a constant *slight* back-and-forth tilting movement of her feet, oscillating between the fronts of the feet and the heels. This is causing stiffening and mild quivering of her leg muscles. This quivering (shaking) is very common for people with a stiffened posture and instability, even when they are standing on a hard surface. It is also an issue that onlookers and therapists frequently miss. Take special note. Frequently, this happens even when the person's leg-muscle strength is quite adequate. Also frequently, this shaking can be relaxed away with stability.

Two important complicating issues result here.

1. The postural stiffening reaction weakens the leg muscles' ability to continue pushing the needed stabilizing pressure into the feet. This reaction adds another cycle of increasing stiffening and instability.

2. Subconsciously, people stop pushing pressure down into their feet because the uncontrolled movement of the pressure in their feet constantly pushes them in unexpected directions. This reaction also fuels the next cycle of increasing stiffening and instability.

So, with a restrictive posture, how can this cycle be stopped? The best and easiest way is to squat. Squat to force the leg muscles to work, to flatten the feet, to increase pressure in the feet, and to stop the instability cycle. Then, with a more relaxed posture, slowly return to standing, while remembering to apply the things we covered on this topic in previous chapters.

In picture 6, Sue has moved her shoulders slightly forward to put the pressure back in the middle of her feet to find stability. Flat feet. However, she does not relax the stiffness in her body. Because her knees are too stiffened to flex, she then continues to turn her shoulders (re-creating some of the instability) and straightens her knees (pictures 7 through 9). Compare the flexing and forward position of her knees to the short, red vertical lines in pictures 4, 6, and 9 to see the change.

Yes, Sue, you did *turn* your upper body enough to see the chair. However, in that posture, you could just barely see it. No other purposeful movement was possible, because you were again on the edge of instability with decreased and shifting pressure in your feet.

Her second example of attempting the rotational movement (Figure 13.9) is a sharp contrast to the previous example. To fully stabilize herself on the spongy carpet, she first lowers into a squat. Then she pushes her left knee forward to rotate her hips and upper body (pictures 7 through 9) as she stretches her right arm out to grab the chair with her hand.

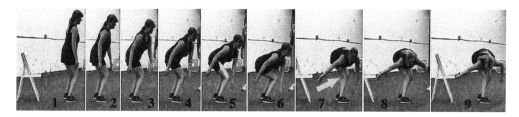

FIGURE 13.9: The proper setup posture allows the movement. One, squat to increase the pressure and stability in the feet. Two, move the left knee forward to rotate the body to the right to reach for the chair.

In the first example, she had multiple thoughts about what she should do. This successful second attempt was done with *one focus*, and that was to make and keep her feet flat and heavy. This is the reason you see her squat first and rotate second. As she becomes more comfortable, she will learn to squat and rotate at the same time, just as people with natural ability do.

Now, to tell you of the one little ploy I used in this second example. I purposefully moved the chair farther away to force Sue to extend her reach, and to capitalize on her competitive nature. With the chair moved farther behind her, the only way she could possibly reach it with her hand was to do exactly what you see her doing. Flex the knees. Squat.

Feisty Sue accepted the challenge. This took her out of her thinking mind and put her into a "just do it" mind-set to prove to Jerry (her husband) and me that she could. Without going through the mental steps of what she thought she should do, she simply went back to what she already knew. She solved her instability problem the natural way, by relaxing, stabilizing with increased downward pressure, and letting her stabilized body do the movement. What was complicated, the proper setup now freed her to do very easily. This simply took her thinking mind out of the process and allowed her natural ability to emerge, which allowed her to brag to us that reaching the chair was "a piece of cake." Hooray!

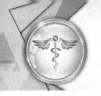

This is a very important point. Many of those with problematic movements *do* have the ability to do better, but they do not understand how to access that better ability. The information in this book provides them with much of this required understanding. Now their job is to learn how to apply what they've learned.

THE FREEDOM OF MOVEMENT

Every movement we do has a posture that prepares our body to begin and follow through with the movement. This is "that" movement's setup posture, and it is vital *because it is the very beginning of the movement.* With it, the movement goes as planned. Without it, the movement becomes an unintended movement.

Static and Dynamic Postural Control

Standing is static and fairly simple. Movement is dynamic and complex. In natural movement, we must have the ability to relax and control our posture when standing still, in order to have the ability to relax and control our posture during movement. Those with a tensed posture frequently are unstable while standing, so how can they then magically be stable during movement? They can't. *The requirement for first achieving static postural control is too frequently overlooked.*

Because it enables the efficient, coordinated counterbalancing act of our body, relaxed dynamic postural control is required for natural movement. This is the primary component that allows thoughtless, automatic movement. It is the only way our cooperative body parts can reflexively (automatically) coordinate their combined movements and hold the pressure on our feet exactly where the body needs it to be. In contrast, movements controlled with thought result in the self-induced slowing of the physical components of movement.

So, what is the foundation for the natural basics of postural control? It is controlling the pressure in the feet and relaxing into it. Our natural and coordinated balancing act on our feet is not something that comes from thinking about how we think it works. It comes from the feelings of the pressure we recognize, trust, and use.

Our natural movements happen when muscles directly communicate with other muscles and respond reflexively through the pathways that link them together. Through these neurological reflex communication pathways, muscles tell other muscles what they are doing. Through the natural flow of these signals going very rapidly back and forth between them, the muscles relax or contract exactly the right amount at exactly the right time. This is a major part of our movement "autopilot system," and our body must be relaxed for it to work.

Thus, our thoughtless natural movement ability is based largely on what our body is telling itself, and not what our mind is telling it to do. This reflexive neurological level of muscle-to-muscle communication does not use or require *conscious* input from the brain.

This is the body determining and doing what is required to keep itself stable on its feet. This is creating the feeling you get in any movement or posture that the mind interprets as, "*This is the correct posture* for what I want to do."

PRACTICE. PLAY. USE IT.

In Figure 13.10, Nate is doing well with his mildly moderate physical level of impairment, which is due to a degenerative neurological disorder. He is working on relaxing, staying down with flexing knees, and

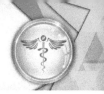

pushing his body into rotation with his right foot as he drops and then hits the ball. But two things are visible here that he can improve on:

1. He has increased pressure in his heels. This pressure keeps his right heel on the floor (pictures 5 and 6) and limits the rotation of his hips and knees. The yellow arrow points to the heel on the floor, when it should be raised.

2. The rotation of his upper body to the left begins in picture 3, but forward movement of his knee and the rotation of his hips don't begin until picture 6. This is backward. He pulled the hip and knee into movement with his upper body in picture 5.

   Done correctly, the forward movement of the knee pushes the hips and upper body into rotation. People with a movement impairment often have a rather large learning curve with complex movements like this.

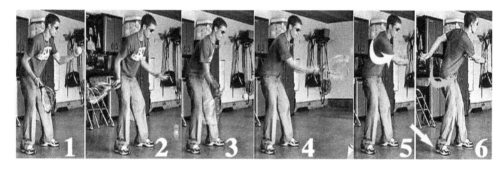

FIGURE 13.10: Dropping the ball, then hitting it when it bounces up. The movement of hitting the ball with the racket is very much the same as swinging a golf club to hit a golf ball on the ground, and many other activities.

What Nate needs to do to improve hitting the ball in the air with the racket is the same as what Tom needs to do to hit the golf ball on the ground with the golf club (Figure 13.11). The movements are very much the same, even though the activities are different.

From a practical-use perspective, our natural movements are not complicated. Yet we so often complicate them in our minds. The movement of swinging a bat, a racket, a fly swatter, or a golf club, or just turning to look in another direction, all involve this same movement. Because our muscles and joints *always and only* work in the limited way they are designed, in different activities we use the same few repetitive movements and stances.

So how did Tom do with his rotational movement in Figure 13.11? He did very well, considering he also has a moderate movement impairment due to a degenerative neurological disorder. That is why his golfing ability in this example is a far cry from the excellent ability he enjoyed for most of his life. However, this example also shows that Tom has not lost all the good aspects of that ability he once enjoyed.

After teeing the ball, he begins in a ready stance with knees flexed (picture 6). In picture 8, both knees are slightly flexed, but then in picture 9, they are straightened. But he still keeps his head down and over the ball in picture 9. This is important to note. Many golfers with natural ability have difficulty keeping their heads down during the swing. This tells the observer that Tom has hidden ability.

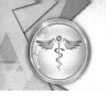

In a natural golf swing, the left knee naturally straightens in the forward swing (pictures 9 and 10). But Tom's knees are both stiffened and resist flexing in those pictures. And there is something else wrong in pictures 9 through 11.

The other problem is his very stiff feet. His feet stay rigidly flattened on the ground. This prevents his right knee from pushing forward to rotate his body, to follow through with the movement.

Flexible feet with increased pressure in the ball areas are necessary for this movement. This pressure allows the knee to be more easily pushed forward, brings the heel up, and allows the foot to pivot on the ball area of the foot. This produces the body's rotational movement.

In picture 8, Tom does have a bit of weight shift onto his right foot with minimal forward left-knee movement. As a result, there is a slight rotation of his hips and shoulders to the right. This

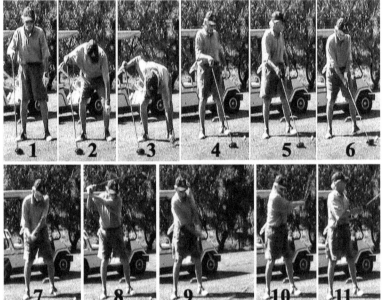

FIGURE 13.11: Tom's dream was to be able to tee up a golf ball, swing the club, hit the ball, and play the game once again.

is good for his restrictive posture. However, in pictures 10 and 11, because his knees and feet are held stiff, there is no weight shift to the left foot.

For much of his life, this was Tom's favorite thing to do, and his memories were filled with the correct feelings from the decades of perfecting his game. The very same is true for many of you with your memories of activities you once enjoyed and perfected. These memories are the most valuable pieces of you, and they must be used to help you wade through your present doubts and confusion. Use them to your advantage. Play to use them as much as you can. Use them to help you rediscover the better part of you. Use them as a primary component of your personal movement therapy.

BUT BE VERY CAREFUL. Why? I say this because some of you will always insist on playing with the same quality of movement you had before your movement problems began. This always leads to a great deal of frustration. The recurring disappointment in yourself will depress and eventually pull you away from the one thing that can help you the most.

If and when you understand how to be content with the ability you do have, to play at a less-perfect level with enjoyment, you will begin to discover much more ability. How? Finding some enjoyment is what helps you develop the patience to practice with the skills you have. Then the activity won't be a chore. With the enjoyment of what you ARE ABLE TO DO, you'll begin to feel a component of accomplishment that will encourage you to repeat the activity. This productive process may be rather slow for many of you. But your progress will lead you to work on improving the basics of the postures and movements to your advantage, to gain more satisfaction and enjoyment.

■ ■ ■

CHAPTER 14

THE PUSH IS THE MOVEMENT

Understand what does, or does not, happen in your feet,
to gain a much better understanding of your movements.

When a person with natural ability walks, the distance the foot moves forward and the width their feet are apart are consistent and evenly spaced in each stride.

But when a person with balance issues, movement problems and a tensed posture walks, the pattern of their advancing foot placement is characteristically not the same in each stride. The distance the foot moves forward and the width their feet are apart in each stride frequently vary.

When a person with natural ability is walking, their body movement is consistently smooth and flowing. In contrast, the body movement of a person with balance issues, movement problems and a tensed posture is irregular and often jerky.

Ultimately, the foot that is being used to power and control the stride is responsible for these movement differences. However, the posture determines how the controlling foot can be used, and where the advancing foot will be placed.

The issues for a person with balance issues, movement problems and a tensed posture are:

1. With each stride, the location of the pressure in the pushing foot frequently varies.
   The location of the pressure in the alternating pushing foot changes, and that changes where the next advancing foot will be placed. This creates the irregular strides and irregular movement.

2. The ability to add stabilizing pressure into the pushing foot varies between stronger and weaker. Because the pressure used to push the body through the movement varies, this also causes stride length and width to vary.

3. When the pressure in the pushing foot is increased, instability is often created on the advanced foot. This occurs when the movement of the body is unexpectedly more than what the previous stride created. This also changes the location and amount of pressure moving into the advanced foot, and the pressure often moves into an unstable part of the advanced foot.

4. Instability prevents the complete transfer of body weight to one foot.

Natural movement depends on the ability of one foot to fully support and control the movement of the body during each stride. Full-body support requires a complete transfer of body weight onto that one foot, to enable that foot to control the movement.

When the transfer of body weight to one foot is incomplete, the pressure will not be centered in the foot to allow it to fully support and control the body's movement.

In previous chapters, all the postures and movements were using two feet while standing in place. We began with standing upright using simplified static postural control. The next chapters introduced dynamic postural control while standing, squatting, sitting, and rotating the body. The remainder of the chapters will build on this basic foundation as we proceed into increasingly complex movements. In these advancing-ability movements, it will be necessary to use one foot to support and control the body while transitioning back to two feet or onto the other foot by itself. This demands a more relaxed and cooperative posture.

When we're using only one foot, everything must be more precise because it's easier to make a mistake and more difficult to correct it. With the precision of natural ability, we have options and choices in our postures and movements. Without the natural ability, our postures and movements are restricted, offering few choices.

How It Works

Per physical law, our natural movements work as nature has designed them to work. In 1687, Sir Isaac Newton described movement in his Laws of Motion. His Third Law states: *For every action, there is an equal and opposite reaction.* This applies to our movements as well.

We direct the increased pressure in the foot at an angle into the floor. This is the force we use to move our body. This is our push. We push this pressure into the floor in one direction, and that moves (pushes) our body in the opposite direction. Thus, for the body to move in the direction as planned, the pressure must be located in a very specific location in the foot and directed in a very specific direction.

Previous chapters discussed adding stabilizing pressure to the feet while standing on two feet. All of this works the exact same way for the exact same reason when using just one foot, only it must be done better, and more pressure has to go into that foot. For many people with balance issues, impaired movements and a tensed posture, supporting and controlling the body when standing on one foot is difficult.

This creates two problems. First, they have difficulty controlling the location of the pressure in the foot. Second, they have difficulty adding and holding increased stabilizing pressure in the foot to stabilize the body. The significance of this is seen in their movements. When they are unable to stabilize on one foot when standing, alternating from foot to foot during movements results in erratic advancing foot placement and movement patterns.

Standing still on two flattened feet uses the entire surface of both feet for support. But advancing movements very frequently depend on just a portion of one foot for the same amount of support. Let the meaning of this sink in.

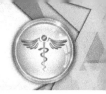

During natural movements, much of the time we are on only one foot, and much of that time we are on only a small portion of the forward part of that one foot. What does this mean? When we're walking, much of the time we're using only the forward part of one foot to completely support, push, and control the movement of our body.

When you find it challenging to stabilize while standing on two feet,
stabilizing on one foot is **very difficult**.

When it is difficult for you to balance on one foot,
it is extremely difficult to use just the forward portion of one foot,
and most times it is **next to impossible**.

This is the fundamental problem for nearly every person with balance issues, movement problems and a tensed posture. That is why it is a challenge for many of them to stand completely balanced and stable on two feet. So, standing on and using just part of one foot is very difficult or nearly impossible for them. For this reason, when they're relearning how to transition to using one stabilized foot at a time, they often feel as though they're starting over from the very beginning. In many ways they are correct. They must now learn how to create the same supporting foundation and employ the same movement basics using just one foot as they did on two feet.

Therefore, this chapter and the next will provide pertinent background details on the concept and application of the pressure, push, and associated body posture required to stabilize, balance, and control the body using just one foot.

THE UPPER BODY AND PRESSURE IN THE FOOT

The three panels of pictures in Figure 14.1 show a comparison of upper-body positioning and the difference in the outcome for the same intended movement: walking. The results demonstrate how a very small change in the position of the upper body at the start of the movement creates a very big difference in the outcome of the movement. Note that a **natural** walking stride is achieved only in panel C.

In panel A, there is no forward movement into the stride. Instead, the movement is immediately backward when the left foot lifts off the floor. Note how the back of the shirt is slightly out of the inserted green zone of stability in picture 1. This shows that the posture is held back and creates pressure toward the heels. As the left foot lifts off the floor, the increased heel pressure in the right foot begins pushing the body backward. As the upper body continues to move farther backward in pictures 2 through 5, the pressure in the heel is concentrated into a smaller area. This further increases the backward push of the body.

In panel B, when the left foot lifts off the floor, the body's forward movement is initially delayed, and then slowly begins *after* picture 2. The movement of the body in picture 1 is delayed because the pressure in the right foot is evenly distributed throughout the foot. With the foot flat, the even pressure holds the body in place, leaving the person standing still on one foot. In picture 2, the left leg is extending

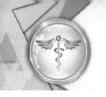

forward. This moves the pressure slightly forward in the right foot, and the foot then begins pushing the body forward in picture 3.

In panel C the body immediately moves forward into a walking stride when the right foot lifts off the floor (picture 1). This is because the increased pressure in the left foot is in the ball area of the foot. This is shown by the front of the shirt being out of the zone of stability.

Note how the posture is the same in all the pictures in panel C. This is a natural posture we use when beginning and continuing walking with the same stride length. Contrast this to the changing postures in panels A and B, taking special note of the resulting upper-body movement with the lifted leg and foot in those examples.

A walking stride is possible only in panels B and C. However, the stride in B is significantly shorter than the stride in C. The size of the inserted red block in picture 4 of both panels is the same, and is the length of the stride in panel B.

In panel C, there is space between the heel of the advanced foot and the red block. That extra space is the added length of the stride in panel C, clearly

Location of Foot Pressure

A   HEEL AREA

B   EVEN

C   BALL AREA

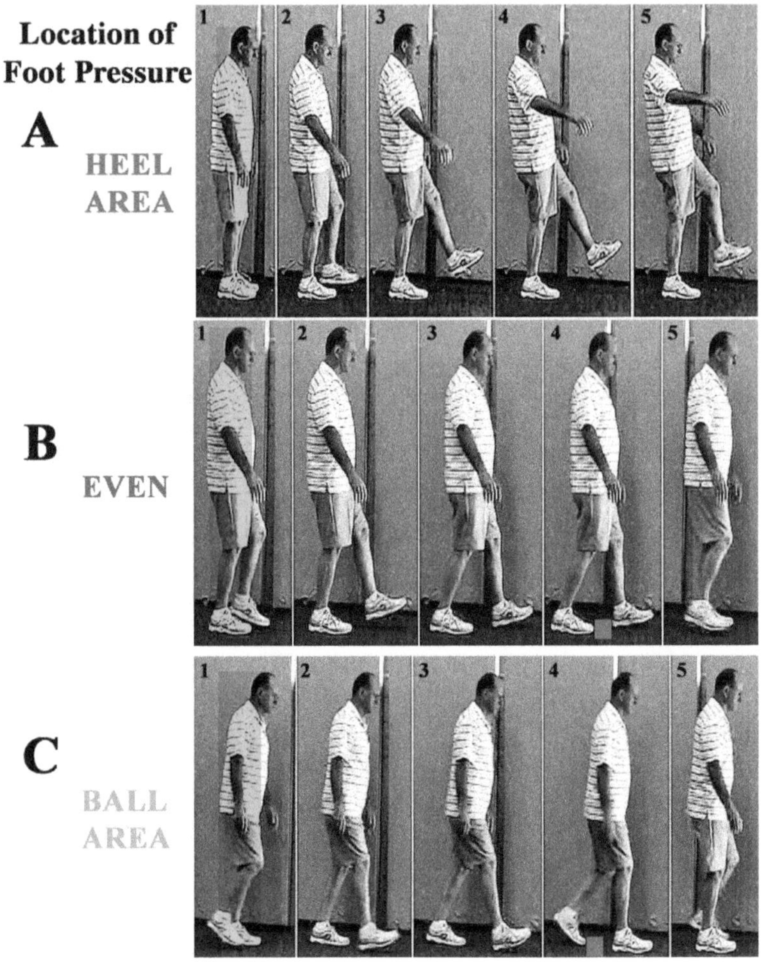

FIGURE 14.1: The posture in these three panels is relaxed, but the stride length and movement of the body in each of the panels are very different. The changing location of the pressure in the foot being used is the one very simple explanation for those differences.

showing it is noticeably longer than the stride in panel B. This difference in stride length is a result of the slight change in upper-body posture that is seen in the first picture of each panel. The difference in the quality and length of each stride is the direct result of the slight difference in the location of the increased pressure in the pushing foot.

Using the increased pressure, the push from the foot
determines the direction of body movement and the length of the stride.

The part of the foot we are using is the only part of us touching the floor. Therefore, that part of the foot must have the ability to control and stabilize everything: our body weight, posture, and movement.

THE ADVANCING FOOT

I cringe when I hear someone give the instructions: "To walk, take a step forward by extending your foot out in front of you and place it on the floor. Then move your body onto that foot." Not only is this advice patently wrong, it frequently puts many people with balance issues and movement problems in a very awkward and potentially dangerous situation. This is especially true for people with a restrictive-posture movement impairment. Heeding this poor advice, they create additional problems for themselves. Why? Review panel A in Figure 14.1:

1. It sets the wrong pressure in the relaxed body for the movement they're intending to do.

2. It puts the focus on the wrong foot: the one that is **not** being used to do the movement.

3. The person fails in their attempt, and the conclusion is that their condition is to blame for the failure.

Especially when their posture is tensed, when people with balance issues and movement problems extend their leg to take a stride forward, the forward movement of their body is significantly altered. But, people with natural ability, good balance, and stability can extend one leg and foot forward without experiencing the effects shown in Figure 14.1. They can do this even when the pressure in the foot on the floor is not located where it needs to be for the movement they want to do. They can do all this because they can easily and quickly change their posture and the pressure in their supporting foot, and then complete the intended movement with little to no problem.

For example, when a person with natural ability is explaining and showing how they begin the movement by extending a foot forward, they begin by balancing on one foot, and then they will adjust their posture without realizing it to begin the movement. Their thoughts are doing one thing while their body is doing something totally different. This contributes to the misconception of how our natural movements work.

All movement is a balancing act on our feet, or foot, and is made possible through fine postural adjustments of the body. So again, when a person with balance and movement issues is challenged when attempting to control the pressures in both feet while standing, they should not be ill-instructed to stabilize and balance on one foot, or a portion of one foot, for walking therapy or practice.

But it happens every day. What is the thought process here? These people tip and fall on two feet, *"but magically we will show them the ability to walk"* using just one foot. Wishful thinking. Bad results.

PRESSURE IN THE FOOT

1. With two feet remaining flat on the floor, your body will only move up or down as you bend and straighten your knees. The same thing happens when standing on only one flat foot.

2. The location of the increased pressure in your foot is the place where you feel the most pressure. When used for pushing, it determines the direction your body will move.

3. The pressure in your foot comes from two sources: One is your body weight. The rest comes from the working muscles in your legs.

4. To understand how to control your movements, you must understand how to use and control the pressure in one foot.

5. Having the ability to feel the pressure in the foot is a plus. Otherwise, it's more difficult to achieve a practical and functional understanding of the working relationship of the upper body and the use of the pressure in the foot.

6. In preparation for movement, the upper body adjusts and maintains the location of the pressure in the foot. The lower body adds to and uses the pressure to do the movement.

7. During movement, the upper body constantly adjusts to counterbalance the movements of the lower body, arms, and head. This holds the pressure stable and in the same location in the foot, and is a requirement for the movement to continue as intended.

8. The increased pressure in the pushing foot is the pushing pressure. When the location of the pushing pressure in the foot changes, the movement also changes.

FEET: FLAT OR NOT FLAT

Much of the time when we are standing upright and stable, the pressure is not evenly distributed throughout our feet. For example, routinely, many people stand with more pressure in their heels than in the ball areas of their feet. This is because the heel area is structurally the most stable part of the foot.

Having done this most of their lives, most people think they are standing on "flat feet" when they are actually standing with increased pressure in their heels. Is this a problem? No, not for those with the natural ability to control it and quickly move the pressure to where it needs to be for any movement they wish to begin.

The point to be made here is that many of the thoughts and assumptions we have grown to accept and understand about most of the things we physically do are actually only *partially* valid. This is because they are based on half-truths.

The true part of what we know is based on the things we actually do. These are the movements and activities we routinely perform, and for which we have a good *working understanding* of what we need to do physically or process mentally to easily repeat them.

The false part of what we accept as true is the web of thoughts and assumptions we spin in an attempt to explain what our working understanding actually is or might be. For example, in many of the activities we enjoy and repeatedly do, there are basically only two things we know:

■ One, "This is my starting posture."

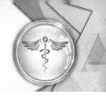

- Two, "This is my ending posture."

- The part we frequently do not know is what happens between the start and the ending. This is what leads to the array of assumptions and thoughts that fill the large spaces where known facts do not exist.

"How did you do that?" someone asks.

"I really don't know. I just do it," most reply.

For each of us, in our movements we adapted to what is "normal" simply because it's the way we learned to do them. In the example of people routinely standing with increased pressure in their heels, their brain has calibrated that pressure distribution to be interpreted as: "My feet are flat. My feet are flat because this is the 'normal' way I stand, and my body is stable." With natural ability, all of this works perfectly fine. But, as natural ability fades away, problems arise.

Many of our movement habits come about this same way. Through repeated use, when we do something the same way long enough, what once felt like the wrong thing to do changes into the correct thing that must be done. Many of the new activities we learn in life work this way. To do better in the activity, you must perfect the required movements and the feelings that are associated with doing it correctly. Next, because of the good results, you learn to trust the feeling. Then the feeling is all you use to do the movement. This is how the feeling becomes a good (adaptive) movement habit.

Forming bad (maladaptive) movement habits happens the same way. Our physical conditioning deteriorates, or something within us changes that makes movements challenging. Our body does not move like it used to. Once good and easy-to-do movements become not-so-good movements. As these things happen, we cope the best we can while learning, "This is the way I must do these things now." We change from our "normal (natural) feelings" because we can no longer reproduce them.

In the natural-ability world of movement, there is no absolute right or wrong as to what our starting postures must be for the basic movements we are about to do. In fact, the only requirement for people with naturally relaxed postural control is that they are comfortable doing what they want to be doing.

■ ■ ■

CHAPTER 15

FOOT + PRESSURE + PUSH = MOVEMENT

*The lessons learned from our mistakes
often provide us with the best guide toward a better understanding of our movements.*

ZONE OF STABILITY

As I worked to understand the relationship of the pressure in our feet to our posture, balance, stability, and movements, I needed something that could help me visualize what I was beginning to describe mentally and feel physically. I needed a way to see this graphically, to prove or disprove my thoughts about it. Then, as I worked with the video and pictures of people I had worked with for this book, I happened to develop the concept of a zone of stability.

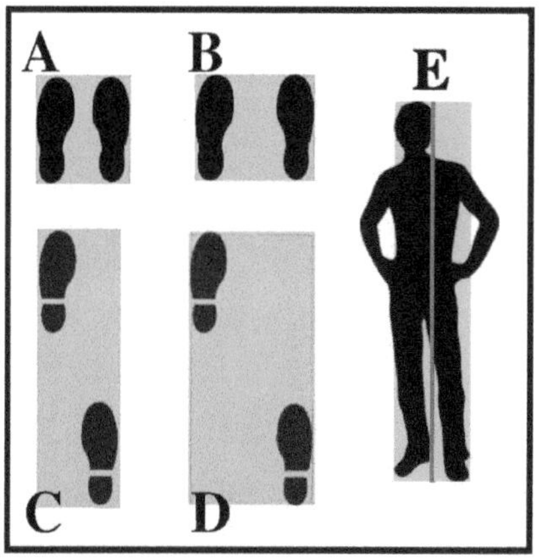

We control our body with the pressure in our feet on the floor, so on the floor is where this zone begins. Thus, the imaginary zone is a graphic representation of the areas of our feet, or foot, that are in contact with the floor and are being used to support our body. This imaginary zone of stability then projects upward from the outer edges of the portions of the feet that are in contact with the floor with pressure, and extends upward to the top of our head. The outline of this zone, colored green, is shown in image E of Figure 15.1.

The solid black shoe prints in illustrations A through D show the feet are flat on the floor, meaning there is equal pressure in all areas

FIGURE 15.1: The size of the zone of stability, the green area, is determined by outside edges of your shoes or feet that are in contact with the floor.

of each footT. hey also show how the size of the zone of stability changes on the floor with the positioning of the feet. Note that the sides of the zone are always at the outside edges of the feet, or shoes, that are in contact with and applying pressure to the floor.

When our body is centered within this area, we are stable and balanced. When our body is not centered within this area, our stability begins to diminish.

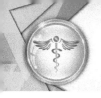

For example, in silhouette E of Figure 15.1, the person is close to being centered within his zone of stability, and therefore stable. Look closely at this figure to see the information that supports this statement. (Note: The person is facing us.)

There is more pressure in his right foot than in his left. This is shown in two ways:

1. His body is off center, shifted to the right, and that is moving all of his right arm outside the zone. Also note that his right hip is slightly outside the zone and his left hip is within the zone.

2. His upper body is angled to the left to counteract his hips, which are to the right.

3. The red vertical line is centered within the zone of stability, but the body is not centered in the zone. More of the body weight is to the person's right, and that puts more pressure in his right foot.

Size Matters

In general terms, the larger the zone of stability is on the floor, the more stable the person will be. However, because there are exceptions and unwanted variables, be careful with assuming that bigger is always better. An obvious exception is placing the feet so far apart that they slide out to the sides. Also, when the feet are spread widely apart, it becomes physically more difficult to move from one foot to the other. A very wide stance requires more strength, added flexing of the knees, and a relaxed posture in order to be useful.

Still, within the limited context of our discussion pertaining to basic movements, we will use the general assumption that a larger zone created by our feet on the floor provides added stability. However, this limited context is **only** being used to refer to the *comfortable stances* we routinely use on a non-slippery, smooth, and firm floor.

As we change the position of our feet, the size of the zone of stability on the floor also changes. With natural ability, as we change the position of our feet, we remain stable by constantly adjusting the required pressure we push into them. This means we can stand upright with feet close together and be nearly as stable as when standing with feet spread farther apart, until something pushes us to one side. However, when a person with a restrictive-posture movement impairment moves their feet closer together, moving from a larger zone of stability to a smaller one, they most often become less stable. The reason: They are not pushing enough stabilizing pressure into their feet.

When the size of the zone of stability on the floor decreases, the downward pushing pressure into the feet, or foot, must increase to maintain the same support and stability the wider stance was providing.

This is a very important concept to understand from the applied-physical-forces perspective. As we walk and move about, our feet are constantly flexing, meaning different areas of each foot are in contact with the floor at different times during our movements. Therefore, as the foot flexes, the smaller area of it that remains in contact with the floor must provide the same support for the body as the entire foot or both feet were providing. To accomplish this, increased pressure is pushed and concentrated into the smaller part of the foot. This is why the size of our zone of stability is constantly changing during our movements.

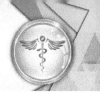

Much of the time during natural walking strides, the zone of stability becomes very small because all our body weight is supported by only the ball area and toes of one foot. That very small area of one foot is *supporting, controlling, and moving the body.* This is possible because a large amount of increased pressure is being pushed into that small area.

Another important concept is the *"pushing point of pressure"* in the foot. The pushing point of pressure is simply the increased pressure we create in the area of the foot that is being used to push our body through the movement. As we walk with natural ability, the body moves smoothly forward without interruption, even though each foot is constantly alternating position with the other foot. This is because the flexing action of the feet continues without interruption. However, the pushing point of pressure moving through each foot *is interrupted.*

In a natural walking stride, the advanced foot first contacts the floor with the back of the heel area, moves to a flattened position on the floor, then to the ball area, and finally to just the toes before the knee lifts the foot away (shown in Figure 15.2). Beneath the foot, I have inserted an area of green that represents the changing size and the corresponding representative depth of the relative pressure of the zone of stability that we exert into the floor. Thus, immediately *after* the entire heel contacts the floor (picture 3), the increasing pressure being pushed into the advanced foot moves forward through the foot until it gets to where it needs to be to take over pushing the body.

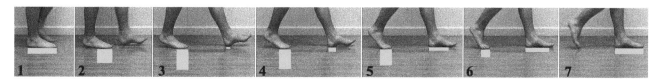

FIGURE 15.2: A representation of the relative pressure our feet exert into the floor as we walk.

In pictures 1 through 3, the lighter green areas show the changing surface area of the zone relative to the changing depth of the zone being created within the supporting and pushing foot. In pictures 3 through 7, the lighter green areas show the transition of pressure from the pushing foot to the advanced foot, as well as the relative amount of pressure each foot is contributing to the total zone, which includes all the green areas.

As shown, the total surface area of the zone on the floor is largest when both feet are in contact with the floor (pictures 3 through 6). It is smallest when only the ball area and toes of one foot are in contact with the floor (picture 2).

For the body to remain stable in the movement as the zone's surface area decreases, the concentrated pressure we push into the smaller area of the foot we're using must be substantially increased. Think of it as if this concentrated pressure in the smaller area of the foot being used is being pushed farther down into the floor. In this way, the *increased depth* of this concentrated pressure provides the same foundation of support as the larger surface area the entire foot provides with dispersed pressure.

When we have the ability to keep our body stable and balanced during our movements, which means we are staying within our constantly changing zone of stability during the movements, we have the ability to relax our body into the perfect posture for very controlled and purposeful movements. This is one interpretation of the "staying in the zone" phenomenon athletes often speak of when they are commenting on their peak performance level.

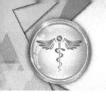
There has always been a mystery to this talk of "being in the zone." However, once it is understood what the physical parameters of this zone actually are, the mystery is no more. In one sense, *staying in the zone* only means that we are keeping our body relaxed and counterbalanced within our personal zone of stability, where our physical balance and control are optimal.

LOCATION OF INCREASED PRESSURE

When you understand the relationship of posture to pressure in your feet, you will have the ability to look at any person and explain with confidence where the pressure is located in their feet. In other words, this allows you to visualize where their body is within their zone of stability and predict with accuracy how stable they are.

Study the eight silhouettes in Figure 15.3 and determine where the pressure is located in their feet, so you can then explain how stable or unstable each person is in that posture.

1. The playful soul labeled number 1 is likely teetering backward due to the increased pressure in the heel of the one foot on the floor.

2. The pressure is concentrated in the ball areas and toes of person 2, and he is likely stable.

3. The handstand artist has increased pressure on the thumb side of his hand and is tipping to *our* left.

4. With hammer in hand, the man is driving nails while standing on his heels, but he is very stable with the slight flex in his knees.

5. Person 5 is very stable in a forward-leaning lunge with increased pressure pushing into a flattened leading foot. Also, look at his back knee and imagine how much increased pressure there is in the ball area and toes of the back foot.

6. Casually, this woman has pushed her hips forward with shoulders held back and is standing stable with increased pressure in the forward foot, and because she is wearing a higher-heeled shoe, she likely has increased pres-

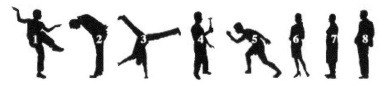

FIGURE 15.3: Where is the increased pressure in their feet, and what is the result of that pressure?

sure toward the ball of the foot. The side of the big toe and ball area of her back foot have increased pressure to ensure that she stays balanced over the front foot.

7. With her upper body leaning backward, the woman labeled number 7 is standing with increased pressure in her heels and light pressure on the ball areas of her feet. This is a common posture for people with a movement impairment and restrictive posture. However, it appears that her feet are close together, and that suggests she does not have an impairment.

If her knees are slightly bent under her dress, that would indicate that she is pushing enough pressure down into her feet to be standing comfortably. If this is the case, there is also pressure on the balls of her feet, but still not as much as there is on the heels.

8. The same is also the case with number 8. The pressure appears to be increased in his heels, but notice he is pushing his hips forward. He is very stable.

Looking at the figures, do you see what I've described? Some of it is fairly easy to visualize. However, without a visual reference, some is not. So, in Figure 15.4, I have inserted the zone of stability each person is creating. Now test your answers and my explanations.

1. The back of his body is outside the zone. This creates increased pressure in the heel.

2. His body is shown to be centered over the balls of his feet. Roughly equal amounts of body weight are on opposite sides of the zone of stability. Remember, in this posture

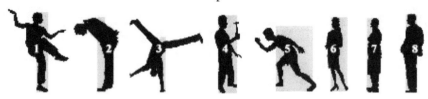

FIGURE 15.4: Our posture sets the pressure in our feet. The zone-of-stability overlays help to more easily identify the location of the pressure.

he is pushing a great deal of stabilizing pressure into this small area of his feet using his calf muscles.

3. More of his body is out of the zone to the left. The very small surface area for this zone of stability makes balancing on the one hand very challenging.

4. His body is leaned to the back edge of the zone. This creates increased heel pressure, but the slight flexing of his knees moves the pressure forward toward the center of both feet. This helps stabilize his body while he hammers.

5. In this forward-lunge posture with the shoulder, knee, and toes close to vertical alignment, the front foot is flattened. In the back foot, there is increased pushing pressure in the ball area and toes, which is holding him in this position.

6. Because she is pushing her hips forward to the front edge of the zone, she has increased pressure toward the ball area in the front foot. But she is also holding her shoulders back, and that maintains pressure on the inside area of the back foot. The pressure in the back foot is important pressure here, because it is stabilizing and holding her over the forward foot, which is supporting her body. She is very stable.

7. With straightened knees, she is leaning and tipping backward, and would be unstable. If she is flexing her knees under her dress, that is pushing stabilizing pressure into her feet and shifting some of the pressure forward out of her heels. That would make her more stable.

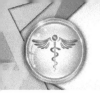
8. He is very stable, standing with a slight backward lean with hips pushed forward, which likely centers the pressure in his feet. Still, because so much of his back is outside the zone, there appears to be slightly increased heel pressure.

To better understand what your eyes are telling you, you should test some of these postures yourself to feel and know it is true. So, stand up and adjust your posture into as many of these stances as you are safely able to do. Using a mirror to see if you are in the posture you think you are in is helpful. Then simply feel where the pressure is in your feet, and also how comfortable and stable you are. Next, slightly change your posture and feel how the pressure in your feet also changes.

You Need to Know How It Feels

All that I've written in this book is what I have proven and trust using every day. However, *before you can believe and trust that what I'm saying is true, you must have the ability to feel and repeatedly reproduce it for yourself.*

Use my words about what you are to do on these pages as a starting point, and then convert my words into your words based on your feelings and experiences. This is vitally important to do. Find your words by feeling the actual pressure you create and feel in your feet, both in the setup for movement and then during movements. Then your words will serve as your personal guide for what is true for you, which is true for all of us.

Why is this so important? It is because you are learning how *your* body and movements work, and not how I relate to or do mine. You are restoring your way of doing things according to what feels right for you, and only you know what your right and wrong feelings are. Only you know what goes through your mind when you feel them. Only you know what images and words you use to relate to and remember them.

This concept of "feeling" what the posture, pressure, and movement are is often very different from what you have thought the posture and movement are, or should be. Understanding the actual feeling of what you do tells you the simplified truth. You must know the difference.

Stability

The more points of supporting contact you have with the floor, the bigger your zone of stability will be. For example, if you're lying on the floor, your zone is basically an outline of your body. If you're crawling on the floor, your hands, knees, and toes are creating the zone, like the crawling baby in Figure 15.5, picture 4.

What happens when you're using a chair? Picture 1 shows that the tips of her heels on the floor make two points of contact, and the four legs of the chair she is pushing into are the other points of contact with the floor. While sitting on the chair in picture 2, most of the man's body weight is being applied to the floor through the four legs of the chair, with a small amount going into his feet. In picture 3, when a person stands with one foot pushing down on the center of a stool, all of the stool's legs are helping to support her, and the other part of her body weight is on her other foot.

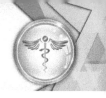

When you're using anything for support, it can help support you only when you are using it appropriately. When you are pushing pressure straight down onto it, it can be very supportive. When you apply pressure at an angle, the object is often less supportive, especially when it is movable.

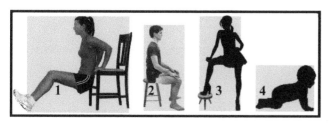

FIGURE 15.5: Increasing the size of the zone of stability.

This includes walkers, and especially those with wheels. Why? Pushing pressure onto it at an angle causes it to move, the exact same way your body moves when pressure is applied at an angle with your foot.

In the stances and postures covered in previous chapters, the message was to stand on flat feet with even and equal pressure in both. The reason for this was to keep your body centered and stable within your zone of stability in order to focus on improving the control and relaxation of your posture. In the following chapters, the focus will be on remaining stable within your zone of stability when standing and during movements without flat feet, using only a portion of one or both feet.

INTERPRETING FOOTPRINTS

If the people in Figure 15.6 were standing on a soft surface that easily molded to the pressure and outline of their shoes, would the imprints of their shoes (feet) look flat, or would they be angled? For example, what would you expect to see if they were standing in soft, moist sand on a beach?

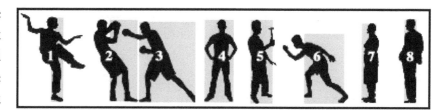

FIGURE 15.6: The flatness, or the functional angle at which pressure puts our foot to the floor, is determined by the distribution of pressures that we create in that foot.

1. Not flat. The footprint is angled, with the heel deeper down into the sand than the ball and toes.

2. Not flat. The boxer is falling backward and to his left. His back (right) foot appears to be pressing deeper into the sand than his front (left) foot. Due to the upper-body-induced fall from the blow that number 3 just delivered, pressure is being pulled off number 2's front foot. The area of highest pressure in both feet is in the heels, with the back heel having much more pressure than the heel of the forward foot. The impression of both feet will be at an angle, with the back foot deeper in the sand.

3. Not flat. With his shoulder behind his front knee and that knee behind the tip of his shoe, the boxer's front foot has increased pressure in the heel. This means his punch was not as powerful as it would have been if he had moved his body farther forward while throwing the punch. Why is it not as powerful? The heel pressure is pushing his body backward while the back foot is pushing his body forward.

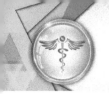
The print of the back foot is made by the toes digging deep into the sand.

4. Not flat. The person facing us (toes are pointing toward us) is standing with more of his body weight over his left foot than his right. The marks of his feet on the beach will be the left foot leaving a deeper impression than the right.

    Also, the inside of his left foot has slightly more pressure than the outside. The same is true for his right foot.

5. Not flat. This man is hammering while he is leaning slightly back and to his left. (I base this on his barely noticeable dropped left shoulder.) His slightly bent knees move some of the increased heel pressure forward in his feet . . . and I will wager this guy is getting tired.

    Why? To accurately and forcefully drive nails, and resist the impact of the hammer strike, the pressure needs to be forward in the ball areas of the feet. Standing in this posture, he loses much of the strength and power from his legs and is creating more work for his upper body. The imprints of his shoes are angled with the heels deeper, and the left heel deeper than the right.

6. One foot is nearly flat, the other not. His shoulder and knee, and the toes of the front foot, are in very close vertical alignment. This makes the forward foot almost flat, with slightly increased pressure in the ball area due to the weight of his head and arm. In this stance, his back foot is pushing from the ball area and toes and the heel is lifted, making the back foot very angled in the soft sand.

7. Not flat. With straightened knees, her heels are buried so deep in the sand that any ant crawling out of the depression has a long, steep climb to the top. Look at the tips of her shoes. They are pointed up.

8. Looks like a yes to flat, but most likely not. This posture has him slightly heel heavy. Therefore, his feet are also at a slight angle in the sand. But if this is true, how is his head almost in the middle of the green zone? Remember, he has moved his hips forward to compensate for his shoulders being farther back. This is a common standing posture for many people. It is also a not-so-attractive, lazy posture.

Functional Flatness versus *Physical Flatness*

Functional flatness is *very* different from physical flatness. The physical flatness of your foot on the floor describes only how your foot *appears* on the floor. For example, if the bottom of your foot or shoe is completely on the floor, then your foot is physically flat because the floor is flat.

The *functional flatness* of the foot is determined by the equal and even distribution of pressure in the foot.

The *functional angle* of the foot is determined by the area of increased pressure in the foot (feet) that is being applied into the floor.

The functional angle of the foot determines the direction of the resulting movement of the body. The force of the movement is determined by the amount of pressure being applied into the area of the foot with increased pressure.

Very importantly:

1. The **physical flatness** of your foot or feet tells you **nothing** about your posture, movements, and stability.

2. The *functional flatness* of your foot or feet *tells you everything* about your posture, movements, and stability.

To illustrate the differences between these two concepts, we'll use the two stepping platforms that are resting on the flat hardwood floor in Figure 15.7. Both are physically flat on the floor, but *only one* is functionally flat.

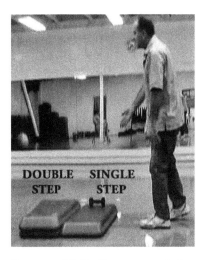

FIGURE 15.7: Because of the added weight on the far end, the single step would leave an angled impression in soft sand.

To judge the flatness of the platform, it's common to compare the line of the bottom of the platform with the surface of the floor. When the bottom line of the platform is parallel to the floor, our eyes see and our brain interprets that the platform is physically flat on the floor. However, this method of determination tells us nothing about the functional flatness of the platform, which is the potential angle and movement of the platform due to the distribution of weight within it.

In this example, the double step platform is both physically and functionally flat on the floor. This is because the pressure it exerts on the floor is evenly distributed throughout the entire step. Thus, the entire imprint of the double step platform in moist and soft beach sand would be the same depth: flat.

The single step platform on the right is also physically flat on the floor, *but only because the floor is very hard.* So, what would the imprint of this platform be in soft, moist sand?

The imprint would be angled and not physically flat. Why? There is a five-pound weight on the far end of the platform. The far end is five pounds heavier and will make a deeper imprint in the sand than the lighter end. The five pounds pushes that end of the platform down with more force, *as it also applies that same force into the floor.* Therefore, the single step as shown is *functionally at an angle* on the hard floor. This same concept applies to how the increased pressure in our feet changes the functional angle of our feet, to create the stability or instability and movement of our body.

> *For movement purposes, it doesn't matter what your feet look like on the floor.*
> *What matters is where the pressure is located and how that pressure is being used.*

The location and quantity of the pressure in the foot determine the functional use of that foot. In Figure 15.8, there are four separate footprints.

- Picture 2 is the imprint of a functionally flat foot. The heel and the ball area were equally pushed into the sand while this person was squatting.

- When your feet remain functionally flat, all of the pressure in them is pushing straight down into the floor. Holding that pressure while squatting or standing, your body will move only straight up or straight down with the bending and straightening of your knees.

- The footprints in pictures 1, 3, and 4 are not functionally flat. These feet were functionally angled because one part of the foot was pushing deeper into the sand.

- The person making the imprint in picture 1 was walking slowly with increased heel pressure.

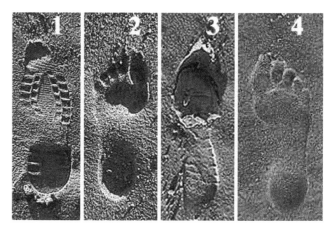

- The person making the imprint in picture 3 was leaning forward while walking, and pushing a great deal of pressure into the ball area and toes of the foot.

- The person making the imprint in picture 4 was standing with slightly increased pressure in the heel.

FIGURE 15.8: According to pressure distribution, the foot in picture 2 is functionally flat. The feet in pictures 1, 3, and 4 are not.
1. Increased heel pressure.
2. Evenly distributed ball-area and heel pressure.
3. Increased pressure in ball area.
4. Slightly increased heel pressure.

In the soft sand, it's easy to see the tilting footprint that the unequal pressure creates. On a hard surface, no tilt is seen unless the entire surface moved.

Which came first, the chicken or the egg? Are the pressures in your feet creating your posture, or is your posture creating the pressures in your feet? True, a rational explanation can be made for either one creating the other. However, *from a natural use perspective*, there is only one correct answer.

The pressure in the feet determines the posture. This is the process every person with natural ability uses in all postures and movements. We learned how this works as toddlers, perfected it, and continue using it throughout our lives.

Basically, we set the pressure in our feet and then relax our posture into that pressure.

This natural use changes only when something forces the change. For some, the forced change comes as a result of certain disorders and conditions that render this natural order of use challenging. It essentially begins with added guarding in their posture. This creates a challenge for relaxing the posture and controlling pressure in the feet, which then creates difficulty in using the pressure. The result is instability. This begins the transition into the reversal of natural use, forces the introduction of excessive thought, and sets in motion the unnatural use of the body.

■ ■ ■

CHAPTER 16

TRANSFER-OF-BODY-WEIGHT MISTAKES

*To stand balanced on one foot, all your body weight
must be centered over and stabilized on that one foot.*

With or without movement difficulties, it is very common for many people to have minor issues
with transferring body weight from foot to foot. For example, the footprints in Figure 16.1 were
made by people with natural ability as they were walking on the beach.

1. The footprint in picture 1 came from a foot that
   had even pressure throughout. The depths of
   the impressions of the heel and ball area appear
   to be the same. This shows that a centered and
   complete transfer of weight was on this foot.

2. The footprint in picture 2 shows slightly increased
   pressure on the inside of the foot, with the body
   weight nearly evenly distributed between the heel
   and ball areas. The minimally displaced sand
   at the shoe's tip shows that the foot was flexing
   minimally as the person walked very slowly with
   an incomplete transfer of weight to this foot.

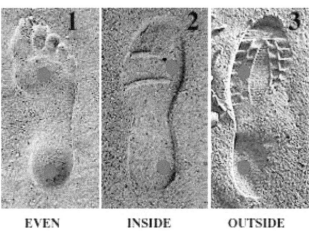

EVEN   INSIDE   OUTSIDE

Location of Increased Foot Pressure

FIGURE 16.1: Footprints on the beach. Red dots show the
locations of increased pressure.

3. The shoe print in picture 3 was made by a person walking with increased pressure in the outside
   of the foot. This is shown by the deeper imprint of that side of the print. This pressure distribution
   caused the person to walk with a slight upper-body sway from side to side. The slightly distorted tip
   of the shoe imprint shows that the foot was flexing very little.

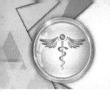

It is not necessary to see the people making these prints to visualize and understand what their postures and walking patterns were. When you understand the effects of the pressure in the feet, you then have the ability to understand the posture that made it and the movements that pressure produces. For example,

1. Because there was a complete transfer of weight, the person in picture 1 was using very little effort to lift a knee and a foot while walking. This person would have been walking with feet close together, moving straight ahead with a uniform stride length.

2. The people in pictures 2 and 3 were putting more effort into their walks, because they were not completely stabilized on one foot. Person 2's transfer of body weight to the foot was incomplete. This creates more work to lift the other knee and foot, to then move the foot forward in the stride. Person 3 was also working harder to remain stable with excessive upper-body movement. The print shows the exaggerated transfer of body weight with increased pressure to the outside of the foot.

    Possibly person 2 could have been walking in a straight line, but the space between their feet would have been slightly wider and their stride lengths shorter than person 1's.

    Person 3 was *not* walking in a straight line. The footprints would wander as a result of excessive shoulder movement.

UPPER-BODY- VERSUS LOWER-BODY-INITIATED MOVEMENT

With natural movement ability, when moving from one foot to the other, a person accomplishes the movement *completely with the lower body.* The upper body only "supports" the movement.

Naturally, *the upper body sets the correct pressure in the foot, and then the lower body uses the pressure to push the body through the movement.* Unnaturally, people with a movement impairment often use excessive upper body movement in an attempt to compensate for the dysfunction of their lower body.

When the upper body is used for more than setting and holding the pressure in the foot, the created movement becomes an unnatural pulling movement. For example, as the upper body leans farther to one side, pressure is pulled from one foot and transferred onto the other foot. This is shown in Figure 16.2. The bigger problem is that this type of transfer creates instability in both feet.

In picture 1, as Chan shifts his body to the right and pushes pressure into his right foot, the increased pressure is in the inside portion of the right foot, as indicated by the red arrow. In contrast, in picture 2, labeled "pulling," when he leans his upper body to the right, the pressure of the transferring body weight moves toward the outside of his right foot, as indicated by the red arrow. This creates problems.

The outside of the foot is the weaker part of the foot, and because of this inappropriate transfer, it is now responsible for supporting and stabilizing the body.

In the foot opposite the lean—the left foot in this example—the pressure is moved to the inside of the foot, *as* the total pressure in the foot is also being decreased.

When the upper-body leaning movement becomes exaggerated, the excessive side lean pulls the opposite foot completely off the floor. For the vast majority of people, standing balanced on the outside area of one foot is not an easy task. For the movement impaired, it is nearly impossible. The resulting instability frequently causes them to react with increasing postural guarding and stiffening throughout the body as they tip and fall to the side.

The pressure moving into the outside of the foot also pushes the body in the same direction the upper body is leaning, which creates additional instability. The more the upper body leans, the farther the pressure moves toward the outside edge of the foot. As the pressure of the body weight moves outward across the foot, it is concentrated into a smaller area, which increases the outward pushing force. As the pushing force increases, it becomes more likely that the person *will be pushed into a fall*.

BUT, the resulting "fall" is *NOT* a fall. It is rightfully **a push**. The force of the pushing pressure in the outside of the foot pushes the person off balance.

Leaning the upper body to transfer body weight is counterproductive because:

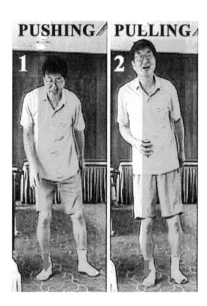

FIGURE 16.2: Picture 1 shows transferring body weight with a push down into the foot. This is a very different posture and movement than leaning the upper body to transfer body weight (picture 2).

1. It moves the pressure to the side of the lean in both feet and pulls pressure from one foot.

2. It decreases the useful surface area and the support of both feet.

3. It reduces or destroys the *purposeful* pushing pressure of the supporting foot, and replaces it with nonpurposeful pushing pressure.

4. Upper-body leaning increases instability while restricting and destroying purposeful movement.

The use of upper-body leaning is a major cause of many of the problems people with balance and instability issues, movement difficulties, and/or a tensed posture create for themselves. Consistently, they make three common mistakes:

1. A minimal upper-body lean pulls pressure from one foot to "help" transfer body weight and increase the downward push into the supporting foot. The created instability in the supporting foot is most often minimal and usually easily corrected. However, the instability *is* there and makes it more likely that there will be a problem. How? Postural guarding and stiffening increase the likelihood of a mishap.

2. As their posture continues to guard and stiffen, they use their legs less and upper body more.

3. Then they begin to stiffly "rock" their body from side to side on their feet, using side-to-side upper-body motion to initiate their movements. Often, they hold their knees straightened with widely spread feet.

    This rocking of the upper body does work for those people who depend on using increased pressure on the inside of the feet for support, because the increased pressure stays in the inside portion of the foot they rock toward. However, this only works when their feet are more widely spread. Also, to mainain their stability, the transfer of body weight onto the foot is always incomplete.

Now let's consider the issue of stability. Initially, it is surprising for some to hear that people who rock excessively from side to side, due to upper body lean, are relatively more stable than those who only rock minimally from side to side. This is because the person who is using a smaller amount of upper body lean typically does not stay on the inside portion of each foot as they move from foot to foot. The reason. Their feet are commonly closer together, and that allows the pressure in the foot to move toward the center and outside of the foot during the transfer of body weight. Those with excessive upper body movement, rocking back-and-forth with their feet widely spread, are more stable because the pressure in their feet stays to the inside.

In this comparison, the difference in stability directly relates to the location and quantity of the *effective* stabilizing pressure in the foot.

1. The inside of the foot is structurally stronger than the outside of the foot.

2. When standing with feet spread farther apart, increased pressure on the *inside of one foot* pushes the body back toward the inside of the other foot.

    What is the effect? Both feet are pushing and holding the body toward the center of the stance. Just using body weight, this physically creates increased stability that is not dependent on the need to add additional pushing pressure into the feet from the legs. This is the reason people do it, because it is easy and stabilizing.

3. Increased pressure on the *outside of the foot* pushes the body to the outside, where we do not have another foot to use for support. Feeling the created instability of increased pressure on the outside of the foot, the person works to reduce that pressure to lessen the outside push. However, to decrease this pressure, they also decrease much of the stabilizing pressure that is necessary to support the body.

    These are the reasons the "rocker" and the "leaner" of the upper body use their legs less for pushing additional downward pressure into their feet. For the people rocking their shoulders from side to side, staying on the inside of the feet "compensates" for the missing additional pressure coming from the leg muscles.

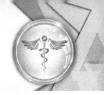

When a person is standing and using rocking movements, the pressure on the inside of the feet works as a stable, self-centering force. However, it also greatly restricts all other movements and does not allow for a natural walking pattern.

4. The greatest support, stability of the body, and movement-enabling pressure in the foot happens when the strong pushing pressure is centered and directed straight down into the foot.

In Figure 16.4 Cyndi is consistent with postural alignment on each supporting foot. This is because she is not using upper-body movement to transfer body weight. However, she doesn't trust her ability. This is due to two basic factors: One, Cyndi's lack of trust in her legs' ability to stabilize her body. And two, the increased pressure she is applying into the walker through her arms and hands.

Psychologically, Cyndi is more dependent on support from the walker than she is from her legs. Thus, the pressure she pushes into the walker through her arms and hands "steals" pressure that would otherwise be going into her legs and feet. Her stiffened arms leaning on the walker essentially hold her upper body in place between them and restrict all movement of her entire body.

Note the position of Cyndi's head with relation to the inserted red line. This shows that she is remaining centered over her feet more than she imagines. Yes, this is partly due to her restrictive use of and dependency on the walker. But, it also reveals her movement ability is better than she realizes.

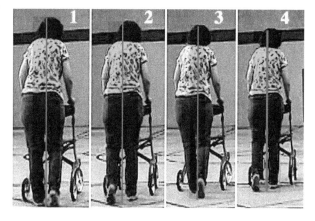

FIGURE 16.4: The effect of a stiffened upper body stealing stabilizing pressure from the feet.

1. Cyndi is consistent in each stride with the placement of the pressure toward the center of the foot. This also limits the sideward movement of her upper body. There is something in the pictures that supports this statement.

   If the pressure in her feet was not consistently toward the center, with each stride the walker would be pushed off the straight line in which she is pushing it. For example, if her feet were wider apart and she was using pushing pressure on the insides of both feet, her walking path would be in a zigzag pattern. With each stride, the walker would be pushed to the other side. The right foot would push it to the left. The left foot would push it to the right.

2. Her legs are relatively relaxed as she stays more centered over each foot, but will stiffen quickly when she is not.

3. Cyndi creates stability in her upper body by leaning with stiffened arms onto her walker. However, this creates instability in her legs with a weakened downward push into her feet.

145

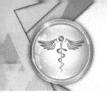

AWKWARD STIFFENING TRANSFERS

When a person with natural movement abilities has a tensed posture, their movements become awkward, but are fairly easily correctable. However, when a person with balance, instability and movement difficulties has a tensed posture, their movements become very awkward and unstable, and very difficult to correct. These issues cause the development of their fear response. As their apprehension and fear increases, they spend long moments thinking about a movement that needs to be done—until they can no longer avoid having to do it. But importantly, they are not thinking about the mechanics of the movement. Instead they are overwhelmed with anticipation of another fall.

Charlie is one example of this (Figure 16.5). We had worked on the first three stances in previous sessions. Then, in these pictures, I was introducing him to transferring body weight between his feet in preparation for working on sideward movements.

Without moving his feet, Charlie was practicing very limited sideward transfer-of-body-weight movements, but the tension in his posture increased each time he shifted toward either foot. Because of this, he required constant reminding to relax his hands and arms, to help in his efforts to relax and flex his knees, just as the vast majority of people with like impairments need the same reminders.

A stiffening/tensing posture restricts bodily movements, especially of the knees and legs. At the same time, the stiffness encourages and often forces erratic and exaggerated upper-body movements, which complicate the person's ability to control the location of the pressure in their feet.

For stability, remember that people with a tensed/restrictive posture most commonly use upper body movement to shift from one foot to the other. They will also be seen to have their feet spread wider apart while they are using the pressure toward the inside of their feet.

Now note how close Charlie's feet are together in pictures 1 and 2. Because the pressure is more centered in his feet with his feet closer together, his stability is more dependent on adding stabilizing downward pressure into his feet from his legs. This is especially important when moving onto one foot. Why? The surface area of the foundation that one

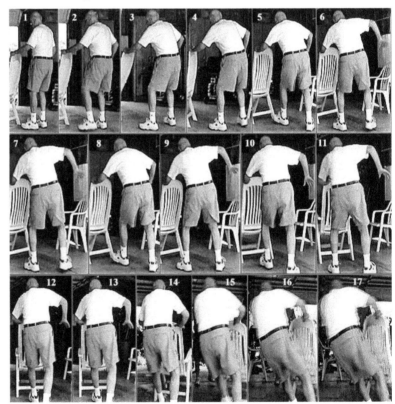

FIGURE 16.5: A person with a mildly stiffened posture standing with increased pressure in the heels. He transfers body weight to one foot while keeping the increased-heel-pressure posture. With all his body weight then pushing into one heel, the resulting instability causes a further postural stiffening response as the concentrated pressure pushes him backward into the fall.

foot creates for supporting the body is suddenly reduced to half of what it was when standing on both feet. So, adding increased pressure into the foot he is transferring to, to compensate for the decrease in foundation surface area when moving onto it, is what he is learning to do again. But unfortunately he was not applying it in pictures 1 and 2, because he forgot it while learning the "new" activity.

Then, beginning in picture 3, he cannot add any downward pushing pressure for two reasons. One, in picture 2 he begins the movement with slightly increased heel pressure, which essentially doubles in the right foot when he moves all of his body weight onto it. Two, the immediate instability caused by the increased heel pressure forces the productive work the leg muscles are doing to change to holding the legs stiffly in survival mode.

As Charlie attempts to correct this mistake and stabilize in pictures 3 through 5, he inadvertently puts increased pressure in the outside portion of his left heel in picture 6. This pressure then pushes him faster into the backward and leftward "fall" that is happening in the remainder of the pictures. He cannot stop the "fall" because he cannot stop applying the pressure that is pushing him into it.

The chair he was using in front of him was only for limited support, and it shows how well he had been doing. It was there for him to rest his hands on, to help remind him to keep his posture forward while focusing on keeping his feet flat. This brings up an important, previously discussed point about working with movement-impaired people with stiffening postures.

Many people with a restrictive-posture and impaired movements do not trust having increasing pressure in the ball areas of their feet when they are standing. Remember, many of them have long favored standing on their heels with very light pressure in the ball areas of their feet. So now, when they begin standing with flattened feet on the floor, they are adding pressure to the ball areas that they have not been accustomed to feeling. So they habitually remove it.

Going, Going, Gone

These backward falls are pushing accidents, and are frequently in a backward-angled or backward-turning movement. The initiating movement is a sideward transfer of body weight to one foot, and the backward component is from increased heel pressure. With their feet closer together, they easily move onto the outside half of the foot they are moving toward, with increasing pressure in the heel area. The sudden increase of concentrating pressure in that area of the foot forcefully pushes them into an angled backward fall to the outside. A complicating factor is their exaggerated fear-filled postural stiffening reaction, which exhilarates the awkward movement.

People with these movement issues can also enter into a turning backward fall to the inside. This happens when their feet are spread wider apart and their transfer of weight is incomplete. Again, with their shoulders held back, or moving back during the movement, the increasing pressure is in the heel area, but on the inside portion of the foot they are moving toward. Then, as the other foot is lifted from the floor they enter into backward angled pushing "fall". Both are extremely difficult to stop.

There are three additional things to understand about this backward-moving accident:

1. This is the most common "fall" they experience.

2. It is a very, very easy transfer-of-body-weight mistake to make.

3. It is easily avoidable.

Much of the time, falling is an avoidable accident.

FEET STUCK ON THE FLOOR

In Figure 16.6, Donna stands with her feet held apart while catching a ball that is bounced to her, and then she bounces it back. In these pictures, her posture, flexibility, and movements are good, but her feet seldom move on the floor. Study the series of pictures. Note the wide stance with feet angled outward and the slightly flexed knees that do not change.

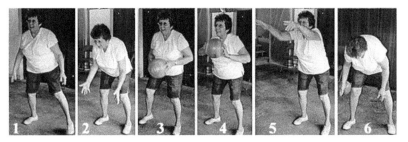

FIGURE 16.6: Donna's movement impairment is mild. Note the intermittent stiffening of her hands and arms, held out as she is waiting for the ball. This self-induced stiffening issue makes catching objects and holding things with our hands difficult.

Now look at her arms and hands. When she's not holding the ball, her arms are away from her body with hands and fingers open. All of these things show residual guarding stiffness in her legs and feet, and mild intermittent guarding and/or stiffness in her arms and hands.

This is common. For example, this intermittent guarding/stiffening of the hands and arms is another reason people with a mild impairment experience additional problems using their hands and fingers for fine motor skills like writing, handling smaller objects, and catching things. In so many activities and movements that require relaxation, we *unknowingly* ill-prepare ourselves with guarding and stiffening in a vain attempt to have better control. Subconsciously, we gradually learned to do this, and consciously we can learn how not to do it.

To learn how to reduce this unproductive physical guarding and stiffness, beginning with hands and then knees, you must consistently remind yourself to relax. But what must come first? **Stabilized feet.** Then, with the added stability of relaxing, you must continue the process of learning how to let go of the fear and the muscle tightening that serves no purpose. This especially needs to be done in the setup before and during many of your movements.

For catching something, prepare yourself in your stance *before* the object is thrown. Then, as the object you want to catch is coming toward you, relax your hands and fingers even more. This takes time, patience, and a great deal of practice to feel and live the difference. Also, smaller objects require much more focus on keeping your hands relaxed. For whatever reason one wants to blame it on, we have much more difficulty catching and handling small objects.

The exact same reminders are necessary for stiffening knees. You must get in the habit of reminding yourself throughout the movement: *Knees down.* Squat. You must consciously remind yourself to lower

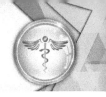

your body with bending knees using words and thoughts that make the most sense for you. But always remember, it's easier to relax your knees after you have first relaxed your hands and arms. This is a must for those of us with restrictive-posture movement impairments.

Previously, we discussed the effects of the widened stance Donna is using. She holds herself stable using pushing and stabilizing pressure from the insides of both feet. However, for those with a restrictive posture, this stabilizing stance also restricts movement of the knees, hips, and body, and often causes the following three things to happen sporadically:

1. With feet spread wider apart, the weight of the body naturally applies pressure into the inside area of both feet and provides stability.

2. Their movements become jerky when their knees are guarded or stiffened.

3. When the feet move closer together, the mild postural guarding and stiffening typically increase. The primary cause of this is twofold. One, the inside-of-the-foot pressure that the person has become overdependent on is decreased. Two, when the person does not compensate for this loss by increasing the use of their leg muscles to increase the pressure in their feet, they become unstable.

    As the posture becomes more restrictive, lower-body movements diminish as upper-body movements increase. This change quickly generates added instability. A primary reason for this is that the positional changes of the upper body are poorly controlled, often exaggerated and at times erratic. This creates another problem. With every upper-body movement, the location of the pressure in the feet moves. Thus, the pressure in the feet is poorly controlled and often erratic as well. So, what do they do to remedy this? They spread their feet wider apart to regain partial control and stabilize their stance.

Standing in a widened stance provides stability, but moving out of it is often a problem. The primary reason? The person must relax their legs to allow their knees to flex enough, then move their body farther to the side to transfer all their body weight onto one flattened foot, and then support themselves on that foot while moving the other foot. This requires additional leg strength.

To center over one foot, they must move sideways a great deal more than they're comfortable with. This creates two basic problems. Either they don't trust their ability to move their body as far as it needs to go, or they lack the leg strength to transfer their body weight onto one foot and stand on it—or both. This topic will be discussed in Chapter 18.

■   ■   ■

CHAPTER 17

FOURTH STANCE:
BODY MOVEMENT TO THE SIDE

Wishing and hoping things will get better is a poor strategy.
However, they can be an excellent guide when the required physical work
is applied to create the desired reality.

I n *Figure 17.1, the width of Carol's stance* is wider than Ron's stance. He has natural movement ability, and his posture is relaxed. She has a neurodegenerative disorder, and her posture is stiffened. He stands with his feet approximately shoulder width apart, while she stands with her feet spread beyond the width of her shoulders.

When Ron begins to walk, the width of the space between his feet will naturally stay small, and the pressure in his feet will be toward the center in each stride. When Carol walks, her feet will remain unnaturally wide apart, and she will be using the pressure that is created on the insides of her feet in each stride.

Movements done with a widened stance are problematic. They require more coordination and strength than movements using a narrower, more natural stance. This is one of the reasons many movement-impaired people tire more quickly. In their widened stance, they are working harder to do the same movements that are easy for other people. This is especially so when their posture is stiffened. Now, consider the fact that movement-impaired people are characteristically weaker than others with natural abilities. Do you see the bigger issue?

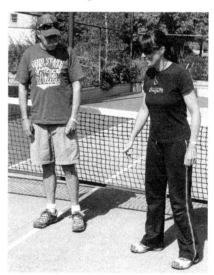

FIGURE 17.1: He is relaxed. She is not.

With a restrictive posture and stance, they must do more work with less strength to achieve less of an outcome than a person with natural ability. What is this saying? The reason they tire so easily is more of a physical issue than an underlying neurological issue.

So what do they do about this situation? Their weakened physical condition is correctable, just as it is for a person *without* a movement impairment whose physical condition is weakened. And how does

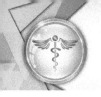
anyone correct physical weakness? Functional exercise: strengthening and stretching the old-fashioned way. And yes, nay-sayers, there are many ways a person with movement impairment can safely exercise and strengthen their muscles.

FOOT PRESSURE AND STANCE RELATIONSHIP

To be clear, when you are standing still, it really *does not matter* how far apart your feet are as long as you are stable, comfortable, and doing what you want to be doing. But *movement is a totally different situation.* The distance between your feet matters a great deal during movement, especially when you're beginning a movement. With feet spread wider apart, the distance your body must move in order to center and stabilize over one foot is increased. The larger distance the body must be moved requires additional leg strength, flexing of the knees, and coordinated pushing with both feet. It requires skills that many people with movement impairment have difficulty with, or simply cannot do. It requires moving off the inside pressure of two feet and onto the centered pressure in one foot. This is scary stuff for many.

For each person in Figure 17.2, the location of the increased pressure in their feet is different. Therefore, the direction that pressure is pushing into the floor is also different. This is shown by the colored arrows below their feet. The purple arrows represent the total pressure, while the blue and red arrows represent how the components (vectors) of the pressure are distributed into the floor.

The size and direction of the arrows are determined by the amount and location of the pressure in the foot, which is determined by the width of the stance.

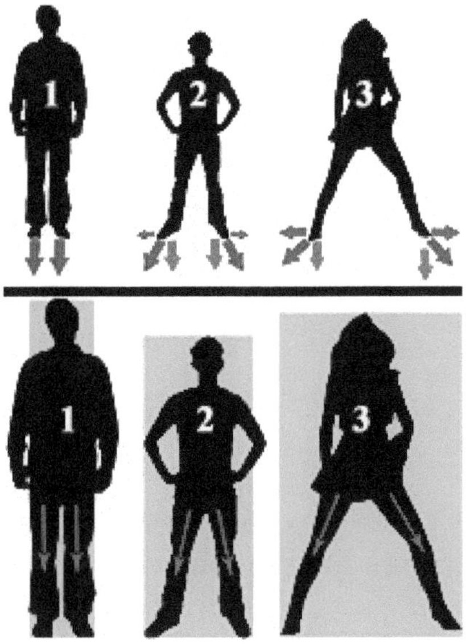

1. The pressure in person 1's feet is very close to being directed straight down into the floor. This person feels the pressure *near* the center of his feet and *feels* that his feet are flat. But they actually are not completely flat.

    There is a *very small* amount of pressure on the insides of his feet. There are no blue arrows shown because they would be too small for this diagram.

2. The pressure in person 2's feet is offset toward the insides of both feet, and is likely halfway between the center and the inside edge of the feet. Because of this, the pressure is split between pushing mildly to the side (blue arrows) and down (red arrows). The result is illustrated by the purple arrows showing the result

FIGURE 17.2: The combination of body weight and the pushing force from the legs creates the stabilizing pressure in the feet. The width of a person's stance determines the angle at which pressure is directed into their feet.

of the force distribution of the pressure pushing at an angle into the floor.

Thus, the purple arrows represent the combined effects of the pushing forces that are created in these stances. This pressure determines your stability but also determines the effort it will take to move out of the stance. Basically, as the pressure becomes more sideward or angled, an increased amount of effort, strength, and body movement is needed in order to overcome it.

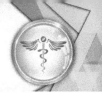

3. The pressure in person 3's feet is farther toward the inside edge of both feet. So, there is a stronger side push, noted with the larger blue arrows. The resulting pressure force is displayed by the purple arrows showing the resultant pressure pushing at more of an angle into the floor than person 2's. This is very stabilizing, provided the feet cannot slip out to the sides. It also often requires more leg strength to comfortably stay in a very widened stance, because additional leg muscles are involved compared with what a narrow stance calls into play. These additional muscles are typically weaker in movement-impaired people because they do not use them as much.

Provided her feet don't slip sideways, this stance creates very strong cross-bracing pressure. Each foot is strongly pushing outward, and that pushes her body to the center of the stance. However, to move out of the stance she must first overcome the pushing force from one foot, to move her body onto it for support, to get into the appropriate posture and position to begin the intended movement. (purple arrows).

With adequate leg strength, a relaxed posture, and flexing knees, centering the body over one foot from this stance is not difficult. However, it can be very difficult for a person with a tensed posture, weak legs, and inflexible knees.

Many people with generalized weakness, balance and movement issues, and especially when they have a tensed posture, *do not* have the ability to move out of a stance as wide as the one shown in this example. They are physically stuck in for two reasons. First, they don't have the ability to transition away from the increased pressure coming from the insides of their feet. Second, their knees won't flex enough to move their body sideward to center it over one foot. Thus, their reliance on the cross-bracing pressure from the insides of their feet in a widened stance is a mixed blessing. For standing, it works very well. For moving, it does not.

Without moving either foot and while staying in the wide stance, could person 2 or person 3 make their feet flat? Yes, they can come very close to doing that, and all they basically need to do is squat and spread their knees.

Prove this to yourself. Stand in a wide stance similar to example 2, and then slowly lower yourself into a squat. As your knees flex and your body descends, feel the pressure on the insides of your feet move toward the centers of your feet. As you squat, allow your flexing knees to spread apart and move outward over your feet. This directs the pressure into more of a straight-downward direction. With the squatting movement, your leg muscles will be doing more work. This adds pushing pressure into your feet and creates added stability, provided you have the strength to stay down in the wider squat.

Person 2 will need to squat less, and person 3 will need to squat very low. The point here is that the easiest and safest way to begin to transition from a wider stance to a narrower one is to first make the foot you want to move onto as flat as you can. The next part is using the stability and support of the flattened foot to move your body over the center of it using flexing hips and knees.

KNEE IN LINE WITH TOES

The postural alignment (front to back) for making both feet flat is one in which the shoulders, knees, and toes are vertically aligned, as covered in earlier chapters. This is also true for creating one flat foot

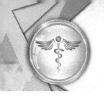

from heel to toe. Yet there is more to creating one flat foot than what we've been doing for two flat feet. But honestly, when we're standing *equally* on two feet, neither one of them is functionally flat, because there is always some increased pressure on the insides of the feet.

This is a reason some people are not very good at balancing on one foot. A common mistake people make when attempting to stand balanced on one foot is not adjusting their posture to eliminate this inside pressure on the foot and spread it evenly throughout the foot. This incomplete body-weight transfer quickly forces them to return the other foot to the floor, as their body moves toward that side.

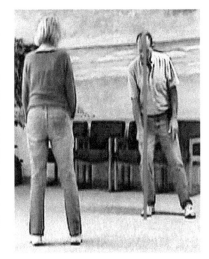

When not in a specific pose and simply standing balanced on one foot, the other necessary postural alignment is that the knee and nipple area be in vertical alignment with the center of the supporting foot (Figure 17.3). In a relaxed posture, this alignment adjusts the side-to-side location of the pressure to the center of the foot. So, in combination with the toe, knee and shoulder side view alignment previously discussed, this additional toe, knee, nipple area alignment sets the pressure to be evenly distributed throughout the foot.

Now the pressure is centered side to side and front to back in the foot, *and this is the only time the one foot is functionally flat*. This is the most supportive the foot will ever be, because the entire foot is being used, and all the pressure is being pushed straight down into the floor. The only other requirements are pushing increasing downward stabilizing pressure into the foot with the weight-bearing leg and relaxing the posture to allow it to counterbalance as needed.

FIGURE 17.3: When your posture is relaxed, you can easily shift your body weight to the side by pushing down into the foot you want your body to move to. Then, when the foot, knee, and nipple are aligned, the foot is flat.

USING ARMS TO CHECK POSTURAL ALIGNMENT

When you know how to interpret what you see and feel, the position of your arms will provide you with a great deal of information. If you can, practice in front of a full-length mirror to see what's actually happening. This will help you to better understand the postures and the feeling you are striving to create.

If you don't have a large mirror, an alternative is to recruit someone to be the mirror for you. They should be standing *at least* eight feet in front of you. The distance supplies both of you with a better perspective. The other person's job is to mimic your posture to reflect what you are doing. But be careful with this! Very often, you will want to disagree with what they're showing you. Stop the defensive thoughts and hold back the urge to argue with them for showing you what they see you doing. This is reason enough to use a mirror. It reflects the truth you can't deny. Another option is to have someone take a picture or video and then immediately review it.

In Figure 17.4, I am in a relaxed posture in the background, while Jack's posture is stiffened or guarded, with the exception of picture 5, in which he does relax. This provides a good visual comparison of restricted and unrestricted body movements in a sideward motion.

In picture 1 of panel A, Jack's posture is stiffened. Because of this, he leads the movement with a slight twisting of his shoulders and follows with minimal movement of his hips. Note that he's holding his arms away from his body (red arrows), and his knees are straightened.

In pictures 2 and 3 of panel A, his goal is to stand relaxed in the middle of the stance, as I am doing in the background. In both pictures, his posture is guarded. In picture 2, he is wanting to be in a ready stance, but he is hunched over in a guarded posture. He has relaxed some from picture 1, and the evidence for this is his arms are closer to his sides and his fingers appear more relaxed. Due to his guarded posture, in picture 2 of panel A he stands upright while intending to be in a ready stance. From picture 3, he moves into picture 4. The red arrow points to the position of his left arm, indicating the amount of guarding he has added in his posture.

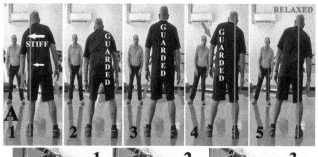

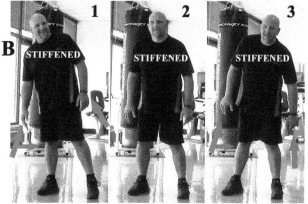

FIGURE 17.4: A comparison of a relaxed posture and a guarded, stiffened posture in sideward movement. The signs are very obvious when you realize what you are seeing and feeling. These are correctable issues.

When reminded to relax his hands in picture 4, Jack relaxes into completing the movement in picture 5. The extra sideward motion shows up in reference to the red lines in both pictures. Note that his left arm is now relaxed against his body, but his right arm is dangling away from his body.

What does this indicate? His shoulders have moved farther to the right than needed, and here his hips have not moved quite far enough to the right, so the arm hangs away from his body. Compare this with my hip and shoulder alignment in picture 5. Basically, if Jack moved his hips a little to the right, and his shoulders a little to the left, his alignment over the flattened right foot would be very good.

In panel B, Jack's posture is stiffened in all three pictures (red arrows). His knees are straight, and in pictures 1 and 3 his right knee is hyperextended. His right hand remains open with fingers held apart and his arms are held away from his body. That is why he used upper-body movement with very little hip and knee movement to move to the side from picture 2 to picture 3.

Any guarding or stiffness in the posture changes the movement! See it in these comparative picture, and you must learn to see and feel it in your body. Watch yourself in a large mirror to know what the posture looks like and what the feeling of relaxing, guarding and stiffening is to you. This is very important.

Remember, a relaxed upper-body posture adjusts and controls the pressure in the feet, and then the legs and feet use that set pressure to do the movement. A guarding posture limits this natural process. A stiffening posture significantly restricts it. A stiffened posture prevents it.

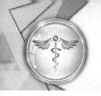
Pushing *into* a Foot, and Flexing the Knee to Center the Body on That Foot

The easiest and most stable way to begin relearning to trust shifting your weight from foot to foot is to keep both feet on the floor and actively use both during the movement. This provides you with increased stability from both feet, making it easier to relax and feel the shifting pressures in your feet as you move.

Begin in a ready stance with flexed knees and hips, and feet approximately shoulder width apart. Your shoulders, knees, and toes (from a side view) should be lined up to make your feet flat from heel to toe. Then relax as best you can. In this relaxed ready stance, adjust your posture so that you feel equal pressure in both feet feet from heel to toe.

Keep both feet flat on the floor. Staying relaxed, gently push pressure down into one foot and note how your relaxed body moves toward that foot. Staying relaxed, as the knee on that side flexes slightly, your hips and body move with the knee toward the increased pressure. The flexing movement of this one knee coordinates and controls the movement of your body. Your goal is to continue flexing the knee until your body centers the pressure in the foot. You will need to feel and know this pressure. You can also "see" it in the mirror by visually lining up the knee with the toe of your shoe and the nipple area on your chest.

If your body doesn't move toward the foot you are pushing more pressure into, there are three potential reasons. First, your knees aren't relaxed enough. Second, you're still pushing too much into both feet. Third, you're not pushing enough pressure into just the one foot. With your knees and body relaxed, your *hips and shoulders will move together at the same time*, and your shoulders will stay in line with your hips, as mine are in Figure 17.3.

For many people with generalized weakness, balance and movement issues, and especially when they have a tensed posture, selectively pushing pressure into one foot is challenging. So, practicing this second way of moving the body to the side will help correct this problem. Standing relaxed in the center of the stance, simply bend one knee, and feel your body moving to the side with the bending knee. Where do you stop bending the knee? When the knee is lined up with the toe, which is when the sideward-moving pressure in the foot is centered in the foot.

Do this in one direction and then slowly do it in the other direction. Keep it simple. Flex the knee down to move toward the foot. Straighten the knee to move back to the center of the stance. Repeat this same sequence with the other knee to move toward the other foot. One knee movement at a time. When you stay relaxed, feel how easily it works with only a small amount of knee movement. Play with it while continually reminding yourself to relax your hands to relax your knees, to stay in a comfortable ready stance.

Now, a special note for those with stiffened postures. You must be much lower in a ready stance than Ann is in Figure 17.3, and Jack in Figure 17.4. Why? You will have a strong tendency not to bend your knees. And then when you do bend them, you'll tend to straighten them as you come back to the center of the stance. To learn how to flex your knees enough and keep them flexed, even just a little, you must start by exaggerating the knee bend. When you do, it will seem that your knees are flexing much more than they actually are. Keeping the knees flexed is the number one challenge for a movement-impaired person with a restrictive posture.

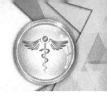

The two most common questions movement-impaired people ask as they begin this movement exercise are: "How will I know how far to move?" and "How will I know when to stop?" There is only one correct answer to both questions. "When the foot you are moving onto is flat, that is how far you move and that is where you stop." When that foot is flat, you will be and feel stable and balanced provided you stay relaxed. This tells you everything you need to know. The feeling in your foot (Mama) tells you exactly what is right. All you need to do is trust the stabilizing and supportive feeling, and double-check your posture alignments as discussed above. The feeling in your feet is always your best guide in all your movements.

Posture and movement rule:

> *Whenever you are thinking about starting a movement, and while you are involved in a movement, and whenever you want to stop a movement, and when you do stop the movement, for all of these things, remind yourself to keep your shoulders forward. Do this to help hold the pressure in your feet where your body requires it to be for that movement.*

PUSHING *FROM* THE INSIDE EDGE OF ONE FOOT TO MOVE SIDEWAYS

In *most* movements, our body is pushed away *from* the pushing foot. So, why did I have you begin doing sideward movements by pushing down *into* the foot you were moving toward? There are three good reasons:

1. To learn how and where to stop your body over a stabilized foot.

2. To learn how to hold pressure in both feet while your body is moving.

3. To get you started using your knees for the movement of your body.

Pushing from a flexing foot is where we're going, but to get there, many of you need to begin pushing from a flattened, non-flexing foot because of your instability issues. Then, when you learn how to stabilize and become comfortable, your posture will begin to relax and your foot will begin flexing.

So, we will begin the movement by using flat feet from heel to toe. This will ease you into the process of learning what the push is and how to use it, while practicing staying relaxed and learning more about the pressure in your feet. For example, during the movement the pressure in the pushing foot will remain in the same location. However, when you are pushing your body into the movement, the pressure will increase. Then, when the push is relaxed your body will move backward toward it.

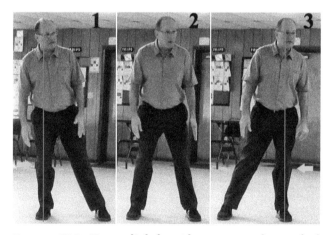

FIGURE 17.5: Use a slightly wider stance to better feel and use the inside pressure in the feet. Push from the full length of the inside of one foot and flex the knee to move your body toward the other foot. To go back to the center, relax the push and allow the inside pressure of the other foot to push your body.

157

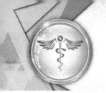

NOTE that I *did not* say "release" the pressure to move back toward the center of the stance.

To begin, stand in a ready stance with your feet slightly more than shoulder width apart and with equal pressure in both feet. This wider stance will put increased pressure on the entire length of the insides of your feet, as shown in picture 2 of Figure 17.5. Then slightly flex both knees and keep both feet flat from heel to toe.

To move from the middle of the stance and center the pressure in one foot, I did two things. One, I increased the pressure in the pushing foot. Two, I allowed the opposite knee to flex. Reading this, many will say this is the same as the previous example. Yes, it is very close to it. However, the difference between the two is what you are using to initiate the movement.

In this example, you are increasing the pressure in one foot to push and move your body to the other foot. In the previous example, you first pushed pressure into one foot and your relaxed body moved toward that same foot. Next, you flexed your knee without increasing the pressure in either foot, in order to use the knee to move your body toward that same foot. The difference now is pushing from a foot and then flexing the other knee adds stabilizing pressure, because both feet are actively being used. This often brings up a question. "What should I do with the pressure in the other foot?" Leave it as it is. Do nothing to change it as you begin the movement, and then feel what happens to it during the movement. Think it through. From a stance with my body centered between my two feet, what happened to the pressure in my right foot in picture 1? It centered in the foot and increased, *and* the left foot is holding the same increased pressure I used to push my body to the right. This is the mechanism for increased stabilization in the movement.

Just remember to relax your hands and elbows to relax your knees. Also, make sure your shoulders stay forward to keep equal pressure on the heel and ball areas of your feet. If you maintain this setup, the rest of the movement will easily happen. Add a little extra pressure into one foot, flex the other knee, and your body will immediately begin to move. The pressure in the foot pushes the body, and the flexing knee *allows* the movement to happen purposefully and smoothly.

Remember, when both feet are on the floor, use both of them. This sounds like a ridiculous statement to some of you, but many movement-impaired people do *not* correctly use both feet during many of their movements. Yes, they are standing on them, but they often are NOT applying the necessary pressure into both of them to provide the optimal support their body requires.

In natural advancing movements, the pushing foot the body is moving away from is directing and controlling the movement. However, both feet are continually providing support when they both are on the floor. Therefore, the focus for doing the movement needs to be on increasing the pressure in the pushing foot while not releasing any pressure from the other foot. The problem: When pushing increased pressure into one foot, many people with a tensed posture mistakenly push pressure into both feet, and/or stiffen their knees while applying the pressure, and then have difficulty with the movement.

To move your body back to the middle of the stance where you began, just relax some of the pushing pressure in the pushing foot that is holding your body over the other foot. So, add pressure to the pushing foot to move your body into the movement, and then relax some of that pressure to allow your body to return. It's as simple as that. The pressure in the pushing foot will move your body exactly where it needs to be, provided your body is relaxed into your stabilizing feet. Practice this in both directions until it becomes comfortable and easy.

This widened stance purposely uses the self-centering stability from the pressure on the insides of both feet to your advantage. The inside pressures from both feet constantly push your body to the center of the stance, and allows you to relax your posture, your knees, and ultimately your feet. So, when standing in this wide-based stance, feel the ease of the movement using only a light added push from one foot. Also note, when you're in a relaxed posture with feet spread slightly more than shoulder width apart, a light push will not be enough to push you too far and onto the outside of the other foot. You will remain within your zone of stability. This is the more complete reason for the comfort you'll be feeling.

A completed transfer of weight centers the pressure in the foot you are moving onto. For those with a widened stance, a good amount of knee flexion is required to enable the body to move the extra distance, as seen in pictures 1 and 3 of Figure 17.5. This will be a challenge for those with guarding or stiffness in their posture. Work and play with it. The goal is to relax enough so the movement goes smoothly, and that requires a relaxed, flexing knee. This is preparing you for doing the movement with a narrower stance, in which more relaxation, control, and pressure stabilization are needed.

The issue: When you're standing with your feet closer together, the angled self-centering downward pressure from your feet *decreases*. As the angled self-centering downward pressure decreases, you must add straight-downward stabilizing pressure.

GOING TOO FAR

With an incomplete transfer, the pressure in the foot you're moving onto stays on the inside of the foot, as in picture 1 of Figure 17.6. In a complete transfer, the pressure is centered in the foot (picture 2). However, when the weight transfer continues beyond the center of the foot, support and stability in the stance quickly deteriorate (pictures 3 and 4).

In this example, Jaesoon is purposefully continuing an upper-body lean to the left while feeling the effects of the pressure moving in her left foot. In picture 3, the pressure has moved into the outside portion of the foot. In this location, the pressure is pushing slightly to the right into the floor and causes her body to tip to the left. As the upper-body lean continues, the pressure on the outside of the foot increases and forcefully pushes her body to the

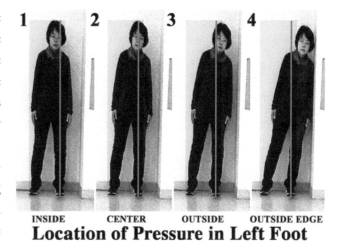

Location of Pressure in Left Foot

FIGURE 17.6: Overshooting the center of the foot in weight transfer quickly causes instability and decreases support. The created increased pressure in the outside portion of the foot pushes the body out of the stance.

wall. In picture 4, the pressure is concentrated in the extreme outer edge of the foot.

The important aspect of this example is what happens between pictures 3 and 4. In picture 3, Jaesoon can recover by moving the pressure back toward the center of the foot. But thereafter it is impossible for her. It's impossible because the push of the pressure is beyond the recovery point. Feeling where the recovery point is, is the importance of this exercise and the reason she's doing it next to the wall. Tipping to the side is very common for people with generalized weakness, balance and movement issues, and

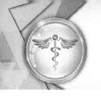

happens more often when they have a tensed posture. Frequently, the tipping they create is at an angle to the side and backward. The primary reason for the sideward pushing tipping is uncontrolled pressure moving to the outside of the foot. The added backward component of the push comes from increasing heel pressure caused by straightening knees and upward-moving shoulders.

Practice this, BUT USE A WALL! The best place is at the end of a hallway, because it provides you with three walls for support when you need them. To begin, first experiment with shifting your weight with your upper body, as Jaesoon is doing in the pictures. As you lean toward the wall, your one focus should be on the pressure in the foot nearer to the wall. As you lean your upper body, feel the pressure building in the outside of the foot, and the tipping tendency of your body. Now pay very close attention to the "breaking point." As the pressure builds, suddenly the body tip becomes a quick body push. This is the big mistake you must learn to avoid. Practice with both the good and the bad pressures. Know them intimately. Create the good and avoid the bad.

With that learned, with feet shoulder width apart or less, do the same practice sequence by pushing your body into the weight transfer using the inside pressure of the pushing foot, rather than using an upper-body lean. Feel and know exactly where you need to stop to have your body weight (pressure) centered in the foot. Feel the comfort and stability. Also, so that there is no doubt in your mind, again compare this good pressure with the not-so-good pressure. Practice using a light push to move onto the center of the foot, as previously discussed in this chapter. Then, practice using a heavier push to feel what happens when you overshoot the center of the foot. It is very important to learn the feeling of both: How to control the amount of push, and how to keep your posture relaxed.

TRYING TOO HARD

With a relaxed posture, all of your body will naturally move cooperatively as one unit as you shift from foot to foot. But with a stiffened or guarded posture, it frequently does not. For example, when the guarding or stiffness is greater in the legs than it is in the upper body, the upper body and hips will move more than the knees. This is why it is very common for people with stiffened postures to use their upper bodies to do most of the weight transfer. Then, the uncontrolled and/or erratic leaning of their upper body complicates the problem. Frequently, this causes them to move too far, and they *overshoot* the center and the flatness of the foot they're moving onto.

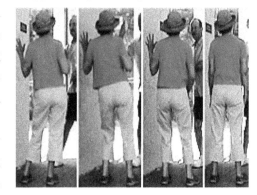

FIGURE 17.7: When the movements of the shoulders and hips are opposite, there is little or no transfer of body weight.

In Figure 17.7, Janette began standing upright centered over both feet, and then she was to shift her body over onto her right foot. In picture 1, she moves her hips to the right and shoulders to the left. Then, in the movement from picture 1 to 2, she uses shoulder movement to move to her left. In picture 2, she has increased pressure toward the outside of her left foot because her shoulders are too far left, but she is not tipping toward the wall. Actually, she is stable. How? The reason is that her hips held to the right are holding body weight and pressure in her right foot.

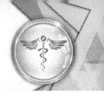

Note: When the movements of the hips and shoulders are equal and opposite, the relative pressure in the feet will not change.

In these pictures, Janette is not as stiff as she appears to be. The bigger issue is, she is trying too hard. She is pushing downward into both feet so much that she causes her leg muscles to become tight, enough that it restricts movement in her knees and ankles. This is common for many people with a mild movement impairment caused by neurodegenerative and other restrictive-posture disorders.

To gain better control and ability, we often overtighten our muscles to improve the stabilizing pressure pushing down into our feet. However, the effect is just the opposite, and "thinking too much" is a big contributor to the mistake. This is trying too hard to do better, and it causes restrictive movements. The solution we should be using is simply letting it be: relaxing into the movement, and limiting our thoughts about how the movement is supposed to be done.

This is a good example of *non-fear-related psychologically-induced stiffening*. Relax this self-induced tightness in your leg muscles to improve the pressures in your feet, to increase the flexibility of your knees and ankles, to improve the functioning of your feet, to find and trust your improved ability. Admittedly, this takes practice and constant reminders to relax the hands first to relax the feet last. With continued practice, you will discover the ability to work this more often from the feet up, which is how we naturally do it.

FLEXING FEET

Natural movement requires flexing feet. Only relaxed feet flex. Stiff feet do not flex. In very simple terms, *the relaxed flexing ability of our feet **is** our natural movement ability.*

For nearly all of our natural movements, we move the pushing (increased) pressure into the ball area and toes of the foot to push the body through the movement. Importantly, the heel area of the pushing foot is lifted off the floor during the pushing movement. This is the next advancement we will now begin to use in sideward movement.

Everything else stays the same, and all of what we have covered must be used. From pushing with the inside of the entire length of the foot, now we'll begin to do the exact same sideward movement while using only the ball area and toes of the foot to push the body. The stopping point for the push will be when the foot you are pushing your body onto is flat. This occurs when the pressure in that foot is centered.

Before starting to use the ball area of the flexing foot to move the body to the side, it will be helpful to do a short review of problems and mistakes that complicate using a flexing foot.

The Heel Will Not Lift or Stay Off the Floor

The most common reason your heel won't lift off the floor is because of the position of your shoulders. When your shoulders are back too far, the heel won't come up because you are pushing and holding pressure into it. With this posture, you'll experience problems shifting from one foot to the other.

1. With increased pressure in your heels, your stability decreases as you shift from one foot to the other. Why? As the pressure increases in the heel of the foot you're moving onto, that pressure begins to push you backward.

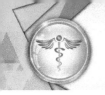
2. Decreasing stability leads to overall reactionary stiffening in your posture and especially in your knees. Frequently, this causes the knees to straighten and pulls stabilizing pressure out of the feet.

3. The result is added instability for two basic reasons: One, straightening knees pull pressure from the feet as the increased pressure is moved toward the heels. Two, the reactionary response to stiffening and straightening knees forces the shoulders to move upward and back, and moves pressure to the heels.

4. With the pressure decreasing in the ball area of the foot, the added pressure in the heel changes the direction of the movement. What began as only a sideward movement becomes a combined backward and sideward movement.

   This unexpected change leads to more instability and more reactionary stiffening as the pressure migrates into the outside heel area of the foot the body is moving toward. As the pressure concentrates in the heel area, the speed of the movement suddenly increases. This chain of events makes it very difficult to recover before a pushing fall occurs.

5. *The correct setup is to have and keep your shoulders slightly forward to move much of the pressure out of your heels and into the ball areas of your feet.*

Ensure that your setup posture is correct before you begin. Before initiating the movement, you need to have a slight amount of increased pressure in the ball areas of both feet. Relax your hands and knees, slightly flex your knees, and move your shoulders slightly forward. Then keep the movement slow and remind yourself to keep your shoulders forward during the movement.

In the correct setup posture, with feet approximately shoulder width apart, the heel of the pushing foot should feel very light. Then, using **only a light push**, push from the ball area and toes of that foot to move your body sideward toward the other foot. When your shoulders stay forward, the heel of the foot that you are *pushing from* will begin to lift as your body moves to the side. The lifting heel is the result of the flexing foot, and that lifting heel is also pushing your body to the side.

Now think back to what was discussed in a previous chapter about the flexing foot. What muscles are we using? They are the muscles in the calf: the gastrocnemius and soleus. The function of these muscles is to push pressure into the ball area of the foot and lift the heel. This is how they flex the foot.

What does this mean for people with small and weak calf muscles? Pushing added pressure into the ball area and flexing the foot doesn't work as well. Therefore, because these muscles are weak, any movements that require flexing feet will be "impaired." Now, consider how many of our natural movements require flexing feet. Nearly all of them do! So, what do these people with small, weak calf muscles need to do to improve their movement ability? They must strengthen these muscles.

Lifting the Heel and Keeping It Up

Do not try to force your foot to flex. The only way to flex the foot is to relax it, which actually means relaxing the muscles that control the foot. This requires you to be stable, comfortable, and relaxed.

When your body is relaxed and your setup posture is correct, your foot will naturally and easily flex in the movement. Importantly, realize that you are not trying to stand on only the ball area and toes of the foot to begin the movement. You are only to put and hold a little extra pressure in the ball areas of **both** feet, and still allow the entire length of both feet to rest on the floor in the setup posture. Also, remember to have your feet at least shoulder width apart to take advantage of the inside foot pressure as you begin this practice.

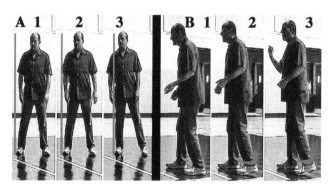

FIGURE 17.8: With a small increase of pressure into the ball area and toes of a foot, the lifting heel moves the body toward the other foot.

The distance the body moves to the side depends on the distance the heel moves upward from the floor. In Figure 17.8, panel A shows the movement of the body, while panel B shows the upward movement of the heel. The increased pressure pushed into the ball area of the flexing foot stabilizes the foot. The stabilized flexing foot lifts the heel upward to move the body.

In this example, I did not flex my knee in the movement as in the previous examples. This exercise is working with one flexing foot only. It doesn't take much heel movement to center the pressure in the other foot, and it does not require flexing the knee.

So be careful and go slowly. If you have stability issues when practicing this, and especially if you are moving pressure into the outside of the foot, use a wider stance while experimenting with the lifting and lowering of the heel.

Warning! It is very easy for a person with a tensed posture to exaggerate lifting the heel with uncontrolled and erratic movements. Keep things small and gentle.

Remind yourself to relax to better control the flexing foot. To move back to the ready stance, *partially* relax the pressure in the ball area of the pushing foot. This will allow the heel to lower, and your body will return. This is simple control of a simple movement, and easy when your posture is relaxed and stays in the proper setup posture.

Heel up, the body moves toward the other foot. Heel down, the body returns.

The amount of pressure in the ball area and toes of your pushing foot will stay the same during the movement, even as the pressure in the other foot increases. This is because:

1. The pressure in the ball area and toes of the pushing foot must be stronger than the pressure on the inside of the other foot, because that inside pressure is resisting the movement. It is pushing back against the movement of your body. This resistance will decrease as the pressure moves toward the center of that foot during the movement.

   Be careful. It will also decrease when your feet are closer together, and also when you flex the knee above the foot you're moving onto during the movement. Doing either of these reduces the amount of pressure needed in the ball area and toes to move the body. Not recognizing this is one reason some people will move their body too far and onto the outside of the other foot, and cause a pushing fall to the side.

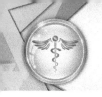

2. The pressure in the ball area and toes of the pushing foot *is the controlling pressure of the movement.* When it increases, the heel lifts more, and the movement of your body increases. When the pressure decreases, the heel lowers, and your body moves back.

When too much of the pressure in the pushing foot is released, the pressure from the inside of the other foot will sometimes push the body onto the outside area of the suddenly non-pushing foot.

HEEL LIFT *WITH* A FLEXING KNEE

As you become more stable, comfortable, and relaxed, it will be easier to stay in the ready stance with your shoulders in position to hold the pressure in the ball areas of your feet. With this, your knees and feet will become more flexible, and the movement will become easier, be more stable, and take less effort. If you are paying close attention during this transition, you'll notice a slight change occurring in the pressures in your feet.

With easily flexing knees, you will be creating and using more power and control with your leg muscles. You will also feel more stable with your feet closer together during the movement. Just be careful not to become too playful, and push too much or too quickly, and overshoot the transfer of body weight to the foot you are moving onto.

With improving ability, your posture and movement will look more like Robin's in Figure 17.9, in which she is alternating flexing her feet. She is at an angle to the camera in these pictures, but the red reference line extending up from the tip of her shoe helps show the movement of her shoulders. In picture 1, her shoulders are slightly back, and note how low her left heel is off the floor, and how far her shoulders are away from the red line. Compare this with picture 3, in which her left heel is now higher off the floor because her shoulders are forward, with the right one now touching the red line. When the shoulders are back, the heel is more difficult to lift. This is because of the added pressure this posture puts into the heel.

But what about picture 2, in which her right heel is lifted higher than her left heel is in picture 3, and her shoulders are farther back? In picture 2, Robin is using more pressure in the ball and toes of the pushing right foot. She extends the knee, and it looks as though she also adds some shoulder movement. In this example, she was also more comfortable in her stance; she wasn't thinking about the movement as much and simply allowed her body to move according to the lifting heel.

So, when you have the ability, what difference does it make if you have a flexing knee or use straighter knees? The simple answer is not much. With natural movement ability, the difference the amount of knee flexion makes is in reference to the function of the movement task you're involved in. It depends on what you're comfortable with and what is needed for the way you are doing any particular movement. So, is there a

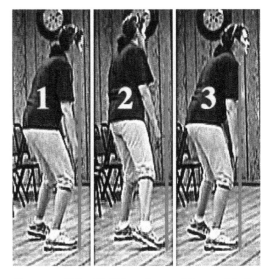

FIGURE 17.9: Shifting from side to side by flexing a knee and a foot.

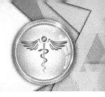

right or wrong amount? Yes and no. Each person decides what amount is correct as they are doing the things they want to be doing.

However, for people with a restrictive posture, the difference between having straight knees and flexed knees is often as different as night is from day. Their straightened knees too easily tend to be guarded or stiffened knees, and their flexed knees too easily straighten during many movements. This one issue leads to many more problems. So, the practice of keeping flexed knees in these exercises is preparation for improving all movements, because easily movable and trustworthy knees are key ingredients in all movements. This is how you redevelop your ability to choose how much knee movement you need to use.

Remember: Straightening and stiffening knees are the number one biggest and most problematic issue that turns natural movements into problem movements.

Do not try to be perfect in your movements. You will always make mistakes.
Use your mistakes as therapy—by learning to understand them.
Realize that a mistake is showing you what you need to work on. Ask yourself,
"Why did it happen, and what do I need to do to correct it?"

When you don't understand why a mistake happens, it is impossible to understand the correction.
*To improve your movement ability, **you must understand both**!*

■ ■ ■

CHAPTER 18

STANDING ON ONE FOOT

Walking requires the ability to stabilize your body on one foot.

I n general, the longer you live with a disorder or condition that negatively affects your movements, the more problems you will likely develop in your movements. This statement seems obvious. But it is also significantly biased, because it speaks only of the disorder or condition while dismissing the individual. To be honest, in too many cases a negative attitude and inaction by the individual significantly contribute to the problems that accumulate. On the other hand, those with a positive attitude and proactive lifestyle often significantly decrease and delay movement problems.

The quality of our life ultimately hinges on how we physically and mentally adapt to the issues and problems that our life's situation brings with it. So, with that said, we must take the initiative to do the best we can to help ourselves. Writing and saying this is easy. Doing it is the tough part.

WHAT IS REAL AND WHAT IS PERCEIVED?

Know the truth about what is real and what is not. It is very important for every individual living with the problems to have clarity in understanding the difference. It is just as important for the people close to them.

The movement issues and problems that you appear to have now are not necessarily predictive of the corrected and improved movements you may eventually regain. Why? Frequently, your physical issues and problems are different from your perceptions of them, and from the perceptions and opinions of others.

In truth, your issues and problems today simply represent your starting point from this day forward. Begin to test them honestly with this added information you are learning. Honestly and consistently work on and challenge your assumptions to find the abilities you can improve upon. Many of you will then be pleasantly surprised by the results. I know this to be true because I live it.

Simply try your best—but your best must be based on true and factual information. This means the negative junk that has become trapped in your thoughts needs to be replaced with useful and productive thoughts. Question everything. Experiment. Work *your* program according to the truths you uncover about yourself. Allow the better you to venture out of the darkness, to expose hidden abilities that will lead you to a better life.

Jenny

I first saw Jenny as she was "walking" toward me in a parking lot. Her movements were forced and unstable, her progress slow and laborious. Her posture likened to a caricature, masking and trapping the vitality of a not-so-long-ago normal young woman. This appearance affected my initial perceptions and assumptions. Truthfully, my initial perception was filled with doubts as to whether I could help her. But later, as I watched to evaluate what was happening, I began to see the truth hiding behind the misperceptions.

The point: When you don't force yourself to look beyond appearances and opinions, the perception of what you think you see is based primarily on the previous opinions. This too often convinces you they are real and truthful, when, in fact, they may not be. When you assume that what you are told or read is true, from that moment on, everything you do or don't do is based on the opinions, assumptions, or perceptions of the previous evaluators. This is a *not*-so-good thing for many issues, and also a not-so-good thing when it comes to movement. Why?

It is not so good because there is so much that is not known about the basics of our movements. First, there are many unknowns each of us have regarding how our movements physically work. Second, you assume that the opinions, assumptions, and perceptions of those with more knowledge about the subject are more correct than your own thoughts and perceptions. Your thoughts become, "Who am I to refute the findings of the experts?" as they use bigger and more technical words to convince you.

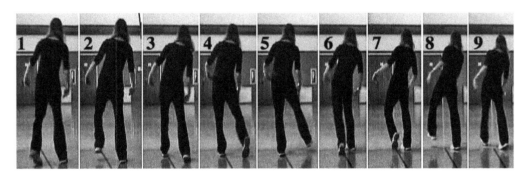

FIGURE 18.1: Jenny's complicated walking posture when I first met her.

The medical issues and problems afflicting Jenny had devastating effects on her posture and movements. To make matters worse, she acquired additional physical problems in dealing with the effects. She developed significant scoliosis (lateral curvature of the spine), shown in Figure 18.1 by her curved torso. Then she developed right foot drop and was fitted with a muscle stimulator to wear on her right leg to correct it, which she is NOT wearing in these pictures.

Knowledgeable physicians and therapists advised, "These issues are most likely due to the progression of her neurological condition" and entered this into her medical records. Now clearly recorded, they are forever the "proof" other medical professionals will use to understand Jenny's medical history and physical presentation. I did not have access to those records, as is the case with all the people I work with. (Jenny's mother and physical therapist told me about the diagnoses.) Thus, I must evaluate what I'm seeing on its own merit without interference by predetermined assumptions. In this example, with unbiased observation I quickly came to doubt that Jenny had these two conditions.

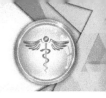

As with nearly everyone I've worked with, Jenny had more function and ability than previously assumed. Like the others, she had developed many maladaptive behaviors that were further complicating her underlying, very real condition. Thus, some of the postures and movements she developed in response to her condition are only "real" for as long as she continues to use the learned maladaptive habits that cause them.

Jenny did not have right foot drop. This is clearly seen in picture 5, in which she is holding the front of her right foot up. What she was doing, prompting many to think she had foot drop, is shown in picture 4. Here she is forcing the front of her foot down and lifting the heel excessively, using the gastrocnemius muscle in the back of her lower leg.

Previously, people watching her movements had incorrectly assumed that she could not lift the front of her foot. They watched the toe of the shoe pointing sharply down at the floor as she finished the stride and began to move her right foot forward. She was also swinging her right leg outward to bring the foot forward. These are the two things a person with uncorrected foot drop typically does. Thus, she was fitted with a muscle stimulator to activate the muscles in the front of her leg so she could lift the front of the foot. This, of course, complicated her movement issues even more, because those muscles were now unnecessarily being overstimulated—and competing with the overstimulated calf muscles.

The stimulator was activating muscles to forcibly lift the front of her foot. At the same time, she was unknowingly pushing the front of her foot down with her calf muscles. Consequently, when the stimulator was activated, all purposeful movement of her foot stopped. This is exactly what a stiffened posture does. Rather than correcting a problem in this example, the stimulator added a new and more complicated one.

What is real and what is not is the question you must continually ask. This is especially so when discussing things pertaining to one person's situation based on what someone else has said. Remember, what one person says about what someone else told them is too often misquoted. Be very careful. The information is often very misleading. This is especially true when the information chain is lengthy. A good example is, "My mom told me that my dad said that his therapist told him that the doctor wrote . . ."

Jenny did have a marked curvature of her body, so the scoliosis diagnosis would seem to have been correct. But no, factual evidence shows that it was questionable, at the very least. The curvature of her body shown in Figure 18.1 is not present in the pictures in Figure 18.2, nor was it as we continued working. She was able to maintain this posture, and when reminded she was not, she corrected her posture. These pictures were captured from a video taken two weeks later. Yes, scoliosis can be compensated for, but over what period of time and to what degree are the issues here.

Jenny's maladaptive movement behaviors only made it appear that she had scoliosis and foot drop. She was misusing the muscles in her legs, resulting in prolonged extension of her knee and ankle during a portion of the stride. To compensate, she arched her upper body to the side to be able to swing her leg and foot forward.

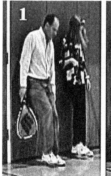
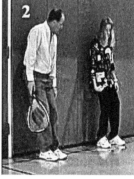

FIGURE 18.2: Two weeks later. No evidence to suggest scoliosis. There is no foot drop. Jenny is self-correcting the use of muscles in her legs to properly use her knees and feet.

Picture 1 of Figure 18.2 shows the truth of both conditions. She is easily holding the front of her foot up without any issues while **standing straight** and leaning against the wall, flexing her knee. How did this transformation happen? She was taught the proper function and use of her muscles, knees, and feet. Then she was taught how to push stabilizing pressure into her feet to relax and self-correct her posture. To sustain these improvements, she will constantly need to work on changing the maladaptive behavior she had accumulated to an adaptive behavior that she is now learning. She must also strengthen weakened muscles to continue the improvement.

This short introduction to Jenny's situation is a very good example of how terribly wrong a perception and missed observation can be. It also shows how the proper understanding and use of the natural basics of movement do have dramatic effects. So again. Stop believing everything you hear, especially the negatives. Test what you hear. Prove it correct or incorrect.

A Relaxed Foot

What does a relaxed foot look like when it is lifted off the floor? In pictures 2, 5, and 7 of figure 18.1, the foot Jenny has lifted off the floor is not relaxed because she is holding the front of it up. When a *relaxed knee lifts a relaxed foot*, the heel of that foot will be the first part of the foot lifted from the floor. The front tip of the foot will be the last part to rise from the floor. It naturally happens this way because the ankle is attached to the foot just in front of the heel.

When the knee moves upward, the heel also moves upward because it is directly connected to the ankle. However, when the muscles controlling the foot are relaxed, the front of the foot does not immediately move with the heel. When the muscles in the lower part of the leg remain relaxed, the ankle remains relaxed and the front of the foot droops, as shown in Figure 18.3.

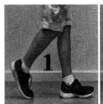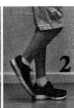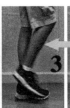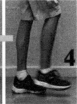

FIGURE 18.3: A relaxed ankle allows the front of the foot to droop downward when the knee has lifted the foot off the floor. Then muscles in the front of the leg lift the front of the foot during a stride. The blue arrow points to where these muscles are located.

In picture 1, the tip of the foot is pressing down into the floor at the end of the stride it was responsible for, as the transfer of body weight and pushing pressure into the advanced foot is completed. In picture 2, the knee has lifted the foot off the floor, and the heel of the foot moves directly with it.

Here the front of the foot is low because the muscles that lift the front of the foot (location indicated by the blue arrow) are completely relaxed. As the foot continues to move forward in pictures 3 and 4, the muscles in the front of the leg begin to pull the front of the foot up, in preparation for it to be returned to the floor as the stride continues.

Therefore, when the knee lifts the foot and the front of the foot stays up, it is because the person is holding it up. The only other reason for the foot to stay up is a problem with the ankle causing it to be held straight.

So now you know why the front of the foot would point upward when the knee is lifting the foot. The person is pulling the foot up with the muscles in the outside front portion of the lower part of the leg. People with this bad habit frequently have additional movement problems from instability and postural stiffness. When standing, they have increased pressure on their heels and will more often remain on their heels during movements.

A few people develop the opposite bad habit of constantly pushing the front of the foot down. Most of them wrongly learn this in an effort to "help" lift that foot off the floor. The problem is, this does not and cannot work. The foot is not capable of lifting or helping to lift itself off the floor.

Like Jenny, Carole in Figure 18.4 has developed this bad habit with her right foot. Instead of pushing her body forward with it, Carole pushes her body upward and sometimes backward, which she compensates for by holding her shoulders forward. Without the forward push from the foot, the person must use other ways to move the body and advancing leg forward. This is another reason for Jenny's abnormal posture in Figure 18.1.

The red arrow pointing to the back of Carole's leg shows the location of the gastrocnemius muscle we are now discussing. The other arrow at the foot shows the effect of using it.

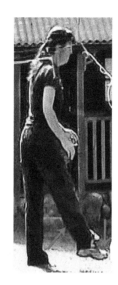

FIGURE 18.4: Inappropriate use of the gastrocnemius muscle forces the front of the foot down.

Why do some movement-impaired people inappropriately overuse their gastrocnemius muscles? Naturally, we use these muscles to stop us from tipping too far forward on our toes, so we don't fall forward on our noses. For this reason, and because they don't know how to correct their posture to stop the tipping, people with a frequent forward tipping problem use these muscles so much they adapt to using them all the time. They become overdependent on them and use them when they should not. This is a very difficult habit to unlearn.

To begin correcting bad use habits with the feet, it helps to first learn how to relax the muscles that control the feet and are causing the problem. The process begins with muscle identification while sitting in a chair.

1. With both feet flat on the floor, lean forward and place your hand and fingers on the front *outside* portion of your lower leg (indicated by the blue arrow in picture 3 of Figure 18.3), and then lift the front of the foot while keeping the heel on the floor. As the front of the foot lifts, you will feel the muscles under your fingers tighten. Relax the muscles and the front of the foot goes down.

   This tells you that these are the muscles that lift the front of your foot, and that is all they do.

2. With both feet flat on the floor, lean forward and place your hand and fingers on the back of the lower part of your leg, the calf area. Now push the front of your foot down. When you push it down, the heel comes up. As you push down and the heel comes up, feel the muscle on the back of your lower leg tighten.

   This tells you that this muscle pushes the front of your foot down and lifts your heel, and that is all it does. This is how we flex the foot.

3. To lift a foot, first push down into the other foot to transfer body weight off the foot you want to lift. Now, beginning with both feet flat on the floor, you are to feel what happens when you attempt to lift a foot in these three different ways:

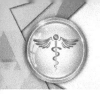
- Lift the foot while holding the front of that foot up.

- Lift the foot while pushing the front of that foot down. (Doing either one of these first two makes it difficult to lift the foot from the floor.)

- Lift the foot while not using these muscles. Just keep them relaxed. (The foot is easy to lift.)

4. When you lift the knee and keep these muscles relaxed, what position is the foot in when all of the muscles are functioning properly?

- If the foot is level to the floor or the front of the foot is pointing up, you are using the muscles in the front of the leg to hold it in this position.

- If the front of the foot is sharply pointing down like Carole's, you are using your calf muscles. To the untrained eye, this may look the same as a drooping foot, because the higher lifted heel has gone unnoticed. Also, when the leg is visible, the outline of the gastrocnemius muscle in the calf is clearly seen.

- If the front of the foot is angled down like the foot in pictures 2–4 of Figure 18.3, both muscle groups are relaxed.

Until the overuse and incorrect use of these muscles is recognized and corrected, standing, transferring body weight, balancing on one foot, and a variety of movements including walking will be challenging and problematic.

Lifting a Foot

Most people with natural abilities have little reason to pay attention to what they are physically doing in their movements. This has led us all to incorrectly assume things about our body and movements, and how the two work. The same is true when people begin to lose natural ability. Since we have more assumptions than facts in our knowledge base about our natural movements, we make additional assumptions about our problem movements and how to deal with them. This *assuming* process only leads us farther away from understanding what natural and unnatural movements actually are.

When standing, the natural way to lift a foot involves two basic steps. First, body weight is transferred. completely to one foot, as increased pressure is also pushed into that foot. Second, the other knee is lifted after the foot supporting the body has been stabilized.

People with generalized weakness, balance and movement issues, and especially when they have a tensed posture, have difficulty completely transferring their body weight onto one foot. This leaves pressure in the leg and the foot they want to lift, and that pressure is working to hold the foot on the floor. The result is that the "not so free" foot is more difficult to lift, and it is pushed back down when it does lift.

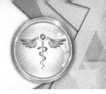

Many of you will repeatedly make these same mistakes when practicing shifting your weight between your feet, and then attempting to move to the side or stand on one foot. With this problem, it is important to stop focusing on the foot that is not the problem. Stop focusing on lifting a foot when you should be heavily focused on pushing pressure down into and stabilizing on the other foot. Why? The foot you are preparing to stand on is the important foot. It is the foot supporting your body while the other foot is doing nothing, as shown in Figure 18.5.

This is a reminder of the extremely important first thing that is required in every movement. Every movement begins and continues with a strong push down into the foot you are using to support and power the movement. When you do this and accomplish a complete body-weight transfer onto that foot, the other hip will easily lift the knee, which will lift the foot that's not bearing weight.

Always focus on pressurizing and stabilizing the foot you are supporting your body with, and not the one that's about to be lifted into the air!

PROBLEMS STANDING ON ONE FOOT

1. **Under- or overshooting the weight shift.**

    a. Undershooting means an incomplete weight shift. Overshooting means the weight shift went too far. Most commonly overshooting is due to the shoulders, and sometimes the shoulder and hip, leaning and/or moving too far to the side, toward the outside of the supporting foot.

    b. Another common overshooting mistake is pushing (moving) onto the foot too quickly with too much force from the pushing foot. This will very easily cause an overshoot, especially when the feet are closer together when beginning the movement.

    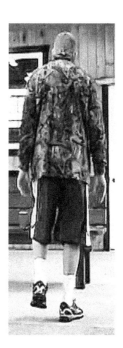

    FIGURE 18.5: Standing on one foot demands a higher level of relaxed control in cooperative and coordinated body movement.

    The problem Ant is having in Figure 18.6 is the incorrect use of his upper body to move his body onto the foot he wants to balance on. In both panels, he leans his upper body to the side to shift onto one foot and then lift the other foot off the floor. In panel A, he is attempting to transfer to his left foot by raising the heel of his right foot, but he is leaning his upper body to lift the heel. Finally, in pictures 3 and 4, the heel of his right foot is up, but note how much upper-body lean is required. Curiously, though, even with this excessive lean, he appears to be stable.

    In panel A, the reason he remains stable is because his bottom is resting against the wall behind him. This also partly explains why he is using this much upper-body lean. There is too much pressure on his bottom restricting the sideward movement of his hips, and his backward-leaning bottom puts pressure in his heels.

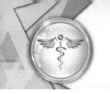

Now compare the movement of his hips in both panels. In panel B, his bottom is not against the wall, so when he leans with his upper body, all of him quickly tips into the cabinet and countertop beside him.

In both examples, he is attempting to balance on his left foot using upper-body movement. Because of this, he is not using his legs and feet very well. He is not pushing pressure into the ball area of his right foot to power the movement, nor is he pushing enough pressure into his left foot to support his body weight. His foundation is weak, and the increased postural stiffness in panel B is evidence of this. Instead, he is pulling the pressure out of his right foot and moving pressure to the outside of his left foot.

His posture remains more relaxed in panel A only because his bottom on the wall restricts the sideward movement of his body.

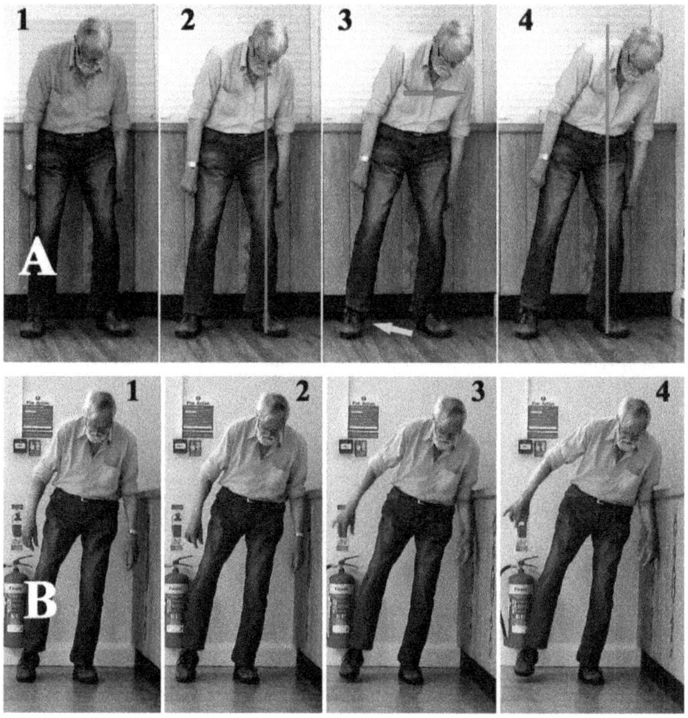

FIGURE 18.6: In both panels, Ant leans to the side to shift to one foot to "help" his legs and feet. Because of this, he overshoots the center of his left foot and puts pressure in the outside of the foot. Note that in panel A, he remains stable, and the heel of his right foot is up only in pictures 3 and 4. But in panel B, he falls into the wall as the foot lifts from the floor. In panel A, his bottom is on the wall and putting pressure in the heels of both feet.

c. If moving onto the outside of your foot continues to be a problem, widen your stance a small amount to gain some benefit from pressure toward the insides of your feet. What is this telling you? When you keep moving onto the outside of the foot, you are not quite ready to be in a narrower stance. Watch yourself in a mirror to see what you are doing, to know what corrections you need to apply.

2. **Unsteadiness when standing on one foot.** *Knees, knees, stiff knees.*

   a. To help correct this, mildly flex your knees more than what they are, to apply more pressure into both feet before beginning the weight shift to one foot.

   b. Remember to use your thigh and core muscles the same way you did to stand up from or sit down into a chair.

   c. As you flex your knees to move into a lower ready stance, remember to keep your shoulders forward. This is a one-flat-foot ready stance that works the exact same way as it does when squatting on two feet.

d. Weak legs make it difficult to remain stable while standing on two feet. So, when you have this problem, do not expect that you will have the ability to stand stable on one foot. You will not. One weak leg will not support what two weak legs are having difficulty with.

3. **Tipping forward or backward.** *Shoulders and knees.*

   a. Before standing on one foot, always begin in a ready stance on two flat feet, and stay in the ready stance as you move onto one foot.

   b. Tipping likely means you are not relaxed. Using only one foot will challenge you to stay relaxed, to keep your shoulders in position and your knee slightly flexed.

   c. The most common mistake is not moving off your heels when you're on both feet. This is often difficult to correct when you move onto one foot. Keep your shoulders forward in the setup.

   d. The second most-common mistake is starting with two flat feet and then letting your shoulders fade backward as you transfer to one foot. Remind yourself to keep your shoulders forward as you begin the movement.

   e. The third most-common mistake, while in the setup, is straightening the knee while moving your shoulders forward, causing you to tip forward off the toes of stiffened feet.

4. **Shaky legs.**

   a. If you have the strength to do at least ten squats on both legs without stopping, then your shaking problem is likely tensed-up, fear-driven, postural-stiffening-induced shaking.
      Yes, stiffened-posture shaking is real. But much of the time you are making it real. You create the shaking with weakness and stiffness, which causes you to fight with yourself. This means you also can stop it, and you will when you learn to relax in a balanced stance and have the strength to easily support your body weight.
      With adequate strength, you can control and stop the shaking.
      Without the strength, the shaking remains uncontrollable.

   b. *If your legs are not strong enough to relax and support you without shaking, then you do **not** have the stability and control required to **comfortably** do the remaining movements covered in this book.* Without adequate strength and the ability to relax, you will be constantly frustrated and possibly injure yourself while attempting to do things your body is not ready to do.
      If this is you, should you give up? Absolutely not! This is not someone telling you what you cannot do, nor is it saying you've failed. This is your body telling you what it needs you to do in order to improve your chances of achieving better movement abilities.

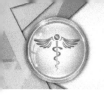

c. When your legs are shaking, listen to them. They are telling you they are weak and/or not relaxed and it's very likely you're not using them correctly. They are telling you that if you want the rewards of improved ability, you must do the required work to strengthen them.

Functionally Flat

Have you ever walked in mud so thick and deep that it sucked the boot off your foot when you tried to lift it? To get your boot up and out of the mud to take another step, the foot you are standing on in the mud must be very stable. The pressure and stability in that foot is exactly what you want to feel in this exercise.

Try to imagine you are in six inches of mud as you shift your body from foot to foot. Remember, mud is slippery, so keep your feet closer together to keep them under you. Because the mud is slippery, the foot going down into it must move straight down, flatten, and be stabilized on the bottom with pressure. Focus on this foot in each stride. Center and support your body on a secure, steady foot as you push a super amount of pressure into it, so it can hold you up and keep your face out of the mud.

For those who used to skate when you were younger, use those memories. Imagine you're walking while wearing **roller skates or ice skates** and there are obstacles on the floor you must step over. Roller skates, ice skates, slippery surfaces when you're wearing smooth-bottomed shoes or when comfortably walking . . . there is no difference in what you must do. For example, when wearing skates, if you begin to walk when *not* standing directly over the skate wheels or blades, they roll or slip out from under you, and your bottom abruptly greets the ground. The same is true when you walk in shoes or barefoot among scattered toys on the floor. Pick whatever you want, because the situation doesn't matter. When the movement demands that you must support and balance your body on one foot to move to the other, it is done the exact same way for the exact same reasons.

Feel It in Your Pinky Toe

Most of the time, we use the inside and center portions of our feet during advancing movements. Whenever we are on both feet, this is where our divided body weight is located. The weakest part of the foot is the little-toe area, and it is very weak in those with generalized weakness, balance and movement issues. With a tensed posture and increasing pressure in this area of the foot, these people are often tipping and falling at an angle to the side and forward. Therefore, they especially do not like to feel pressure in the forward outside area of the foot, even more than they don't like feeling pressure in the entire forward part of the foot.

Balancing on one foot works best when **all** of the foot is used. This sounds very obvious, but many people with natural ability are challenged to stay balanced on one foot in different poses. Most people with balance and movement problems find it extremely difficult to stabilize standing on one foot. For all these people, the one big reason is that they are not using the entire foot for support, because they are not completely centered and stabilized on that foot. They are not making the foot functionally flat.

I know that standing balanced on one foot is difficult or impossible for many of you when you are not holding on to or leaning on something. So, use your hands when you need them. Use a wall or

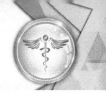

something similar that is very stable to help you through the process of learning what you need to be doing. Be careful and be honest with yourself. To the best of your ability, limit how much you lean on what you're using, and gradually reduce the support to learn how to better use your leg and foot for the total support of your body.

In Figure 18.7, Charlie is using the support of his son's hands. Notice that he and his son are using only the ends of their fingers. This provides Charlie with minimal external support while encouraging him to increase the use and support of his leg and foot.

This is a very, very important part of this process. Standing balanced on one foot requires

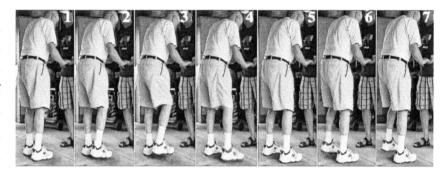

FIGURE 18.7: When you need support, use it. The importance is the focus and practice of putting increased pressure into all areas of the foot, and then relaxing the body into it. This is practicing completing the transfer of body weight onto a stabilized, supporting flat foot and balancing on it. The focus is on the foot you will be standing on, and not the one you are lifting off the floor.

a complete transfer of body weight and much more additional pressure pushing down into that foot than most people with a balance and movement problems are accustomed to applying. So, because of their physical and psychological challenges with this, they stop doing many things. Then, strength, motivation, and ability fade away as they stop doing many of the activities they were previously doing.

Supporting and balancing your body on this much smaller foundation of one foot demands more strength, motivation, effort, and ability. Why? In most cases, when moving to one foot, the total surface area of your supporting foundation is quickly reduced in total area to one-third or less of what you've just been using. In itself, that reduction of surface area is destabilizing. Therefore, downward stabilizing pressure must be immediately increased and concentrated in the suddenly smaller foundation area as the surface area decreases.

To create the same support in one foot that was being shared between two feet, the effective pressure pushed into this smaller area made by the one foot must be increased, to maintain the support and stability of the body, as described in Chapter 15. What is the other requirement for this added pressure? It is the slight change in the direction in which the one foot is applying pushing force into the floor, as described in Chapter 17.

When we're standing on two feet, there is always a stabilizing pressure that is pushing into the floor at an angle. This angled outward force from the inside area of each foot is pushing and holding the body toward the center of the stance, and helps significantly in supporting and stabilizing the body.

But when we're standing balanced on one foot, there is no angled stabilizing pressure. Therefore, all of the body's support and stabilization on one foot comes from the concentrated, single, straight-downward pressure. Working alone, this pressure must be greater to produce the same support and stability that the two feet were providing.

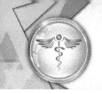

OTHER KNEE- AND FOOT-POSITION ISSUES

Let's assume you're doing things correctly but are finding it difficult to stay standing on one foot for even a couple of seconds. What and where is the problem? Before attempting to answer that question, first ask this question: Which way do you tip off the foot? We've covered tipping to either side, so you know why that happens. But what if you tip backward, like Ann in Figure 18.8, and don't understand what is causing the increased heel pressure that pushes you backward? And you are holding your shoulders forward, just like Ann is. So, the question: What causes her to fall backward?

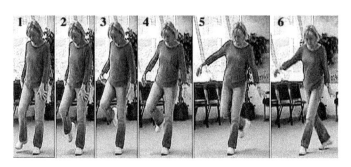

FIGURE 18.8: Attempting to balance on one foot but tipping backward. In picture 2, Ann complicates the movement with excessive movement of her shoulders. That is what causes the imbalance and adds postural stiffening.

The position of her right leg and foot combined with postural guarding causes it. In picture 1, she is balanced. But then in picture 2, she begins flexing her right knee, which moves her leg and foot out behind her. This causes two things to happen:

1. The weight of her lower leg and foot moving backward moves more pressure into her left heel, and the increased heel pressure pushes her body backward. Note that she lifts her knee by flexing her right hip. However, she is also over using the muscles on the back of her thigh, the hamstrings. A job of these muscles is to flex the knee, and that is only minimally needed for this movement.

    Do you see what else is happening in picture 2?

2. Ann is pushing the front of her lifted foot down in picture 2. This means she is also inappropriately using her calf muscles (the gastrocnemius and soleus) to push the front of her foot down. These muscles also have nothing to do with lifting the knee. This is the same mistake Carole made in Figure 18.4.

    We use the muscles in the front of the thigh (quadriceps) to flex the hip to lift the knee and foot. Ann does this in picture 1. However, she then uses the muscles in the back of her thigh (hamstrings) to begin flexing her knee and extending her hip. This is why her leg moves backward, and is the reason for the increasing heel pressure in the foot on the floor.

MOVING TO THE SIDE, ONE FOOT AT A TIME

Controlled, advancing-sideways movement combines the skills learned in this and the previous chapters. Mary demonstrates it in Figure 18.9. For the recovering movement-impaired person with a restrictive posture, it is very important to practice moving from one flat foot to the other flat foot. This provides the optimal support and stability that affords the best opportunity to relax the posture.

Another tactic is to keep the length of the sideward stride small, like baby-step small, when you are experiencing any form of stiffness or instability. The small stride makes it easier to move from flat foot to flat foot. Because the movement of the body is small, the sideward movement of pressure in each foot will be very small. All of this keeps things simple, more stable, and more comfortable. This translates into a higher success rate with complete transfers of body weight.

You have choices in how you push your body into the movement, as explained in Chapter 17. When you are feeling stiff, push down into the entire foot you want to stand on and move from. Then, when you are relaxed, practice pushing your body into the movement from the ball area and big toe. Feel both methods and become as comfortable as possible with them. Many of you will also need to frequently remind yourselves to relax hands and arms to relax knees and feet. This means you will also likely need to remind yourselves to keep your shoulders forward to hold the pressure constant in your feet.

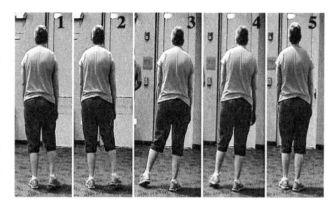

FIGURE 18.9: Advancing-sideward movement. Stand on a flat foot, then push your body sideward with that foot to stand on the other flat foot, and then bring in the foot you began with to stand on both feet. Moving from a flat foot to a flat foot provides the stability you require to become comfortable with the movement.

Keeping your knees relaxed and flexed is a big problem when there is guarding or stiffening in your posture. Often, when you seem relaxed, you aren't as relaxed as you think you are. Be very aware of this!

CONTROLLING THE FOOT

Ultimately, the movement of the body determines and controls the movement and placement of the advancing foot. However, the knee directly controls the movement of the foot according to the following:

1. The upper body sets the location of the pressure in the foot.

2. The pushing pressure in the foot determines the direction and distance the body will move. The body moves the knee, and the knee moves the advancing foot. Therefore, the push from the foot on the floor determines where the advancing foot will land.

3. In a relaxed movement, the body will naturally place the lifted foot on the floor *exactly where the body needs it to be* for the best support in the continuation of the movement or stance.

4. Therefore, if you change the position of your upper body during a movement, or if you change the amount of pressure you are applying into the pushing foot, then you will also change the location where the advancing foot will contact the floor.

Read that again, because it is so very important to understand. Directed by the push from the supporting foot, the lifted knee will deliver the lifted foot to exactly the right spot on the floor where the relaxed body requires it to be for support. *This will happen each and every time, provided there is no interference from your thinking mind.*

Therefore, except in specific circumstances that require it, DO NOT attempt to place your foot where you think it should be. Your body knows exactly where that foot needs to be, and you must learn to trust it. How do you do this? Focus on the foot you're standing on. Focus on the foot that is controlling the movement. Focus on the pushing foot and relax your body into it.

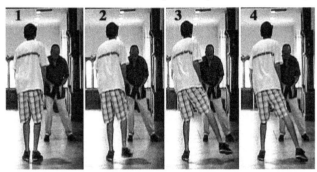

FIGURE 18.10: In the background, I am pushing my body in one movement. In the foreground, Alex steps, causing two movements. He leans his body to the left to lift and move his right foot. Then, after placing the foot, he still must move his body to the right. By thinking about controlling his right foot, he complicates the movement.

In the previous example, Mary *pushed her body through* the movement. This is evident by her relaxed and flexing foot. In Figure 18.10, Alex is *stepping into* the movement. Closely compare the sequence and postures in both.

Alex complicates the movement. In picture 1, he begins on a flat right foot and leans his body to the left to lift and move his right foot. This lean was necessary to counterbalance the extending leg. The next part of the movement that is not shown is moving his body over to the right foot. Sometimes in life we must do a movement just like this, but for most purposes, this only makes things much more difficult for the movement impaired. Look again at Mary's movement. Easy, relaxed, and simple.

Pushing into the movement is a very different action from stepping into the movement with a focus on placing the extending foot in a particular spot on the floor. When pushing, the body moves together as one unit, and the advancing foot is placed where the body requires it to be.

When stepping, the placement of the extended foot is controlled by where your mind wants the foot to be placed. Yes, this almost always works well when a person with natural ability does it. However, when a person with a restrictive-posture movement impairment does it, the results are often disastrous.

Why did Alex do this? He was watching and listening to me explain the movement. What you see is him thinking about, interpreting, and confusing what I am saying. He then attempts to mimic my movement using what he sees, hears and thinks he needs to do.

This is a classic example. The change in the performance and outcome of the movement is strikingly different, because just thirty seconds before this he was moving naturally through the movement. This demonstrates what many people with problematic movement issues experience. Through doubts, fears, and a restrictive posture, they think themselves into worsening movements. Some may be surprised that this same thing happens when people with natural ability overthink their way through some of their movements.

■ ■ ■

CHAPTER 19

KEEPING YOUR KNEES FLEXED

When your movements are forced and awkward, check your posture.
Frequently, your knees will be a big part of what is wrong.

Often, when people with a stiffening posture and impaired movements move down into a ready stance with flexed knees, it feels odd. This is especially true when they try to keep their knees flexed during a movement.

DROP AND CATCH

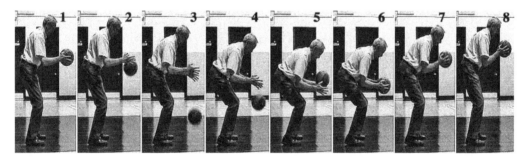

FIGURE 19.1: Relaxed postural control. Relaxed knees control the movement of the body. Relaxed hands and elbows control and handle the ball.

Because of their size, weight, and texture, a basketball or school-yard (playground, foursquare) ball is a perfect choice for this next activity. Both have good surface texture, making them easier to handle, grasp, and catch. A properly inflated basketball or foursquare ball works well because the weight of the ball keeps it stable when bounced. Also, when slightly underinflated, these become more controllable because they rebound less. This means the ball's return movement will be a little slower and not as high. This serves another important purpose. It forces the person to move and stay lower in their stance with flexing knees, which is exactly what many people need. A simple exercise is dropping and catching the ball as shown in Figure 19.1.

Beginning in a ready stance, hold the ball with flexed elbows and relaxed fingers, as Bob is doing in picture 1. Then drop the ball by only slightly opening your fingers. As the ball begins to fall, immediately squat

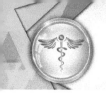

to catch it when it rebounds upward (pictures 2 through 5). The objective is to catch the ball while you are lower in the squat and then return with the ball to the ready stance (pictures 6 through 8). Take note of the location of Bob's hands in relation to the ball in picture 5. The ball has bounced up above his hands. Your goal is to catch the ball the same way. So, lower yourself quickly into the squat with flexing knees to position your hands below the height of the rebounding ball, so it then drops back down into your relaxed hands.

This is a good exercise to use for working on improving dynamic postural control. It requires coordination of the movements of the upper and lower body. It depends on relaxing the elbows and knees, flexing the knees, and moving the shoulders forward appropriately while holding the pressure stable in the feet.

This is a simple exercise, yet there will still be many things that will want to occupy your thoughts. So, try to limit your focus as much as possible. There is one basic focus that will help you keep this simple and allow the movement to happen more naturally. Push down into your flattened feet to squat, and then push down into your flattened feet to stand up. That is all. Move down into the stabilizing pressure, then move up from the held stabilizing pressure.

In Bob's example, he is doing very well, but his fingers still have some mild stiffness in them (pictures 2 through 5). Relaxing stiffening fingers is a challenge for many, but it is necessary in order to enable the rest of the movement to happen more naturally. Also, focus on holding the ball with only your fingertips, with relaxed hands. Try to avoid having your full hand on it, because this encourages applying added pressure onto the ball.

The Exercise

Holding the ball as shown, relax in a ready stance with *slightly* increased pressure in the ball areas of both feet. This slight forward shift of pressure in your feet results from your partially extended arms and the weight of the ball.

This is where you need to keep the pressure, but for some, keeping it there will be challenging. *In preparation, they correctly stabilize and adjust their posture in a ready stance on flat feet*, but then become unstable when they extend their arms forward with the ball in their hands. The reason they become unstable is most always stiffness, especially in the knees and feet. Another factor is extending the arms out too far forward.

When you maintain a relaxed posture, the bounce-and-catch exercise is easy to do. Therefore, when you notice it's not easy, the most likely reason is that you're not relaxed enough to allow it to be easy.

1. Begin in a high ready stance on flat feet. Take a moment to relax your hands and knees. Then bend your elbows to raise the ball in your hands to chest height.

    The pressure in your feet should move slightly forward. If it doesn't, only slightly lean your upper body forward while moving into a high squat. Why doesn't the pressure move to and stay in the ball area of the feet? It's common for people with a movement impairment to move their shoulders back when they bring the ball up.

2. Release the ball. You're striving to release it by doing nothing more than relaxing your fingers. With relaxed fingers, let the ball slip away. When you are using just your fingertips, it will slip out easily.

If you have the palms of your hands on the ball, it probably won't drop when you relax your fingers. Then you must pull your hands away from the ball to release it, and many people exaggerate this movement. Often their hands will quickly move widely apart when their arms and hands are stiffened. Some people will be confused and throw the ball to the floor. Others will throw it so it bounces higher up, so they don't need to squat. Resist this urge. The purpose is to learn to stay relaxed and flex your knees.

3. As the ball drops, immediately *squat with bending knees to lower your hands* to just under the height where the ball will rebound. Do not stoop forward to lower your body and hands. Many of you will need to practice **not** starting the squat with your shoulders moving forward, to stop the habit of stooping forward instead of bending your knees.

    Also, **DO NOT** lower your arms and hands with extending elbows to reach down for the ball. Many of you will want to do this instead of squatting. Watch your elbows and hands, and keep them close to where they were in the starting position.

4. In the squat, your goal is to catch the ball *gently and quietly* with relaxed hands and fingers, and then return with relaxed hands to where you began in the ready stance. When your hands are spread widely apart because of your stiffness, often you will hurriedly slap them back together on the ball to catch it.

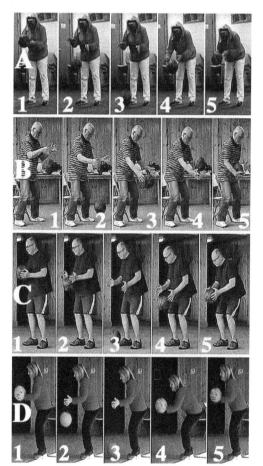

When you do this exercise correctly, you will be down in the squat waiting for the ball to fall back into relaxed hands that are close together. However, this easy movement quickly fills with problems for a person with a restrictive posture and uncooperative, stiffened hands, elbows, knees, and feet. The people in the four panels in Figure 19.2 demonstrate many of these common problems.

Panel A. Compared with the others, Lynn has the most stiffness in her posture. Her knees flex very little, and not until picture 4. Then, in picture 5, they're already straight again. To drop the ball, she uses a stiffened left wrist to move her hand. Instead of squatting to catch the ball, she stoops forward to lower her stiffened hands and elbows, but does not lower them far enough. When the ball returns in picture 5 it is bouncing off the tips of her stiff fingers. To her credit, Lynn does do something correctly in this example. She stays stable on flat feet.

Recall, when a person with a stiffened posture stoops, the forward and downward motion of their upper body often quickly moves increased pressure toward the ball areas and

FIGURE 19.2: The task is to drop the ball and then squat down to catch it while keeping the arms and hands in the same position. The lesson is learning to relax fingers and knees.

toes of their feet, causing them to tip forward. So, how did Lynn stay on her flat feet? Simple. She learned to counterbalance the forward movement of her shoulders with the backward movement of her hips. She pushed her bottom backward as she bent forward. She did well to stay on stable feet, but not so well with the movement she intended to do.

The other issue with stooping with straightened knees is the increased back pressure it applies to the knees. The added pressure pushes the knee backward and holds it in a straightened position, which is what is happening in picture 5. Lynn has been using this bad habit in her movements for many years. That makes it a very difficult habit to break.

Panel B. Dan's posture is more relaxed than Lynn's, but stiffer than Gene's in panel C. Dan begins in a high ready stance, but his knees flex very little as he tries to lower himself into a squat. This forces him to extend his arms downward to catch the ball. Then he has trouble grasping the ball with his stiffened fingers, hands, and arms. So, he uses his body to trap the ball. In the process of trapping the ball, his shoulders and head move slightly backward (picture 5) and cause him to become unstable with slightly increased pressure in his heels. Also note, bringing his arms and the ball closer to his body also causes pressure to move toward his heels. He remained standing, but it took him a few very long seconds to relax his posture enough to return to stable flat feet.

What allowed Dan to remain standing and not tip back onto the chair when the pressure moved toward his heels in picture 5? His knees stayed flexed, and he held downward pressure in his feet. This helped him compensate for the effect of the pressure moving toward his heels.

Panel C. Gene's posture is mildly stiffened. His shoulders stay back a bit too far, so he has slightly increased pressure in his heels. This limits his ability to squat. His knees flex minimally, so he must extend his elbows to lower his hands. He then catches the ball with his hands toward the top of it.

Panel D. Carol is showing the correct way to drop the ball, squat, catch, and stand. Her posture stays in alignment (shoulders, knees, and toes), her arms stay in position, and she remains relaxed with slightly increased pressure in the ball areas and toes of her feet. She releases the ball with a little excessive movement of her fingers and wrists, and then squats with flexing knees to catch it with little effort as it bounces up. To catch the ball, she only has to close her fingers and wrists a small amount.

Now compare all of them. What do you see? From top to bottom, the stiffness decreases and the level of function increases. In A, moderate postural stiffness. In B, mildly moderate postural stiffness. In C, mild postural stiffness. In D, mild postural *guarding*.

Importantly, from bottom to top, these examples show the typical *advancement of difficulties* people with neurodegenerative disorders develop as their situation deteriorates. In large part, their increasing movement difficulties arise from the maladaptive behaviors and bad habits they acquire. This brings forth the stronger point that needs to be made here. Physically, Lynn, Dan, and Gene have the hidden ability to be doing very close to the same as Carol is. What is hiding it? Stiffness. Fear.

REACTING VERSUS ANTICIPATING

In the bottom panel of Figure 19.3, Gene intends to drop, squat, and catch the ball just as Bob does in the top panel. Compare the differences in their movements. Gene drops the ball, hesitates while it bounces on the floor, and then squats to catch the ball. Bob drops the ball and immediately squats to be in position to catch it. This highlights two important points:

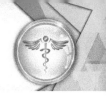

1. Gene has guarded stiffness that Bob does not.

2. Gene moves with a *reactionary mind-set*, while Bob moves with an *anticipatory mind-set*.

Bob is anticipating the movement of the ball. Trusting his ability, he moves where he knows the ball will be without hesitation.

Gene is reacting to the ball's movement. Yes, he knows where he needs to be to catch the ball when it bounces up, and he knows the squatting movement. The problem is the learned mind-set he has acquired, which has developed out of his postural stiffening. Because he doesn't trust his ability to remain stable in his daily movements, he has learned not to move until he's forced to move. This is why he delays starting the squat.

Many people with a restrictive-posture movement impairment delay their movements with this reactionary process. When a situation presents a reason for them to move, they often stay standing in place, hoping they won't have to move. Then they move only when they are forced to react to something or someone. They wait, hoping the object or other person won't force them to do something they don't trust doing. In reality, this is about fear and a restrictive posture. I lived with this destructive issue for years.

When faced with a situation that requires them to adjust their posture or move, especially if they must change their location, people who don't trust their movement abilities will always do it very cautiously. So, instead of moving to avoid a potential problem, they stop, watch, and timidly wait, hoping they won't need to move. They wait until they have no choice, but in their waiting, they seldom prepare for the forced movement they fear they must do.

There are contributing issues.

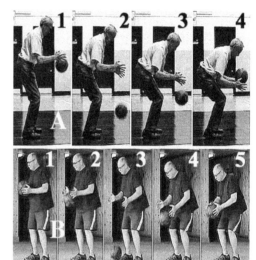

FIGURE 19.3: When Bob (in panel A) drops the ball, he immediately squats to be in position when it bounces up. Bob anticipates where the ball will be. Gene (in panel B) reacts to the ball. He hesitates when it drops, and then he must hurry to get to it when it bounces up. A restrictive posture causes the person to develop this reactionary hesitation.

1. They don't know how to prepare for the movement that would allow them to avoid an interfering situation.

2. They don't want to embarrass themselves by showing their awkwardness and possibly tipping or falling in public.

In people with a moderate or more significant impairment, in that moment when the interfering situation forces them to react, very often their minds go nearly blank. This is why they often "freeze" in place, and very often they cannot see beyond the whiteout of nothingness that suddenly overwhelms their minds. This is why they remain standing still. Fear, anxiety, stiffness, instability, and a lack of self-trust overwhelm them to the point where they are truly powerless to anticipate postures and movements. So, they react by adding more guarding and stiffening to their posture while hoping they won't be touched or need to move.

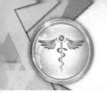

Make no mistake about what this is. This *is not* defensive posturing.
It is *victim posturing; a learned reactionary mind-set of indecision.*

This reactionary or nonaction mind-set develops from their most problematic movement challenges, which are starting, stopping, and changing directions. They are anxious about, intimidated by, and/or fearful of these because these are the junctures when they are most likely to have a problem and fall.

With a restrictive posture, the most common mode of **starting** a movement is a tipping action done with the upper body. The tip might be to the front, back, or side. But, surprisingly to many, this tipping of the upper body is frequently done in the opposite direction of the movement the person is initiating. This leads to postural corrections and overcorrections with an increasingly uncooperative body, resulting in frequent, unpleasant, embarrassing outcomes and falls.

For example, when they come close to the place they want to **stop**, they extend their arms out with fingers wide open to catch themselves as they tip forward. But characteristically they do this with withdrawn shoulders. They subconsciously withdraw their shoulders to slow their tipping-forward movement. As a result, they then often begin to tip backward because they frequently exaggerate and overcorrect the movement of their shoulders. When this happens, they will commonly do one of two things. They will exaggerate shoulder movement forward to essentially fall forward onto an object or person to stop their fall, or they will continue to tip and often fall backward.

Yes, some don't withdraw their shoulders as they are stopping, but this is typically when their movements are slow and small, and they have better control of themselves.

With natural movement abilities, people use an **anticipatory mind-set**. They know where they want to go and what they need to do, and their trusted ability works instantly without concern or fear. Their body is relaxed and prepared, or very quickly becomes prepared for almost any situation. With natural movement ability, they are **not** focused on their movements. Instead, they are *focused on the purpose* of the movement. They are focused on the game they're playing, the place they're going, the situation they're moving away from, or other thoughts completely unrelated to the movement their body is doing.

With natural ability, when something looks as if it might interfere with our intended movement, we instinctively do something to avoid the interference. Because we can easily adjust our posture, we instantly change or stop the movement to avoid it and then proceed. We have no reason to doubt our ability, because it simply works when we want to use it. Our body stays in relaxed postural control, or easily moves back into it, in a perfectly coordinated balancing act on our feet, or foot. Our knees and feet remain flexible. Without fear, our mind remains clear to see and hear what's happening around us. We are constantly subconsciously and consciously anticipating. This provides us with many choices.

Living in their reactionary world, movement-impaired people with a restrictive posture have few choices. Their minds are perpetually busy with their bodies' movement issues, so they see and hear less. Their minds are anxious and/or fearful, which makes their bodies reactively guarded or stiffened. This leaves very little space for rational thought. In their world, their psychological and physical dilemmas leave little opportunity for choices. Of note, this issue does not only apply to people with a movement impairment stemming from a neurodegenerative disorder. Anyone who reacts to any situation with postural guarding or stiffening and is anxious or fearful about their movements will display the same behavior. Many examples of this are seen in the elderly population.

Making Sense of the Ball Drop

Remember, you won't gain the ability to make this transition in mind or body until you consistently feel stability, comfort, and trust in your movements. Only then will you be able to give yourself permission to release fears and intimidating anxiety, flex your knees and hips, and allow your mind to focus more on simply *playing* with the ball. When this begins to happen, the small amount of freedom you'll experience will feel like a very big thing. You must find and celebrate this feeling! Without it, you will not advance to gain the added freedom required for improving additional movement abilities.

Also, and very importantly, it doesn't matter what the game or activity is that you use while working on these basic things. It only matters that you *do* something. Work on and especially play at these things with an activity that makes sense to you.

In the ball bounce, become comfortable doing the exercise with one bounce of the ball and then catching it. Then practice letting the ball bounce twice before catching it, and then three times or more. Why? The extra bounces force you to flex your knees into a lower squat to be down where the lower bouncing ball will be. In the process, you'll be improving your relaxed postural control, and coordinated and anticipatory movements.

A tip: Regardless of how many times you let the ball bounce before catching it, the timing of when to lower into the squat is always the same. When the ball leaves your fingers, immediately squat to be in position for the catch. Down in the squat, pause, relax as the ball bounces up between your hands, and then catch it as it is starting to descend again.

Play the game as a child would. Play it just for the fun and challenge. Play the game to enjoy life with improving ability. To a child, the rest of the world stops when they immerse themselves in only that playful activity. Our adult minds frequently block our attempts to have fun, but having fun is so very important.

Like young children, the vast majority of you *do not require* someone to teach you how to walk, squat, or play with a bouncing ball. You already know these things extremely well. Never forget that you became a masterful expert in doing these things many, many long years ago. For most people, that part of you is not gone. Rather, it has merely been misplaced. So, what have you actually lost? The trust in your ability. Therefore, the help you need most is with how to reestablish your self-trust, and that requires first knowing how to stabilize your body on your feet, and then relaxing your body and mind to play. Keep it that simple. Honestly try over and over again to learn how to allow yourself to play again. It can be done.

DRIBBLING A BASKETBALL

This is another great teaching exercise that you'll progress to when the drop-and-catch exercise becomes easier.

- You must be *more* relaxed to dribble the ball than for the drop and catch.

- Do not overinflate the ball. Instead, use a slightly *under*inflated ball, because this requires you to stay in a lower squat. When underinflated, the ball won't rebound as high or as quickly. This forces an increased use of coordinated body movement with flexing knees and hips, while you hold stabilizing pressure in your feet. It also requires a better ability to transfer body weight between your feet as you move with flexing knees *with* the ball's movement.

- To hold the correct pressure in your feet and move your body where it needs to be to continue dribbling the ball, you must keep your upper body's position steady and in the proper coordinated reference to your hips and knees. This is working on *in*dependent and dependent upper- and lower-body control. Moving with the movement of the ball is done with the legs. Later you will also move your feet with the movements of the ball.

- Sometimes your focus will be on keeping your upper-body position stable, and other times it will be on keeping your knees flexed. But always keep a focus on holding the increased pressure in the ball areas of your stabilized feet.

- Dribbling a basketball teaches you how to stay down in a squat, with your knees, hips, and ankles shifting your body to stay in alignment with the ball. This is the *in*dependent control and function of the lower body.

- Hips, legs, and knees functioning properly allow the upper body to relax in the activity. The relaxing upper body then can be where it needs to be. This describes the dependent control and functioning of the upper and lower body.

- *The dependent control of the upper and the lower body is simply the cooperation and proper functioning of the entire body working together as one unit, while both are independently doing separate movements to enable the activity to continue.*

When the Ball—Meaning You—Won't Cooperate

Some of you were once upon a time basketball dribbling stars on the courts, but now it is difficult to do. You can't stay down in a squat. Your arm stiffens. You slap the ball and are lucky if you dribble it more than three times before it bounces away. Learn to stop much of this frustration by reminding yourself how you once did it so well. Think back to what your posture was when you had this ability. See and feel it in your memory, to help you remember what you need to be doing now. Use your experiences and memories as a valuable tool.

In her college days, Lynn was a starter on the basketball team. But today, dribbling the same ball with her moderate movement impairment is very frustrating (Figure 19.4). During a working session, Lynn said, "I think there must be some sort of disconnect between my mind and my hand." This was Lynn

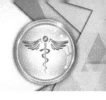

saying, in effect, "My dribbling problem is due to and controlled by my disorder." To a *small* degree, I must agree with her. Her disorder is a *contributing* factor. However, with all certainty, I can also assure you that her disorder is *not* the primary cause of her dribbling difficulties.

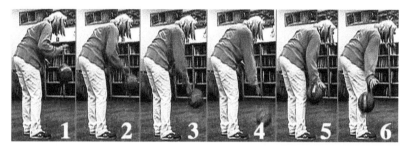

FIGURE 19.4: Lynn is forcing the movement with stiffened knees, elbow, wrist, hand, and fingers. If she were to relax, much of her past ability would still be with her today.

In practical terms of ability and function, Lynn's primary problem here is her inability to release the guarding stiffness from her arms and legs. When you study the pictures, some of this may not be overtly obvious to you. So, I will relay to you what I observed.

Lynn is doing at least three things incorrectly with her arm.

1. She flexes her elbow upward and then rapidly extends it downward to push the ball to the floor, without flexing the wrist. This forces her to push her arm farther downward using her shoulder (pictures 1 through 4), and then the shoulder stays down.

2. The muscles in her arm are tense, which prevents her from using her wrist appropriately. This became apparent as she rigidly opened her hand and fingers.

3. As the ball bounces back up, she attempts to use the palm of her stiff open hand to forcibly push it back toward the floor.

Even with the limitations her disorder causes, Lynn could be doing much better. For example, her arm stiffness and the force of the pushing pressure coming from her shoulder restrict and delay her ability to retract her hand upward using her elbow. Thus, she only minimally flexes her elbow before the ball bounces back up (picture 5). This is not the fault of the disorder.

She could be doing better if she would do just one thing differently. She needs to relax enough to squat, but she continually resists flexing her knees. If she would work on and play at doing only that, then she would likely also gain improving ability to use her elbow and wrist to bring her hand up after pushing the ball down. What is an easy exercise she could use to make flexing her knees and squatting easier? Dropping and catching the ball in a squat. And sitting: going back and working on Chapter 11.

If Lynn would squat with the same stability she presently has, she would have a much better setup to relax into for this dribbling exercise. If she would squat, she wouldn't be interfering with the movement of the ball as much as she is in picture 5, where the ball hits the palm of her stiffly held hand and bounces away. Her knees and elbow would be more relaxed.

The truth: There is no disconnect between her mind and her hand. Honestly, *the opposite is true.* She has *too much* connection between her thinking mind and the movement. This is forcing overcontrol within

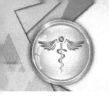

stiffening, and is the primary cause of her dribbling frustration. She knows this dribbling movement extremely well and is physically able to do it. Still, her controlling mind and postural stiffening won't let her use that ability.

There are some good points in what Lynn is doing in this example. The good is that even though her shoulder starts high and then ends relatively low, she coordinates the movement of her upper body to stay on stabilized feet. But she is not on flat feet, meaning her potential ability is more than what is seen. The negative side of this coordination is that she is stooping forward with stiffened knees instead of squatting with relaxing knees, and both of these issues restrict movements.

What else is going on here that supports the claim that Lynn has the ability to be doing better? This good overall postural control shows that she *is* fairly relaxed in other parts of her body. This indicates that she has more ability than she realizes, and is blocking herself from feeling or recognizing it. Many people have this very same issue and blame the disorder to avoid responsibility. It is the baited trap within the doctrine that the disorder is responsible for and controls all these issues. *No!* It does not.

If you're experiencing difficulties with using a basketball for dribbling, try using a larger, relatively heavy and very bouncy ball like the one in Figure 19.5. With it, you won't need to squat as low, and standing in a higher ready stance may make it easier to relax. A big bouncy ball will do much of the work for you, *provided* you are relaxed enough. *And* you still must do the exact same relaxed movements with your elbow, wrist, and fingers.

If you don't have a big bouncy ball, try slightly overinflating your basketball or school-yard ball, and bounce it slower while you're in a higher ready stance. Everything about the movement is always the

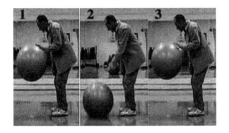

FIGURE 19.5: Whether the ball is big, little, or very bouncy, the wrist and finger movements to dribble it are the same.

same, so find the ball and stance that work for you. Then, as you improve, increase the challenge by removing some of the air from the ball.

But be careful! It's easy to make a mistake with uncontrolled shoulder movement, especially backward movement that can lead to a backward tipping fall, when you are in a more upright posture.

Stoopers

Like Lynn, Howard has a degenerative neurological disorder with a movement impairment that is moderate. How would you rate his technique and dribbling abilities in Figure 19.6? He is doing very well in this example, even though his knees are also stiffened and not flexing very much. He is demonstrating good flexibility with his elbow, wrist, and fingers. So, despite the problems his disorder causes him, Howard still can control and dribble the ball.

There is something else to be noted in these pictures that is quite significant. Most people with a moderate movement impairment and a degenerative neurological disorder don't have the muscle definition in their lower legs that you see in Howard's leg (yellow arrows). So, why is it that his legs have that much muscle definition? The answer is highlighted in the pictures. What is his posture? That gives you the answer.

1. He is stooping. His shoulders, head, and arm are forward with a bit more body weight toward the front of his feet than his bottom sticking out to the back is adding to his heels. This is tipping him slightly forward from the ball areas and toes of his feet.

2. He is stable in this stooping posture because he is using the muscles in his calves to push a strong downward force into the ball areas of his feet. This keeps him from tipping forward, but the stability he's gained comes at a high price. The same is true for Lynn in Figure 19.4.

3. The high price is, the forward stoop puts back pressure on the knees, while the tightened lower-leg muscles add to the stiffening process of the knees and feet. In this setup, Howard and Lynn are only relatively stable. Holding their calf muscles tight to remain in this posture forces them to work much harder than they need to.

    This situation explains why their movements are rather abrupt and forced much of the time. To begin a movement, they typically start with upper-body movement. This initiates the forward tipping and the overuse of the calf muscles, and is a difficult bad habit to undo. It is well ingrained in nearly everything they do. For many, this is a huge negative factor that makes it very difficult for them to relax in advancing or forward movements.

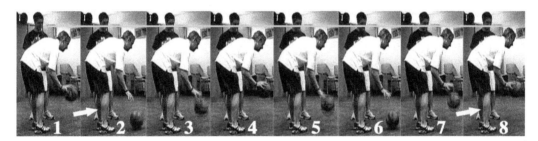

FIGURE 19.6: Howard dribbles the ball well with partial relaxation of his elbow, wrist, and hand, but needs to continue working on relaxing and flexing his knees more. Flexing the knees is challenging and sometimes difficult for those who have long had a habit of stooping forward from the hips.

When they're standing upright and stable *without* a forward lean or stoop, that is about the only time they relax their posture and calf muscles. This is also when their posture appears to be close to the same as that of anyone with natural ability.

Relaxed versus Guarded Stability, and Your Feet

On any given day, John often struggles with his movements. Sometimes he feels awkward and clumsy, and sometimes his movements feel okay. He is bewildered and frustrated, asking, "What happens? My walking feels normal one minute, and then I'm tripping and clumsy the next." Actually, the basic answer to his question is straightforward. Simply put, John becomes unstable when he is not controlling the pressure in his feet.

When our foundation (feet) is unstable, the rest of us is unstable. When we feel unstable on our feet, our natural tendency is to guard against that instability, correct it, and then resume the movement with

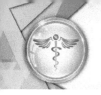

relaxing stability. However, when we don't correct the instability, the postural guarding reaction remains. Then the movement becomes challenging, and typically instability increases.

The good part of what John was explaining was, he was able to make the necessary postural corrections to fend off the instability. The unfortunate part was, he was unaware of what those corrections were. The very important message here is the following. When he learns what causes his instability and how he can correct it, then he will be able to prevent the instability from happening as often, and make quicker corrections when it does. Still, there is one more benefit he'll gain. Understanding the problem and the correction, he won't be as concerned and anxious about it. Those without these types of problems may not fully comprehend how much of an impact this has on a movement-impaired person's daily life.

After discussing the inciting problem and the corrections he needs to understand, I said, "John, you told me that you were good at playing basketball when you were younger. I would like you to tap into that ability today. Take this ball and show me how *you* dribble it."

"But I haven't done that for a long time," he responded while holding and looking at the ball like a long-lost friend.

"Okay," I said. "So, you might be a little rusty at it, but I'll wager that you haven't forgotten how to do it. Show me how the younger John used to dribble that ball."

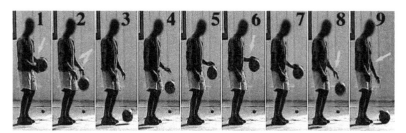

FIGURE 19.7: The ease of dribbling a ball comes from the relaxed action of the elbow, wrist, and fingers. The elbow extends and the wrist and fingers flex to push the ball down to the floor. As the ball bounces up, the elbow flexes to lift the hand up to meet the ball when it reaches the highest point, as the wrist and fingers extend upward to prepare to push the ball downward.

He thought about it for a few seconds, then adjusted his posture and began (Figure 19.7). His old ability had not faded away. His dribbling was easy and flawless. Without thinking about the "why" or "how" of it, he stabilized his posture and feet, assumed the proper stance, and relaxed into something quite familiar in a not-so-distant memory. With natural ability, he dribbled the ball using a very relaxed elbow, wrist, and hand. With them, from his fingertips he pushed the ball down to the floor. Then he flexed the elbow up in sync with the motion of the rebounding ball, put his relaxed hand and fingers on the ball as it reached the highest point of its return, and then repeated the same process many times.

John was stable and relaxed within his memory of the feeling of how he dribbled the ball. This is what Lynn did not do. John, Howard, and Lynn were all stable on their feet the entire time they handled the ball, but only John had relaxed postural control and true stability. Lynn and Howard had guarded postural control with only partial stability.

In picture 1, John relaxes into a flat-footed ready stance, then flexes his knees a slight amount (pictures 2 and 3), shifts slightly to the ball areas of his feet (picture 4), and further relaxes into dribbling the ball.

John used a high ready-stance posture. Being relaxed and comfortable, he had unrestricted movement ability and choices. Lynn and Howard used a guarded stooping posture. This forced the use of tightened

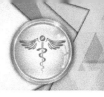

calf muscles to stop the forward tipping movement. Because of this, their movement choices were very limited by restricted movement ability.

How does any of this address John's "why" question? He is in the early stages of his degenerative disorder and, for the most part, maintains good postural control in his movements. But when he unknowingly makes a small postural mistake, his walking movement changes markedly. These are subtle mistakes, but enough to cause bigger changes to the location of the pressure in each foot, and that unexpectedly alters the movement.

Brian was developing issues of stumbling on his feet, but I was having him practice dribbling a basketball. What's the connection? It is actually a direct connection.

He was having difficulty focusing on and feeling the pushing pressure in the ball area and toes of his foot with each walking stride. So, I changed to something he understood and could easily relate to, to better illustrate what I was explaining to him about his foot.

The movement and function of the hand and fingers when we're dribbling a basketball are similar to the movement and function of the foot on the floor as we walk. So, while John was very relaxed and not thinking about how to dribble the ball, I asked him to feel how his hand was moving and what he felt in his hand and fingers when he pushed the ball to the floor.

"The end of my hand goes down," he said, "and I feel more pressure in my fingers as I push the ball toward the floor."

Bingo! That's what your foot is doing on the floor as you walk. Your foot flexes as increased pressure is pushed into the ball area of your foot, and, at the same time, more pressure is going into your toes. Your hand is tilting down in the air, and your foot would be too if it were in the air. But it is on the hard floor. So, instead of the front tilting down as the pressure increases in the front of the foot, the back (the heel) is lifted up to enable the pressure in the front of your foot and toes to be pushed backward at an angle against the hard floor. This is the work of the functional flatness, or functional angle, in the foot we were talking about. Now the job is to focus on feeling and understanding what's happening in your hand, and then apply that same focus to your feet as you walk.

For example, when you don't push the ball down to the floor hard enough, what happens? The weak push causes the ball to be low when it bounces back off the floor. That same type of effect happens in your foot when you stumble. When the push into the floor from one foot is weak, the advancing foot comes down on the floor quicker than it was supposed to, and scuffs on the floor. That is what causes you to stumble. So, how do you stop it from happening? Push better from each foot in each stride. (This topic will be discussed in more detail in later chapters.)

Wrist Flexibility

Dribbling a ball is *not* a different or unusual movement. It calls for the same elbow, wrist, hand, and finger movements that we use in many of the things we do every day. Prove it to yourself. Wave your hand to fan your face, toss a wad of paper into the trash, swat at a fly, comb your hair, prepare food, or gesture with your hands while you speak or exercise. The same muscles and joints repeatedly do the same natural functions in the same patterned movements, per their design. So again, the movements are the same. Only the activity we are involved in, and the sequence and/or the extent of the individual movements during the activity, appear to be different to our eyes and mind.

In Figure 19.8, two women are throwing foam balls to each other. When she is standing using her walker, Cyndi, in the right panel, has a moderate movement impairment. In the left panel, Gay's movement impairment is significant when she is standing with her walker. But when both are seated, *provided they use their legs to stabilize* their bodies, many of their postural instability issues are not so apparent. Having recently relearned how to use their legs to stabilize when sitting, they now have a more relaxed posture that allows them to throw the ball. In this activity, they are playing to learn how to relax their elbows, wrists, hands, and fingers. Because of their instability when standing, this activity is very difficult or nearly impossible for them to learn in that position.

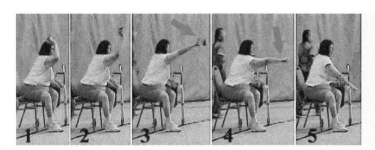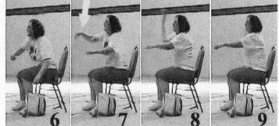

FIGURE 19.8: Sitting comfortably in chairs, Gay and Cyndi practice relaxing their wrists and elbows to throw the foam ball.

Seated in the security of the chairs and using their feet and legs to keep themselves that way, they can relax. Then, through playfully throwing foam balls to each other, they are able to divert their attention away from the chore of the movement exercise and simply allow it to happen. In this fun activity, they provide their own feedback through what they see and feel.

In many activities, a stiffened wrist considerably limits the hand's usefulness. For example, before I swing a golf club to hit the ball, I direct a final focus toward relaxing enough to have very loose, flexible wrists, which is the opposite of what many good golfers advise. So why do I want loose and flexible wrists? It's because with my mild movement impairment, my wrists have some residual stiffness that a person with natural ability does not have. For my game, when I feel my wrists are floppy loose, I have relaxed them to an extent that's more like what the players with natural ability already have in their wrists.

The point: Each person must learn what their body is telling them by feeling what is happening. Seeing what they are doing on video or in a mirror is very helpful. With these disorders, it's common to have a degree of postural restriction that other people don't have. Each affected person needs to know and understand this factor, and everyone attempting to help them needs to recognize it as well.

Our disorder is what it is. Therefore, if we are to have a better life, we must learn to deal constructively with the issues that come with it. However, many people instead resign themselves to fighting a frustrating war in hopes of mediating the effects of their disorder, yet what they're actually doing is only talking about an attitude toward what they think the disorder is and what it's causing. They repeatedly fail to realize how they might physically learn to create some order within themselves, to ease much of their burden. While it might feel better to think you are being proactive in "fighting your disorder," it is useless to fight ourselves.

Importantly, our disorder is not a separate part of us. It is part of our body's order, and it is not going away. It is the order of our neurological system. Therefore, fighting the disorder is fighting and blinding yourself with frustration, anger, and bitterness. Let it go. Replace the fight with learning how to cooperate with yourself.

STANDING STABILITY

The concept of pushing stabilizing pressure into our feet for support and stability cannot be overemphasized. Emily has a mild movement impairment but stays relaxed in posture and mind in Figures 19.9 and 19.10. In the first example, she begins and stays in a ready stance as she shifts, turns, reaches, and catches.

In panel A of Figure 19.9, Emily's reaction to catching the ball is typical for a person with natural ability. She prepares by slightly lowering in her stance and then moves slightly up in her stance as she catches the ball. She keeps her knees flexed. She moves her shoulders forward and down to compensate correctly for the moving force of the ball.

The appropriate distance her shoulders shift forward for the catching movement can be seen in her alignment in the inserted zone of stability in pictures 1 and 4. Also note that in picture 4 she remains in a stable squatting posture with flattened feet (green arrow) and stands with increased pressure in the ball areas. She does very well with cooperative and counterbalanced relaxed postural control in this example.

In panel B, Emily is prepared to catch the ball coming toward her, but she doesn't expect it to bounce to her left. She responds with a very common restrictive-posture mistake. Comparing her position with that of the zone of stability in pictures 1 and 2, you can see that she reacts with a backward movement of her shoulders. This moves the pressure in her feet toward the heels and causes some straightening of her knees as her body is moving to the side. This is why the front of her right shoe is pointed up in pictures 2 and 3, and then the front of her left shoe points upward in picture 4 (red arrows).

Because the front of her foot is up off the floor, the zone of stability in picture 2 is only the small green area. The red area is the immediately lost area of the zone.

Not shown in this series of pictures is her recovery from this movement mistake. She quickly and correctly applied the necessary corrections of downward-flexing knees and forward shoulder movement, which is to say she squatted. She moved down in the stance to reestablish proper body alignment and stability in her feet.

With her mild movement impairment, this is possible because it is easier to remain relaxed. With a *moderate* movement impairment, this mistake often results in a nasty fall to the floor, even

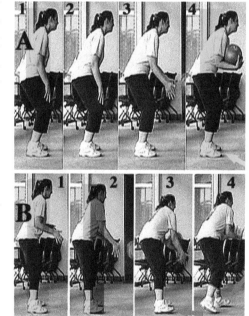

FIGURE 19.9: Panel A: Emily responds and pushes the correct stabilizing pressure into her feet. Panel B: Her backward-moving upper-body reaction shifts increased pressure into her heels.

when you know how to correct the error. This difference stems in very large part from the increased postural stiffness, anxiety, and fear that come with the mistake, and *typically the more movement-impaired person is in a more upright posture at the beginning of the movement.* These factors make the correction more difficult to apply.

Recognizing mistakes by feeling them and quickly applying the corrections is an important goal in improving your movement abilities. Learning how to reduce the limitations of the tightened muscles before the movement begins is the first part of this recognition and corrective process.

FEELING THE RIGHT AND WRONG

Gaining the ability to repeatedly correct many of your mistakes will do more to improve your attitude, movement abilities, and quality of life than anything else you could ever imagine. Having that ability is what "naturally normal" is all about. Normal is doing things without worry. Normal is knowing that when you make a mistake, you can correct it without shattering your world with another disappointment.

In Figure 19.10, Emily has another surprised reaction, this time to the ball bouncing unexpectedly high, over her right shoulder. Aside from her missing the ball, what else do you see in the series of pictures? Look closely at her response in the middle four pictures, in which she quickly turns her head and shoulders, whipping her ponytail to the side. Note that she remains stable with the pressure centered in the ball areas of her feet.

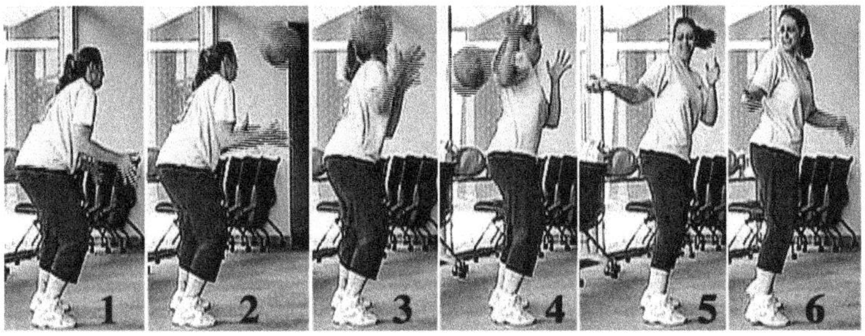

Question: What do you see happening that does not fit with what her neurodegenerative movement impairment is supposed to be restricting her from doing? Or, where is the evidence of her disorder in this example? Or, better yet, rather than looking for a person with a movement impairment having inability or disability, view these pictures with the expectation that they show a person with natural movement ability. Now, another question: Which one do you see?

FIGURE 19.10: There is nothing in these pictures that suggests Emily has a movement impairment, but she does. This is exactly what everyone with an impairment would love to be able to have again: freedom of movement. The ability to enjoy their life with stability and without fear. For many, this is an unrealized possibility. Only each individual person can change their reality. The "how" of it requires personal, dedicated effort and responsibility.

Confused? If you are, instead of focusing on looking for the mistakes Emily is making, focus on what she's doing correctly. Your perception of what you want to look for makes a difference, and *when you are the one living with an impairment, this makes a huge difference.*

Living the disorder makes it so very easy to overfocus on the mistakes, because we are constantly reminding ourselves of them. Through each mistake we feel and show, every day we're living the same drama of repeatedly being reminded of how bad we are, and of the terrible things to come.

The bad overshadows the good things that you still do, and quickly wilts the good away. The negatives are always highlighted. The positives are forever hidden beyond the glow of the negatives' spotlight. You must learn to stop this self-degrading, self-destructive process, because it only holds you prisoner in the darkness, causing you to revert to frustration and internal fighting. To escape from this prison,

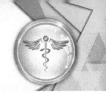

begin feeling, recognizing, and celebrating **all** the good things you do. Even the smallest ones! Don't let any of them pass unnoticed. Declare them to the world, dance, and celebrate the *"Yes, I can!"*

In these two examples, Emily's movements look and are as natural and normal as anyone's. You see a person moving with relaxed postural control, holding her foundation firm and steady, and having some fun. She makes a mistake, then immediately corrects it. She stays stable with coordinated, counterbalanced movement when standing high, looking for the ball over her right shoulder. Her response is naturally stabilizing, pushing extra pressure into her feet with strong legs while holding the pressure in the correct location with her posture.

These show what every movement-impaired person is hungry to have once again:

Free and easy movement ability.

Play, to learn to relax the stiffness from your body,
to calm and ease the fear from your mind,
to allow improving abilities
to come into the light.

It is extremely important to note that for a great many people, there can be a *reversal of the pattern of deteriorating function.* The multiple examples presented in this book highlight this. These examples are individual representations of the **reversal** of only the **indirect** effects the people unknowingly accumulated through years of living with their disorder. Seeing this pattern repeatedly, I am convinced that everyone has the potential to do better than they presently are. The question is, realistically how much can anyone improve. That is relative to each person and is dependent on pertinent factors. In the end this can only be proved by each person, as they do the required work.

■ ■ ■

CHAPTER 20

CREATING AND HOLDING THE PUSH

A person with a movement impairment does more things correctly than incorrectly.
But because of their slanted perception, the incorrect things they do dominate their thoughts.

tomping. This is the next coordinated movement that will help you recombine separate body movements into one flowing movement, Figure 20.1. Stomping involves transfer of body weight, pushing and holding stabilizing pressure into the feet, and flexing the knee and hip as your body lowers in the movement. This represents the natural progression in improving movement ability.

Many people dealing with restrictive postures very often complicate this movement. They do not get into the proper setup posture, and often inadvertently add guarding to their posture by trying too hard. Not using the proper setup frequently causes imbalance and potential falls. So, when you are not as relaxed and your knees are not flexing easily, begin by doing small and gentle stomps to focus on posture and transfer-of-weight issues. Then work up to more aggressive stomps when you are more relaxed with these basic elements.

STOMPING: THE ESSENTIALS

The basic stomping movement begins in a ready stance. Then, completely transfer your body weight to one foot and stomp with the other foot. But how far down in a ready stance do you need to be to begin the movement? And what about at the end of the movement? As always, it is according to what your mama (feet) is telling you. It depends on your ability and is defined by your stability. It depends on how relaxed you are. It depends on how hard you stomp and the positioning of your feet. Therefore, the only correct answer is, lower yourself into the posture that you need in order to feel comfortable and secure throughout the movement.

The next thing you must consider is the effect of the stomp. By this I am referring to your reaction to the forceful impact of the foot hitting the floor. This brings up a key point that will determine whether or not you remain stable.

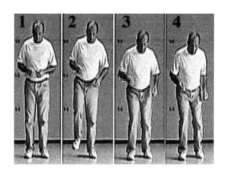

FIGURE 20.1: Stand balanced on one foot to then abruptly stomp down with the other foot. This is the combination of transfer of body weight with increased pressure pushing the foot forcefully down.

199

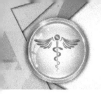
The two most frequent mistakes made when beginning the stomping exercise:

1. The *first mistake* a person with impaired movements and a restrictive-posture makes is failing to flex their knees enough to begin the movement properly.

   Then, when they do flex their knees to start the movement, their knees frequently *will not stay flexed* during the movement.

2. The *second mistake* a person with impaired movements and a restrictive-posture makes is failing to move their shoulders forward into the correct setup alignment.

   Then, when their shoulders do properly move forward to begin the movement, they *do not stay forward* to keep the posture that's required to continue the movement.

Anticipate these problems. Focus on relaxing and moving into the correct posture *before* the mistakes happen, and remind yourself to keep your shoulders forward during the movement.

1. Instead of moving their shoulders down and forward to coordinate the movement of the stomp, many will pull their shoulders up and back in an effort to lift the foot higher. Withdrawing the upper body backward and to the side moves pressure into the outside of the heel of the foot they're standing on and pushes them backward at an angle.

2. They have their shoulders forward when lifting the foot, but then will attempt to stomp down by quickly moving their shoulders up, often with limited movement of the knee. The result will be a weak non-stomp with the heel of the foot likely contacting the floor first. Striking down with the heel first is an excellent way for those with a restricted posture to push themselves backward, and they are already unstable with their shoulders back. Stomping the heel down creates an added backward push to an unrelaxed body.

3. While focusing on stomping the foot, many do *not* have a flexible knee. It may be slightly flexed, but it is not flexible. It is stiffened in anticipation of the exaggerated movement and the stomp.

   When we stomp, some of the force of the impact returns and travels back up the leg. A flexing knee absorbs the force and stops it from continuing into the body.

   When a person stomps down with a stiffened knee, much of the force of the stomped foot moves through the stiffened knee and continues up into the body. Typically, this causes the shoulders to move up and backward, and commonly pulls the knees straighter. This is another reason some have increased pressure in the heels of both feet during and after the stomp.

4. When you are not in the proper position and don't have the stability to hold the stomped foot down, that foot will bounce up from the floor when it has been forcefully stomped. How high the foot will bounce back up will vary with the amount of stiffness in the stomping leg and foot, the stomp's force and quickness, the weakness of the legs, and how much your posture is out of

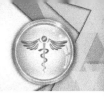

alignment for the movement. The flexibility of the floor's surface may also affect the foot's degree of rebound, but I am specifically referring to this happening when standing on a hard floor without any flexibility.

The foot bounces back up when you fail to hold the forced pressure down with a flexing knee and posture. With a restrictive posture, it happens most often when the knee is stiffened and you stop using the muscles in the leg immediately upon stomping the foot.

This "bouncing foot" happens more often for a person who uses their upper body to "help" with the stomping movement. The foot is also allowed to bounce when the body is not centered over the stomping foot in a squatting movement with the stomping knee.

The best way to circumvent these mistakes is to anticipate them and use some postural reminders to *avoid them.*

1. Remind yourself in the ready stance before the stomp, when you are still on both feet, to move your shoulders forward. Then do the transfer of body weight to one stabilized foot to be in the proper posture to make the stomp. And what else? You must be balanced on that foot.

2. Remind yourself *knees (both of them) down* before the stomp, when you are still on both feet, and keep them flexed and down during and especially after the stomp.

3. If you are having any of the problems described above, try keeping your head down with eyes looking at the floor where you want the KNEE to stomp the foot. This will often help you have your knees and shoulders in a better position.

Helpful Hints

Look down. Pick a spot and watch your foot stomp on that spot—*by controlling your stomping foot with the stomping knee.*

1. Start the movement by shifting onto and standing balanced momentarily over a flattened foot.

2. Keep your eyes down to help keep your shoulders forward, to push harder into the foot you're standing on and more easily lift the other knee. The proper postural alignment improves your chances of having the stomping foot flat when it hits the floor.

3. How high should you raise your knee to stomp the foot? You decide. Your comfort in your abilities will tell you how much without the need to think about it. Most importantly, the stability in the foot you are standing on to make the stomp determines this.

4. To *stomp your flat foot* on the floor, quickly push the lifted knee down with extra force. YES! Focus on stomping with the knee and avoid focusing directly on the foot.

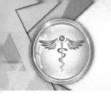
Stomping one foot down on the floor *is not* the completed movement. The completion of the movement is continuing to hold the push down into the foot after the stomp with a flexing knee and posture, having most of your body weight centered in that foot, and stabilizing your body with both pressurized *FEET*.

Hold the pressure of the stomp as if you are trying to forcefully push the foot down through the floor. This is to ensure a nearly complete transfer of body weight onto that foot and to stabilize your body. Move the flexing knee forward and your body downward to help center your body over the flat foot and hold the pressure. And because the movement uses both feet, continue to hold the increased pressure in *both* feet.

Be very careful with this. Not holding the pressure in both feet is something many people with a movement impairment have become very lazy with. This is another reason why many movement-impaired people need to begin with small stomping movements. They need time to play with and feel what is happening, while being aware and very careful of stiffening postural issues and how they are using their legs.

Holding on to something for support will be very helpful for those with stability problems.

Stiffness

In Figure 20.2, Mike does a stomping movement with an unchanging, stiffened upright posture. He achieves a good weight transfer onto his left foot to begin the movement and flexes his right knee upward in pictures 2 and 3. But in pictures 4 through 6, he does not transfer weight off his left foot to his right foot. Note that he's holding his arms in place and is making fists with both hands. These are all signs that he is doing the movement with stiffened postural control.

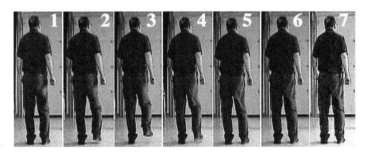

FIGURE 20.2: Mike holds his arms stiffly in place, stays standing upright, straightens his right knee with the stomp instead of flexing downward, and does not shift his body over the stomping foot. This is a common example when the posture is guarded or stiffened.

Mike's posture does not change from start to finish. Yes, he is doing a good job of maintaining his posture, but *that is the problem*. He should be flexing downward into the stomping movement with his upper body, hips, and knees in pictures 4 through 6, as previously described.

His left knee starts stiff and straight and stays that way throughout the movement. This holds him upright. He remains shifted toward the left as he stomps. With the left knee straightened, the only way he can get his right foot down to the floor is by also straightening his right knee. This is a very common problem in people with a moderate movement impairment.

Now, to another point about Mike's stomping. With the information you have, where would you say the increased pressure in his right stomping foot is located, and how much pressure is he pushing into that foot?

1. He is stomping down onto the inside of the heel, and some of the force of it is coming back up through the straightened right knee and into his body. This is pushing him farther back in his stance and

adding instability. This is another reason why he is unable to shift toward his right foot and lower into the stance with his knees.

2. This is also the reason he cannot stomp with too much force. A more forceful stomp would push him into greater instability. In this example, there actually was not a stomp. Mike did do a quicker downward movement with his right knee, but the foot just barely reached the floor to make a rather soft noise.

Right and Wrong

Compare Mike's stomping posture with Ken's in Figure 20.3. With a mildly guarded posture, Ken can flex downward with knees and hips. With a moderate amount of stiffness in his restrictive posture, Mike doesn't. Both do a good transfer to begin the stomp, but Mike cannot shift his upright posture off the supporting foot and onto the stomping foot. Ken begins with and stays in a flexing posture. This allows him to shift his body onto the stomping foot.

Mike's non-stomp consists of extending his right knee to lower the foot to the floor. Ken's stomp is forceful because it is created by flexing joints, working muscles, and a coordinated downward movement of the body, with a good transfer of body weight to the stomping foot. Therefore, these compared movements are physically quite the opposite. Ken directs the force and intent of his stomp downward. Mike's intent is downward, but the force of his stomp is weak and becomes misdirected as the non-stomping foot rebounds upward from the floor.

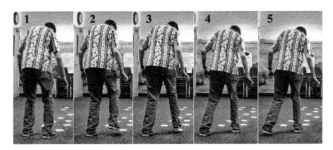

FIGURE 20.3: Mildly guarding posture. Stomping with flexing knees and hips to stay down in the movement. Transferring body weight to the stomping foot, and then holding pressure in both feet to complete the movement.

Foot Placement

Many people with impaired movements and a restrictive-posture will likely experience a problem with how and where the stomping foot comes down on the floor.

1. The *how* refers to which part of the foot contacts the floor first. Sometimes it will be the heel, the ball area, or the inside or outside of the foot, and sometimes it will be a flat foot.

2. The *where* refers to the direction the foot is moving as it is stomped. For example, when you see a spot on the floor where you want to stomp your foot, many times you will have difficulty delivering your foot to that spot.

The objective is to stomp onto a flat foot. What posture do you need to be in to make that happen? You should be using the same starting posture you used when doing the sideward

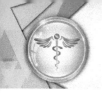

transfer-of-body-weight movements, and adding an exaggerated downward flexing knee over the flattened stomping foot. The stomp is the very same movement you've been practicing, but is much more aggressive.

One way to remain relaxed, and keep the movement smaller and better controlled, is to limit how high you lift the knee. This also helps you limit the amount of coordinated counterbalancing of the body that is needed to balance on the supporting foot. Start by lifting the knee a small amount while practicing flexing the knee downward to stomp the foot lightly, with a small weight shift. As these skills improve, then work into lifting the knee higher and stomping more forcefully with increasing knee flexibility.

Another way to make the movement smaller is to have your knees and feet *comfortably* close together in your setup posture. Your feet should be approximately one shoulder width apart or less. Remember, the sideward shift of your body for weight transfers will be less with your feet closer together. Also remember that you will need to increase the push down into both feet to remain stable. Why? As your feet come closer together, the self-stabilizing pressure on the insides of the feet decreases.

From a stable setup, shift completely onto one foot, and the lifting knee will begin to lift the foot. *The knee lifts the foot, and the knee stomps the foot down.* Stomp downward with the knee, but always realize that the stomping foot is your secondary focus in the movement. So, what is the primary focus?

Your primary focus is on the supporting foot you balance on in the beginning of the movement.

Hearing What You Feel

When your foot hits the floor, what do you feel and what is the sound you hear? As you become comfortable with more aggressive stomping, start listening closely to the sound your foot makes when it hits the floor. Pay close attention to *the changing sound and feeling*, because the different sounds and feelings are coming from the different parts of the foot hitting the floor first. These two things tell you a great deal about what you did or did not do.

For example, what sound does the ball area of your foot make when it is first to hit the floor? How is that sound different from the sound the stomping heel makes? When your flat foot stomps down on the floor, what do you feel and hear? All of them are different. Also, listen carefully as you watch someone stomping onto different areas of their foot to help you understand the sounds and the movement.

Small changes you make in your posture will cause the foot to come down onto the floor differently.

1. Shoulders too far forward, or holding the front of the foot down using calf muscles, causes the ball area to hit first.

2. Shoulders too far back, or holding the front of the foot up, causes the heel to hit first.

3. When the foot hits the floor, a flat foot happens when the shoulder, the knee, and the stomping foot's toe are vertically aligned—provided the muscles controlling the foot are relaxed.

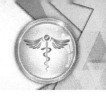

4. Knees and hips not flexing enough changes how the foot is delivered to the floor.

The sound and feeling of the foot hitting the floor tell you what the rest of your body is doing. Pay attention, and stop scolding the innocent foot for a problem it is not creating. The changing sound and feeling of the foot landing incorrectly on the floor are symptoms of a problem with your posture and stability.

Fidgety Feet; Postural Instability

Many people with impaired movements typically use a weaker push of pressure into their feet during movement, and they often prematurely release the pushing pressure. Both issues cause instability. A fidgety foot is a foot that moves without purpose on the floor. When you see it happening, this is telling you something very important. That fidgety foot is providing limited support.

In the following example, Figure 20.4, Camron has a fidgety right foot, and then a fidgety left foot. In pictures 1 and 2, he stomps his right foot on the floor, but then releases much of the stomping pressure. This allows the front of his right foot to move in picture 3, and then he reapplies pressure back into it (picture 4). The shift of the front of the right shoe is small, but is visible when comparing the black tip of the shoe to the black line on the floor. Also, compared to pictures 2 and 4, slightly more of the right foot is seen in picture 3. The angle of the heel to the line has changed. This takes a keen eye to see the changes.

In picture 5, Camron releases pressure from

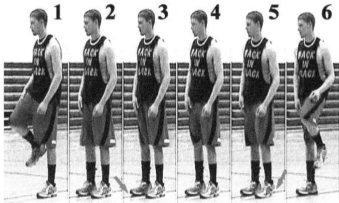

Tip of right shoe in 3 moved outward, then returned in 4.   Left heel in 5 moved inward.

FIGURE 20.4: Camron stomps his right foot, releases some of the pressure, moves the front of it, and then reapplies pressure. In preparation to stomp down with his left foot, he moves the left heel inward and then transfers to his right foot, to lift his left knee.

his left foot, then moves the heel of it inward before he transfers body weight over to his right foot, to lift his left knee. To see this, compare the space between his legs in pictures 4 and 5, and also compare the position of his left heel with the black line on the floor. Note that the space between his legs is smaller in picture 5 than in picture 4.

This raises two questions. Was it necessary for him to readjust either foot, and where was the pressure located in each foot when a portion of that foot moved?

1. The only possible way a part of a foot can move on the floor is when it has little or no pressure holding it down.

2. Look at Camron's knees. Before and after the stomp, they are straight.

3. An unexpected brief pressure force from the stomp on the heel area came back up the leg through his straightened knee. This caused mild instability and forced him to momentarily relax downward pressure from his legs to reposition and stabilize.

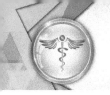
4. The heel movement in picture 5 is a continuation of his restabilization efforts, and tells you he had moved his upper body slightly forward. This moved increased pressure into the ball area of the foot, freeing the heel to be moved. The front of the foot moved in picture 3 because pressure was removed from the front of the foot and moved to the heel. The lack of pressure to hold it in place allowed it to move.

Fidgety feet lead to "**bouncing feet**," another common issue many movement-impaired people with a restrictive posture have when beginning these stomping exercises. To understand the concept of bouncing feet, think of a ball bouncing on the floor.

When stomped, the foot rebounds off the floor when the downward push is not continued. In fact, many people with a restrictive posture immediately release the downward force just before or as the foot hits the floor. This tends to happen more often when there is increased heel pressure and their posture is more upright and *stiffened*. In addition, because this created increased instability will not allow them too hold the downward pressure, they have learned to be timid or stop the downward push in an attempt to lessen the expected instability. Therefore, as they begin to improve in postural control and movement ability, they must also learn to resolve their anxiety and fears.

Bouncing feet can also happen when the foot is flat as it contacts the floor. As an example, I have seen the stomping foot rebound up from the floor much like a rubber ball, in various amounts up to approximately twelve inches. The person either is too unstable to hold the foot down, has forgotten how to hold the push to keep the foot down, and/or subconsciously jerks the knee up sharply once the foot hits the floor. The bouncing foot happens when the person is being aggressive and is unprepared to control it.

The bouncing foot often confuses the person and commonly leads to abrupt postural reactions, increased stiffness, instability, and fear. People with this problem typically have difficulty flexing their knees or don't flex them at all. This means they require constant reminders to relax their elbows and knees and make the supporting foot stable. Then, to improve their ability to hold the downward pushing pressure in the stomping foot, they need to be slowly coached into developing a more relaxed posture and a much smaller stomp. They also need to be coached to exaggerate their flexing and squatting posture.

Creating and Holding the Stabilized Push

When standing centered over both flattened feet and then squatting straight down (pictures 1 and 2 of Figure 20.5), the relaxed body remains centered over both feet. In this squatting movement, the pressure in both feet increases exactly the same amount.

When squatting in a sideward or forward stride movement, because the body has shifted toward one foot, the pressure going into that foot is greater than that in the foot the body has moved away from (pictures 3 and 4 of Figure 20.5). Very importantly, though, the foot the body has moved away from is still being used to partially support the body. It is

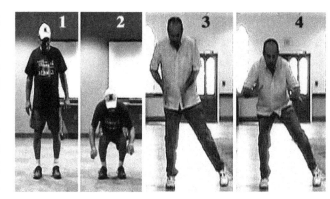

FIGURE 20.5: As our body shifts, the applied pressure in the feet changes. In pictures 1 and 2, the pressure increases in both feet and remains equally divided. In pictures 3 and 4, the pressure increases in both feet but is not equally divided.

also functioning as an anchor to hold and stabilize the body over the other foot. This foot has less pressure in it, but is vitally important to the body's movement and stability.

1. In picture 1, the pressure is equally divided in Chuck's feet. Each foot supports 50 percent of his body weight.

2. In picture 2, because his body remains centered over them, the pressure increases equally in both feet.

3. In picture 3, my body is offset to the right. Therefore, the pressure in my right foot is greater than the pressure in my left foot. For reference purposes, assume 75 percent of my body weight is supported by my right foot in this instance, and 25 percent by my left.

4. In picture 4, the pressure in both feet increases during the squat, and *proportionately* it increases by the same relative amount in each foot. Therefore, the pressure pushing into my right foot remains at 75 percent of the total, while my left foot has 25 percent of the increased pressure.

5. The left foot in pictures 3 and 4 has great purpose. It pushed me onto the right foot, and then it functions as the "anchoring" foot. It powers and controls the movement, and continues to provide a great deal of the body's support and stability at the movement's completion.

6. *Without it, you would be balancing and squatting on one foot.*

■ ■ ■

CHAPTER 21

FIFTH STANCE:
BEGINNING FORWARD MOVEMENT

Frequently, our movement problems are the direct result of failed preparation.

With natural ability, Lucas easily takes a forward stride in Figure 21.1. But for many people with impaired movements and a tensed posture, this movement is much more difficult than expected. The reason? The orientation of the foot during the movement.

During sideward movements, the toes point forward while our body moves to the side. In forward movements, the toes point forward as our body also moves forward.

Forward movements are more complicated because they require improved cooperation, coordination, relaxation, and functioning of, and between, the upper and lower body. Forward movements are more difficult because they bring out some of the biggest fears, worst postural guarding and stiffening, and greatest instabilities that movement-impaired people encounter.

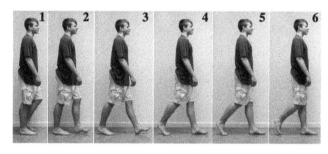

FIGURE 21.1: Forward stride. Pushing the body forward from the ball area and toes of the flexing right foot.

For example,

1. When moving to the side, the pushing pressure in the pushing foot is fixed within the length of the foot. During sideward movement, the increasing pressure moves through the width of the advanced foot, moving from the inside of the foot toward the center.

2. In forward movements, the pushing pressure in the pushing foot is fixed within the width of the foot. During forward movement, the pressure moving into and through the advanced foot does so through the length of it, beginning in the heel area and moving to the ball area and toes.

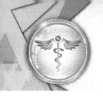

In all our natural movements, our feet always *function* in the same way, because *that is the only way they work*. During a forward stride, the increased (pushing) pressure moves forward through the advanced foot and into the forward portion of the ball area and the toes. This pressure pushes the toes against the floor, and they begin to extend (bend upward) as the heel of the foot is pulled upward. This action of the foot is not peculiar to only forward movement. This same action occurs within the pushing foot when we move to the side, forward, or backward, and for the same reason.

Therefore, since the foot works the same during various directions of body movement, what causes the directional change of the body? *To move our body in a different direction, the concentrated pushing pressure in the ball area and toes is directed into a different direction.*

MOVEMENT, PRESSURE, AND ORIENTATION OF THE FOOT

Moving onto the advanced foot:

1. In **natural sideward** movement, the pressure travels across the foot from side to side, a short distance.

2. In **natural forward** movement, the pressure travels through the length of the foot from the heel area to the toes, a relatively long distance.

3. In **natural backward** movement, the pressure remains in the ball area and toes of the foot. It then only moves from the ball area and toes toward the heel when the movement of the body is stopping or stopped.

4. In **limited natural sideward** movement, control of the movement and the pressure moving through the foot can be maintained with limited flexing of the foot. Thus, a sideward movement can be done well with guarded feet, and fairly well with stiffened feet.

5. However, in **limited natural forward** movement, to maintain control of the movement of the body and the pressure moving through the foot, some *flexing of both feet is required.*

   For this reason, when the feet are guarded and not easily flexible, forward movements are challenging, with sluggish and often erratic body movements, and the strides are shorter.

   When the foot is stiffened and inflexible, forward movement is very problematic because essentially there is no stride being created. Instead, the advancing foot is pushed slightly forward in a shuffling, flat-footed skidding movement, unless compensatory movements are made, like lifting the hip abnormally, to enable the foot to clear the floor.

A **natural forward stride** requires an easily flexible foot, to allow the free and continuous movement of the pressure through the length of the foot. In a forward stride, the first point of contact the advancing foot makes with the floor is the narrow heel area. With a steady pushing force from the pushing foot, the body continues moving forward, and the body movement transfers the pressure into the entire surface of the foot, and then into the ball area and toes. At this point in the body's continuing movement, the advanced foot becomes the new pushing foot.

As the pressure moves from the heel to the ball area and toes, it also increases. When the advancing foot's heel makes initial contact with the floor, it does so with a very light pressure. At the moment the heel makes contact with the floor, that contact pressure is **not** an increased pressure, because at this point in the stride, the heel **is not** functioning to support and stabilize the body, **or** the movement. It is very important that the pressure in the heel remain light and passive, as this allows the pushing foot to continue the uninterrupted forward push of the body, to continue moving the pressure forward in the advanced foot without interruption.

There is a common misconception that when the heel of the advanced foot contacts the floor in a natural stride, we push into it for support. This is absolutely *false*. If anything happens to change the continuous flow of increasing pressure through the foot, the movement of the body also changes. For example, if the pressure in the heel is increased when it contacts the floor, the pressure's forward movement in the foot will either slow or stop. This will slow, stop, or otherwise alter the body's movement.

You can easily see the proof that the heel pressure in the advanced foot remains light by watching people with natural ability walk. How? Their body movement is smoothly continuous. For proof of the effect of increased heel pressure, observe the interrupted body movement of those with restrictive-posture movement impairments. You can hear the contrast as well, in the loud heel strikes of those who walk with jarring movements owing to the increased pressure in their heels.

In continuous forward walking strides, as the advancing heel contacts the floor, the ball area and toes of the pushing foot continue to fully support the body. Very importantly, the transfer of body weight (pressure) into the forward foot does not begin until the light pressure moves forward into the remainder of the foot, as it flattens on the floor.

When walking forward with repeating natural strides, our body moves forward at a constant rate. This happens because our feet are flexing in the same direction the body is moving, and the push from them is continuous.

In addition, the movement of the pressure through the advanced foot and the flexing of the pushing foot are directly proportional to the movement of the body.

The smoothness of our natural walk happens because
*the movement of the body is **precisely synchronized** with the flexing action of both feet.*

However, in **natural sideward and backward movements**, because the feet are not flexing in the direction of the movement, the movement of the body is commonly *not continuous*. Instead, the body's movement is an interrupted, stop-and-go-type movement, unless we intentionally do something to modify the movement within our feet. An example would be crossing one leg over the other to move an advancing foot into position to continue the sideward movement without interruption.

Natural, Relaxed

When the movement of the body is continuous and smooth, the combined movement of the flexing feet and of the pressure in the pushing foot is also continuous and smooth. In a natural, easy, and effortless walk, all three are perfectly matched and precisely synchronized. In this perfectly matched arrangement, the transfer of pressure from the pushing foot to the advanced foot is a process in which the pushing foot does not stop pushing until the advanced foot takes over.

This brings up a complex issue. When the forward-moving pressure in the advanced foot moves into the ball area and toes, as that foot becomes the pushing foot, the movement of the pressure quickly slows, and then stops. However, the forward movement of the body doesn't change. How does this happen when the synchronization of the movement of the body and the movement of the pressure in the foot no longer exists?

The body's movement is not altered because the heel of the foot is pulled upward as the toes bend, as the concentrated pressure pushes the toes against the floor, and this action of the foot continues to push the body. The working muscles in the calf of the leg are responsible for this. As they contract, the pushing pressure increases and concentrates in the forward ball area and toes of the foot. This is required to stabilize and firmly hold the front of the foot in place, and that enables the upward-moving heel of the flexing foot to continue to push the body through the movement. As the foot flexes at the toes and the heel rises, length is added to the leg. Thus, it is the lifting heel that continues to push the body forward through the remainder of the stride when the pushing pressure stops moving forward in the foot.

Comparison: Location of the Pressure in the Advanced Foot

The following discussions in this section refer to taking one single stride forward, and stopping on a flattened advanced foot.

Naturally Relaxed Posture

In *relaxed* **forward** movements, we push our body from the ball area and toes of the pushing foot, and the initial contact area of the advancing foot is the rear area of the heel, as represented by the red target circle labeled "point of contact" in panel D of Figure 21.2.

As we continue to push our body forward onto the advanced foot, the pressure in the advanced foot moves forward with the movement of the body. In this example of stopping on the flat advanced foot, we stop pushing our body forward when it is centered over the foot, meaning when the pressure is centered within the foot. As a reference, the approximate center of the length of the foot is shown by the green line across the foot's width in panel D. The blue arrow represents the distance the pressure moves forward from the point of first contact in the heel.

In contrast, in naturally *relaxed* **sideward** movements (when we do not cross one leg over the other leg), we push from the inside ball area of one foot, and the initial contact area for the advancing foot is also the inside of the ball area, as represented by the red target circle in panel C labeled "push and point of contact" in Figure 21.2.

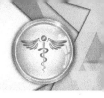

As we continue to push our body to the side to center it over the advanced foot, the pressure in the foot moves sideward toward the center of the foot. In this example, the distance the pressure moves in the foot is the length of the small blue arrow in panel C. The approximate middle of the foot's width is represented by the green line through the length of the foot in panel C.

In **relaxed straight-backward** movements, the pushing pressure is in essentially the same location as when we move forward, in the ball area and toes (panel D).

The initial point of contact for the foot advancing to the rear is also in the forward ball area and toes. Then, as we continue to push our body backward onto the advanced foot, to stop on a flattened foot, the pressure in the advanced foot (which is the one we moved behind us) moves backward from the ball area toward the green line in panel D.

In **naturally continuous backward** movements, often the only part of the foot that is used in both feet is the forward part. Thus, in natural, continuous backward movements, the heel area is held off the floor, or it only lightly contacts the floor during the movement. However, in smaller backward strides with continuous movement, many times the entire flattened foot is used.

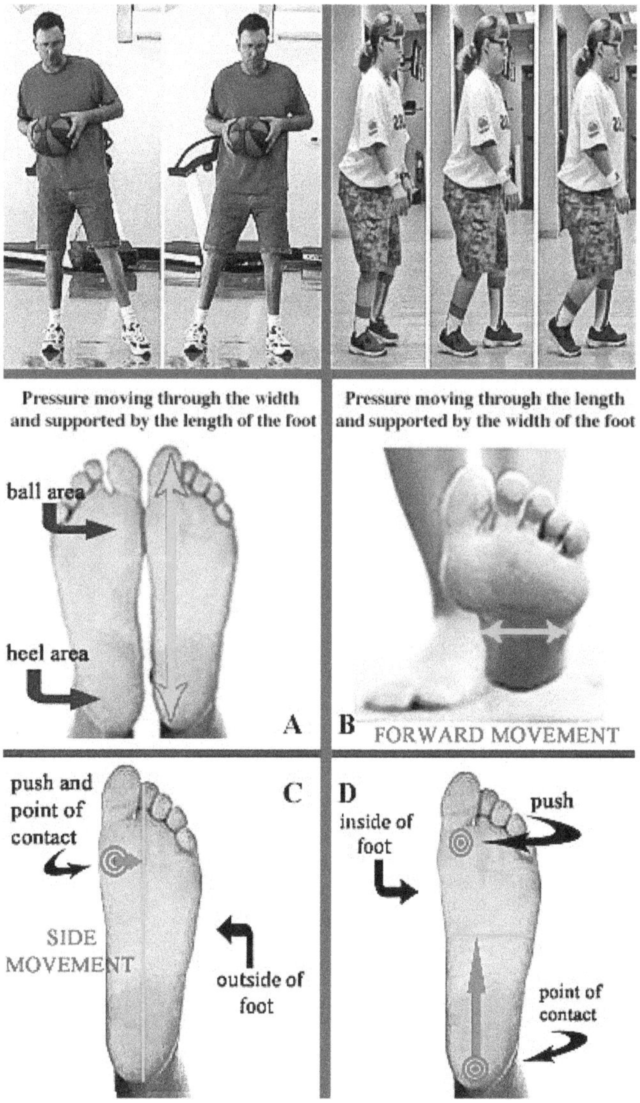

Guarded Posture

People with **guarded postures** have limited ability to flex their feet. This also means they have limited ability to hold increased pressure in the ball areas of their feet, and limited ability to flex their feet to lift their heels. During times when they *do* lift a heel, they often have difficulty keeping it

Pressure moving through the width and supported by the length of the foot

Pressure moving through the length and supported by the width of the foot

ball area

heel area

A

B FORWARD MOVEMENT

push and point of contact

SIDE MOVEMENT

outside of foot

C

D inside of foot

push

point of contact

FIGURE 21.2: In relaxed natural body movement to the side, the pressure in the advanced foot begins on the inside of the foot and moves a short distance toward the middle. The pressure moves sideward through the foot, supported by the length of that portion that is in contact with the floor.

In forward relaxed natural body movement, the pressure moves a long distance forward through the length of the advanced foot, and is supported by the width of that portion of the foot that is in contact with the floor.

off the floor during the movement. Why? People with a guarded posture most often push from the back portion of the ball area of the foot. This commonly leaves pressure *toward* the heel area that resists the heel being lifted, and it also works to push the heel back down to the floor when it is lifted.

This forces them to do more work with limited results, and it causes mild instability. How? They have limited control of the use and movement of the pressure in their feet, and that directly affects the

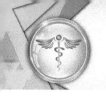

body's movement and stability. So, to help improve their stability, these people have a strong tendency to use the entire length of their feet in many of their movements. But there is a downside to this. It leads to a quicker decline of movement ability. Why? When we don't use them, muscles become weaker, and we learn not to trust them as much. As one muscle group weakens, other muscle groups also lose strength, due to the lack of support and function of the others.

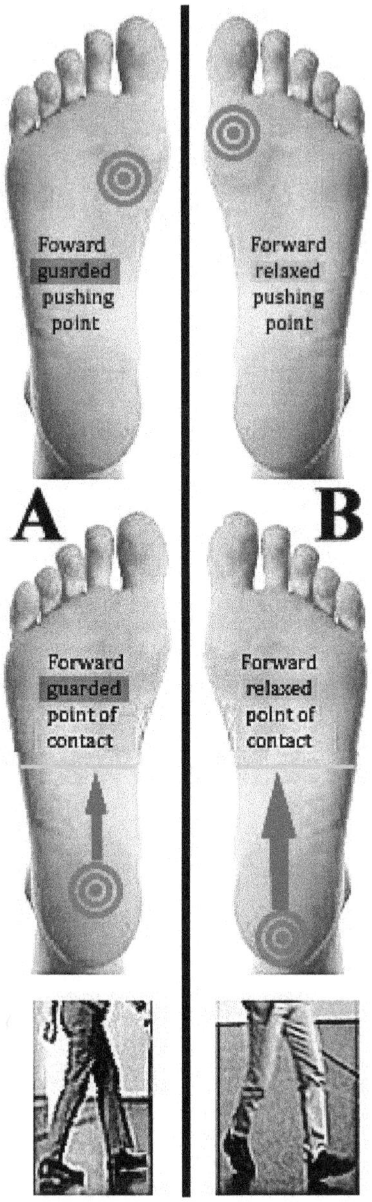

There is another problem that simultaneously arises in this situation and often is not fully realized. Many of the people in this category learn to limit the use of their calf muscles in advancing movements, for three common reasons. One, occasionally they push themselves too aggressively into the movement. Two, they begin having problems with tipping and/or stumbling forward. And three, because of reasons one and two, they are learning to inappropriately overuse their calf muscles to stop their bodies' unexpected forward movements.

Recall that the muscles in the calf push increased pressure into the ball area of the foot and lift the heel, and that pressure adds power and stability to the stride. However, when the feet are not easily flexing, this extra force causes a forward body tip. To counter the tip, people begin using the action of the calf muscles as a forward-movement brake, which, by the way, is part of a natural function. While this helps to compensate for some of the instability, it adds another complicated layer of inability and disability. Use of the muscles for movement decreases. The use of them to stop movement increases. The result is increasing instability, increasing postural guarding and stiffening, increasing fear, and decreasing ability.

In **guarded forward movements**, the push typically comes from the middle to the back portion of the ball area of the foot, and the pressure *does not* move any farther forward in the pushing foot when they are in control of it. When the pressure does move farther forward, it often causes a forward tipping of the body off the toes of a foot that is flexing insufficiently. The result of the repetitive forward tipping is an overuse of the calf muscles as described above.

When a person is using the middle to back portion of the ball area of the foot for the push, the initial contact area for the advancing foot is the forward aspect of the heel, as shown in panel A of Figure 21.3.

Due to the location of the pushing pressure and the limited flexion of the pushing foot, the stride length is much shorter than it is with a relaxed posture and easily flexing foot, for the same amount of applied

FIGURE 21.3: Forward movement.

Top panel: The red target represents the area of increased pressure that is used for pushing into the forward movement.

Center panel: The red target marks the initial point of contact for the advancing foot. The blue arrow represents the distance to the center of the foot.

Bottom panel: The resultant stride length and angle of the foot to the floor.

pushing pressure. Panel A in Figure 21.3 shows the typical location of pushing and initial contact area in the foot when the posture is guarded. The picture at the bottom shows the result.

Compare this with panel B, in which the typical pushing and initial contact areas in the feet are shown when the posture is relaxed and feet are flexible. The picture at the bottom of panel B shows the longer stride. Now compare the feet in the two pictures to see the results of the different pressures and foot functions.

In **guarded sideward movements**, the location of the increased pressure for the push is typically toward the back portion of the ball area, but to the inside of the foot. Because of the foot's limited flexibility and the mild instability, the length of the foot is commonly used for pushing, as shown in Figure 21.4 and depicted by the extended thick brown line.

Provided their postural alignment does not change during the movement, the initial contact area for the advancing foot is in the same location that the push came from in the other foot (shown by the brown "guarded posture" target circle on the foot at left in Figure 21.4).

When postural guarding *increases*, the location of the push and initial contact area for the advancing foot moves toward the heel. This is caused by the upward and rearward movement of the shoulders.

On a good movement day for those with a guarded posture, the above locations are common. However, on the not-so-good and bad movement days, the location of the push and contact areas will typically be toward the heel.

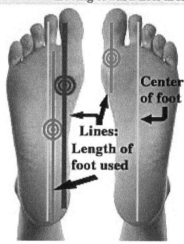

FIGURE 21.4: *Sideward* movement. The flexibility of the body and feet determines where the pressure will be located in the feet, and how it will be used. As the stiffening of the posture and foot increases, the function of the foot and created movement decrease.

Stiffened Posture

In **sideward movements** with a **stiffened posture**, the push always comes from the entire *rigid foot*, because the foot is too stiff to flex. If the push were forward in the foot, the person would tip and fall forward. If it were toward the heel, they would tip and fall backward. The length of the "stride" is very small, and the initial contact area for the advancing foot is also the entire foot. The area of the "pushing" and initial contact area in the feet will be off center toward the inside of the foot, and is represented by the purple target circle on the "stiffened posture" line on the left image in Figure 21.4.

These people are typically in a very upright position with a stiffened posture. Because of this, the slightest amount of sway of their upper body (shoulders) causes big changes in the location of the pressure in their feet. When the upper body stays in place directly over the hips, their movements are methodically very slow and restricted. When the upper body moves, their movements frequently become suddenly very erratic, as the location of the pressure in the feet is also erratic. Thus, these people are very unstable.

A stiffened posture forces stiffened, shuffling movements on stiff, flattened feet, with very limited upper- or lower-body movement, which is their method of forward motion. These people are always on

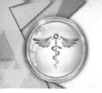

the brink of disaster and always having great difficulty controlling the pressure in their feet. Thus, there is no pushing their body into movement to speak of, because they cannot produce or control it.

Natural Movement, Forward Stride

When beginning a forward stride, we balance, support, and push our body into the movement using only approximately 25 percent of the total surface area of just one foot. This is the ball area and toes. As we continue pushing through the stride, we then momentarily balance, support, and push our body with a slightly *smaller area* of the pushing foot, the most forward portion of the ball area and toes, as we transition onto the advanced foot. The pressure gradually decreases in this area as the transfer of body weight and pressure into the advancing foot proceeds, and then the toes are lifted from the floor as the advanced foot becomes the new pushing foot.

The pushing pressure remains in the most forward portion of the ball area and toes as *the flexing foot* continues pushing the body forward. During this time, in a natural stride the back tip of the advancing foot's heel makes **light** contact with the floor. Therefore, in midstride we are momentarily balanced and supported on the forward portion of the ball area and toes of one foot, and *not* on the heel of the advanced foot. Yes, in midstride during continuous natural movement, the support and stabilization of our body, and control of the movement, are coming from the forward portion of the ball area and toes of the pushing foot, and *virtually no support* is coming from the heel of the advanced foot.

This requires a great deal of stabilizing and pushing pressure in the forward portion of the ball area and toes of the back, pushing foot. It also takes a great deal of coordinated balance to remain stable on that very small area. Only a very relaxed, strong, stable, and easily flexible foot is capable of providing this.

The very light pressure in the tip of the heel of the advanced foot quickly moves forward through the foot, as it is also increasing. As the flexing back foot continues to push the body forward, the forward-moving pressure in the advanced foot increases from both body weight and the addition of downward pressure from working muscles in the advanced leg. Very importantly, the pushing and flexing action of the back foot cannot stop or decrease until the body is pushed far enough forward to move the developing pushing pressure into the ball area and toes of the advanced foot. Thus, in our continuous natural walking movement, there is a steady and smoothly *uninterrupted transfer of the pushing pressure from one foot to the next.*

Any interruption or restriction in the amount of pressure, any change in the location of the pressure, or any limitation of the flexibility of either foot alters the natural function of the feet and changes the intended movement. People with a movement impairment develop a combination of problems in these areas, and these form the root source of the movement difficulties they encounter. These difficulties are always more problematic in forward movements, and they increase as the posture becomes more restrictive.

When we were very young, our improving movements were based entirely on our ability to control, support, balance, and power our movements using a smaller and smaller area of one foot. *People with a degenerative movement impairment gradually undergo a reversal of this natural progression.* For this reason, the critical point of any effective therapy for movement recovery must rightfully be based on an understanding of the diminished functioning of their feet.

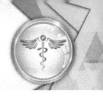

To reclaim a more natural forward stride and improve movement ability, the person must learn to once again trust flexing the foot, and using only *the forward 25 percent of that one foot* for stabilized support, balance, and control while pushing their body. This will not be an easy task, but it's still possible for many.

This 25 percent of the area of one foot is approximately 12.5 percent of the surface area of *both* feet. Let the concept of these numbers sink in for a moment. If a person is having difficulty standing stable on two feet (100 percent), they do not have the ability to stand with stability on one foot (50 percent). What is the bigger implication? Many such people are put into walking therapy and are encouraged to use a very small part of one foot, 12.5 percent of the surface area of their feet, for stabilization and support during midstride. This is not a reasonable expectation.

MOVING FORWARD, STIFFENING PROBLEMS

Forward movement is more complex. It requires a higher level of functioning and ability than sideward movement. For this reason, many movement-impaired people will again experience guarding and stiffening in their posture and feet that previously had been resolving in sideward movements, and many of their instability and fear issues will resurface. This is due to the difficulty of controlling the pressure moving through the length of the foot.

The three people in Figure 21.5 are classic examples of the difficulties experienced when attempting a forward stride with a stiffened posture and feet. With limited ability to begin the movement with their legs and feet, they depend on their upper bodies to start the movement. They tip forward to begin, and then must catch up with the tipping movement of their body with their legs and feet. This always puts them on the edge of a forward fall, and forces a constant internal struggle to move their feet fast enough to prevent the fall.

In panel A, Sangwon's stiffness is extensive throughout his entire body and includes the muscles in his hands and face (red arrows). In pictures 1 through 4, he leans forward onto the ball area and toes of his feet until a foot is freed up to lift off the floor. In picture 5, he has lifted his left knee slightly to move the left foot forward in a very small stride (shown by the green arrows).

An important feature of this is what follows. He must continue leaning forward to continue making these small strides. The problems: First, his upper-body tip necessitates very quickened, uncontrolled, stumbling forward strides, which frequently force him into a forward fall. Second, the part of the advancing foot making first contact with the floor is the ball area of the foot. The result: With each forward-tipping "stride," the push from the ball area is greater than in the previous "stride." So, he is tipping forward while continually pushing his forward-tipping body into a faster movement. How does he stop this runaway situation? Most often, someone catches him, he comes to a wall or heavy object, or he falls in an erratic and uncontrolled accident.

In panel B, Bong Soon looks to be relatively relaxed in pictures 1 and 2, but the opposite is true. She is very guarded in her posture and very stiff in the knees and feet. She is holding on to her son's arm while leaning her upper body forward to take a stride. However, her upper-body lean goes too far and puts increased pressure too far forward into her toes. This causes her to tip forward on stiff feet and pushes her body into a forward fall (red arrows). Fortunately, her son stopped the fall and supported her as she moved back onto flattened feet.

The stiffness of her feet is seen in pictures 4 and 5, while she is tipping forward. The entire length of the foot is straight. There is no movement of the joints where the toes meet the foot, as is seen in a relaxed and flexing foot. Thus, stiff feet are basically nonfunctional feet.

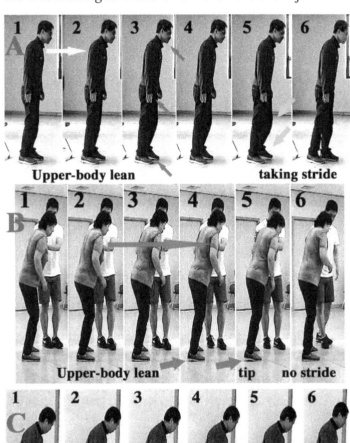

Upper-body lean   **taking stride**

Upper-body lean   **tip**   **no stride**

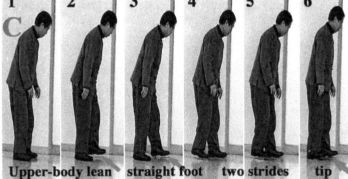

Upper-body lean   **straight foot**   **two strides**   **tip**

FIGURE 21.5: All three are moving into a forward stride with a very restrictive posture, with stiffened knees, ankles, and feet. This forces them to use upper-body movement to begin, but leaning the upper body forward to begin the movement causes tipping and falling forward off stiff feet.

In panel C, Yusoo has total-body guarding with less stiffening in his knees and feet than Bong Soon. This is why he has relatively good postural stability but still has limited control of the pressure in his stiffening feet. The lifted, flattened left foot in pictures 2 and 3 shows how stiffened his feet actually are, as he holds the front of his foot up.

Yusoo leans his upper body slightly forward to take a stride with his left foot (pictures 1 through 4). Then, with the start of the next stride with his right foot, to prevent tipping forward, he begins moving his shoulders back in picture 4. This sets up the next problem. His shoulders continue to fade back in picture 5, which makes him more upright, adding increasing pressure to his heels, which is the reason he is tipping backward on his heels in picture 6. Note that his left knee does not change in pictures 1 through 5 and then straightens in pictures 5 and 6.

Yusoo's knee straightens because of the increased pressure that moves into his left heel beginning in picture 4, which is also why he cannot complete the next stride with his right foot. Note that the advancing right foot in picture 5 is quickly forced back down onto the floor in picture 6. Why? Instability. Increased heel pressure in the left foot is pushing him backward and forces an incomplete transfer of body weight to the left foot. This is a common mistake for people with a restrictive posture.

Stiffening, restrictive postures create problems of instability and posture control. Therefore, people with these postures should begin practicing a forward stride with *very* small advancing ministrides. This means taking baby steps that are no longer than ***one-half*** *of the length of their foot*. This will keep them on flattened feet with better control—provided they are also using adequate body-weight transfers from foot to foot. With practice, moving from one flat foot to the next flat foot provides them with stability that allows them to *begin* to relax. Note: This beginning of "letting their guard down just a little" will happen only when they can feel and reproduce, and begin to trust, their self-made stability. Using baby steps, they will also be balancing only momentarily on the entirety of one flat foot before moving to the next flat foot. This is how they will begin trusting a more complete transfer of body weight, and is what Carol is working on in Figure 21.6.

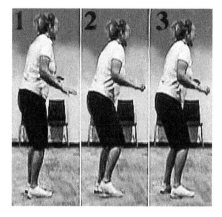

FIGURE 21.6: A ministride is a baby step that is one-half of the length of your foot, or less.

What does this allow people to avoid? They don't need to flex their feet as much while using a relatively flattened foot in each stride. Remember, with a restrictive posture, the greatest degree of guarding and stiffening is always in the feet, and it will not lessen until people feel comfortable enough to reduce their anxiety and fear. Moving forward is scary for them, and their anxiety and fear will not magically go away despite anyone's best efforts or soothing words. They will not begin to relax until they feel and know that the scary problems have gone away, and for them, using anything less than two flat feet is scary. This is why they must begin to resolve the scary issues by moving in very small strides from one flat foot to the next flat foot.

FORWARD STRIDE: SETUP

The proper setup posture for a forward stride is the very same posture used in preparing for virtually any movement: that is, standing in a ready stance with your feet spread approximately shoulder width apart, or less. The next thing to do is to move your shoulders slightly forward until you feel a slight increase of pressure in the ball areas of both feet, while keeping your knees flexed as you hold that pressure.

Now you are ready to transfer body weight to one foot, but this is also where many movement-impaired people begin to have difficulties in forward movements. During the transfer of body weight to one foot, you must have a better ability to hold the increased pressure in the ball area. Then the movement of the body must be synchronized with the movement of the pressure in the feet, and flexing of the feet.

These factors are critical in forward movements, and this is why forward movements are more complex and more problematic to do. This is why the common mistakes in posture and transfer of body weight happen more easily in forward movements, and the consequences of those mistakes are greater.

Mistakes: Two things frequently happen when people with a restrictive-posture movement impairment begin a forward movement:

1. Typically, they are completely unaware that their shoulders are slowly moving backward as they shift body weight toward one foot.

   When the shoulders fade backward, the increased pressure in the ball areas moves toward the heels of both feet. Then, as the person continues to transfer more body weight onto one foot, that

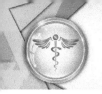

foot will be flat or will have increased pressure in the heel (depending on how far the shoulders have moved back).

2. When the pressure is kept in the ball areas of the feet, and the transfer of body weight is completed, the body will begin to move forward as the other foot is lifting off the floor. Many people with a restrictive posture are not comfortable with this free movement of their bodies, and they are uncertain they can control it. So, in response, they quickly move their shoulders back to stop the forward motion.

   Remember, to them, that easy movement feels like they are beginning to tip forward into a fall.

When the setup for the movement is destroyed, the intended movement doesn't happen. When the pressure moves a small amount and makes the foot functionally flat, the body does not move when the transfer onto one foot is completed. Then what is the person's typical response? One, they move their shoulders back more to help lift the foot they want to move. Two, they move their shoulders forward and then stumble forward on their feet to catch up with their tipping body.

When the shoulders fade backward in the setup and the increased pressure moves into the heels, the body moves backward when the transfer onto one foot is completed. Now they stumble backward on their feet to catch up with their backward-tipping body.

Backward-moving shoulders are the reason many people often feel they are "stuck in the mud" when walking. For example, they move slowly when walking across the street in front of cars, while desperately trying to go faster. They move their knees and feet but barely make any forward progress. And even worse, sometimes they tip backward and fall while trying harder to move forward.

Without realizing it, they change their postural alignment and move the location of the pushing pressure in the foot. They try harder, but what they do in trying harder only makes things worse. What happens in their mind when this occurs? Panic, fear, and worry that their condition is getting worse. But no, it was only another simple and easily explained postural mistake.

There is both a conscious and a subconscious response, as well as a psychological and a physical response, happening. The only way to calm the psychological-sensitivity part is to first work on correcting the physical part. The ball areas and toes of the feet must be physically desensitized to increasing pressure, which only means the person becomes stable, comfortable, and trusting of having and using pressure in this portion of the foot. The other part of it is becoming comfortable with that pressure in this area of the foot while moving the body forward, as the other foot lifts from the floor. This requires time, patience, practice, and playful activity. As the physical problem parts are corrected, the psychological components will begin to fade.

HEEL TO TOE

The flexing pushing foot, and the movement of the body, control and place the advancing foot exactly where and how it needs to be, per the requirements of the movement and support of the body. So, tell your mind and advisors to leave the advancing foot alone. Why?

The advice to focus on placing the advancing foot is exactly the wrong advice. It is wrong because it is the *pushing* foot that is producing, directing, controlling, and supporting the body's forward movement.

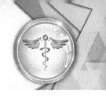

Therefore, ultimately it is the pushing foot that determines where the advancing foot will contact the floor. Where is the advancing foot when all this is happening? It is held off the floor and is moving through the air. What can it contribute to the movement while it is off the floor? Absolutely nothing. This is the reason your primary focus for the movement must be on the pushing foot, the only foot that is making the movement possible. With relaxed postural control, the pushed body and advancing knee will place the advancing foot exactly where it needs to be to support the body and continue the movement.

To the Wall, to Work on Using Flexing Knees

Using a wall for practicing knee and foot flexibility is very useful in forward movement.

1. With feet approximately shoulder width apart, stand with the front tip of the forward foot approximately one length of your foot away from the wall, as shown in Figure 21.7 and picture 1 of Figure 21.8.

2. Next, move your back foot to place the front tip of it approximately one-half of the length of your foot behind the forward foot, and then angle the toe of the back foot outward about thirty to forty-five degrees, as shown in Figure 21.7. This will give your stance additional stability, for those who need it.

   Standing with your body centered over both *flattened* feet, slightly flex both knees and then bring your hand up in front of you as shown in picture 1 of Figure 21.8. In this example, I have my right leg forward and right hand up.

FIGURE 21.7: Foot placement for knee and foot exercise facing a wall.

   Note: The primary purpose of the raised hand **is not** to keep your nose off the wall. That is the job of your feet. The purpose of the raised hand is to have an easy and immediate visual guide to see the results of how your forward knee is working and your body is moving.

   As you hold the hand steady in place with the elbow, when the hand moves straight forward to a reference point on the wall and then straight back, this shows you your flexing knee is moving your body. If the hand tilts down when you move forward, and up when you move back, this shows that you are using upper-body movement and likely little or no knee movement. This means you're bending (stooping forward) at the hips.

3. Standing centered over both flattened feet, prepare by relaxing into a ready stance, with a focus on relaxing your elbows and knees, and slightly flexing both knees.

   Pay attention to this position, because it stays the same as you move forward and backward.

4. Now shift your focus to only the forward knee, and begin to slowly push that knee straight forward toward the wall, as shown in pictures 2 through 5 of Figure 21.8. Many of you will need to resist the urge to push your hand forward with your elbow instead of using your front knee.

   When you do this properly, you will feel:

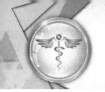

- As your front knee moves forward, your body moves forward over the forward foot.

- Your feet stay flattened when your posture is relaxed enough, you keep your knees flexed, and you are not using upper-body movement to "help." If you begin to tip forward, add more knee flexing. Squat more.

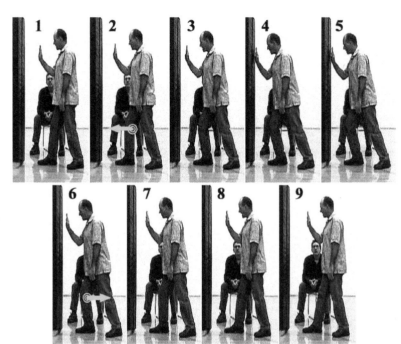

- As your body moves forward, the pressure in your front foot increases as the pressure in your back foot decreases.

- As the knee moves forward, allow it to flex (bend) more, and this will lower your body in the stance. Allow this to happen. When you fight it your knee will stiffen and you'll begin to tip forward. Why? The pressure moves into the ball area and toes of the feet.

FIGURE 21.8: Top panel: Push your front knee forward to move your body and stand balanced over the forward flat foot. With a relaxed posture, your body will lower slightly as the knee flexes forward.

Bottom panel: Pull the knee backward to move your body and stand balanced over the flat back foot.

5. Flexing your knee forward and down moves your body forward and keeps you stable. Let this slowly happen until your hand is very close to the wall, as shown in picture 5 of Figure 21.8. Then, using *only* your front knee, reverse the movement.

6. *Slowly* pull your front knee backward to move and center your body over your flattened back foot. This means allowing that knee to extend (to straighten). Do this slowly and keep your shoulders forward. Why?
   Importantly, remember to stop moving backward before your front knee fully straightens, which will be just before your body is fully centered over the back foot, provided you hold your shoulders forward (shown in picture 9). This helps to prevent you from going too far back and adding increased pressure in the heel of the back foot, to avoid tipping backward.

7. Now repeat and repeat everything. Play and experiment with moving your body by focusing only on moving the front knee. Stay relaxed. Stay down. Shoulders forward.

Problems with the Wall Exercise

When you have difficulty staying in the setup posture using only knee movements in this exercise, the most common reasons are:

1. **Problem:** You're unstable on your feet. Much of the time, this has to do with the positioning of and stiffness in the knees and feet. Often the feet are too close together, and sometimes they're too far apart.

   To correct this, reposition your feet as shown in Figure 21.7. If this arrangement doesn't work for you, adjust the position of your feet slightly to where you're comfortable. What I am showing and describing is a guide. Use it as a starting point, and then adjust to your comfort and ability level.

   Stiffened knees are a big contributor to the unstable-foot problem, and a stiff-knee problem in this exercise often begins with your raised hand. The tendency is, the more impaired your movements are, the more you will unknowingly stiffen your arm while holding your hand up. Be patient. Add another step in the setup: Relax your hand to relax your elbow, to relax your knee.

2. **Problem:** Your hand moves closer to the wall, but the pressure in your feet doesn't change.

   This happens when you lean your upper body forward instead of flexing your knee. This is what Mike is doing in Figure 21.9. His stance is good and his front knee is flexed, but that flexed knee is also being held stiffly in place. Also note that he is holding his back knee stiffly straight.

   Take note of this point: *A flexed knee or elbow does not necessarily mean a relaxed and flexing knee or elbow.*

   As a reference to see the lack of movement of his knees, I am standing behind Mike in the pictures. See how his raised arm moves forward and down to cover my arm in the background. Now look at the bottom of my shirt. His hips move back as his shoulders move forward, revealing more of my shirt in each picture. This is not what he intended to do.

   Now go back to Figure 21.8 and compare my movement with Mike seated in the background. As I move forward, gradually there is less of Mike showing in the background. When I move back, gradually more of him appears. My setup posture remains the same as I use only my knee in both directions. His setup posture changes as he uses his hips and shoulders.

   Another common thing people with stiffened knees do is push their hand forward and then pull it back using the elbow, while at the same time they may or may not also bend slightly forward with their hips.

3. **Problem:** You are stable in the setup, but then become unstable when you begin the movement. The common cause is postural stiffening, and especially stiffening in the knees and feet.

   When your posture is only mildly guarded, typically you will begin the movement correctly, but then your body will begin to tip forward as pressure increases in the forward foot's ball area and toes. This happens when tensed muscles controlling the forward knee restrict its movement, but the movement of the upper body is not as limited in bending forward at the hips. The resulting forward-moving posture will be very similar to Mike's posture in figure 21.9, but *with the knee farther forward.* Remember, with a guarded posture, your feet will easily mildly stiffen.

4. Problem: You are stable in the setup but then tip forward in the movement.

In Figure 21.10, Bob begins stable on both feet centered in his zone of stability, and then begins the movement. Then in pictures 3 and 4, he tips forward out of the zone. He has some mild guarding in his posture that contributed to this outcome.

While attempting to move only the forward (right) knee, he mistakenly moves both, and both of them move farther than expected. This quickly moves increased pressure into the ball areas and toes of both feet, and his reaction is stiffening of the feet in response to the induced forward tip. This is why his feet are straight and not flexing in the last picture (indicated by the red arrow). The amount of forward tipping of his body is clearly visible with respect to the green zone of stability.

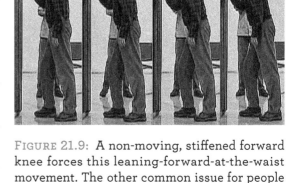

FIGURE 21.9: A non-moving, stiffened forward knee forces this leaning-forward-at-the-waist movement. The other common issue for people with chronic postural guarding and stiffening is being confused as to how to move the knee.

5. Problem: The forward part of the movement goes well, but when you move backward, your front knee straightens too quickly.

When your feet are spaced far enough apart (front to back), the front knee will straighten as the body moves backward to become centered over the back foot. The problem in this example happens when the feet are too close together. When the toe of the back foot is too close to the heel of the front foot, the straightening front knee can quickly push the body onto the heels of both feet.

FIGURE 21.10: Bob flexes and moves his knees too far forward, too quickly. This moves the pressure forward in his feet and creates the forward body tip on the front areas of both feet. Note how stiffened his feet are in reaction to the unexpected tip.

The abrupt increase of heel pressure and tipping of the body occasionally pull the front foot off the floor. This puts more pressure in the heel of the back foot, and commonly pushes the person into a backward tip or fall. This situation is more likely to happen when the posture is moderately guarded during this movement, because the movement of the knee is often erratic and difficult to control.

When the posture is stiffened, the person's knees are most always too straight with little flexibility, but they will still have this same tipping and falling-backward problem. Their excessive upper-body backward movement causes it, and the stiffened knees make it more likely to happen.

6. Problem: You are confident that you're doing everything correctly, but you can't move your hand to the wall, and you feel too much pressure in the ball area and toes of your front foot.

When this happens, check the position of your front foot, because it is probably too far away from the wall, as seen in Figure 21.11.

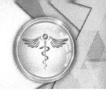

Practice using just the knee in this movement until it becomes easy and comfortable, and you remain stable without any tipping. The most common tipping will be forward into the wall. The most common cause is non-flexing knees that do not lower the body enough to stabilize into the feet. Many people will need to use an exaggerated correction of squatting farther down during the forward movement. To many, this feels odd and "way too much," but when seen, it is typically *almost* enough.

FLEX THE FOOT TO PUSH THE BODY

In the next exercise, you will **not** be using your forward knee to power the movement of your body as you did in the previous exercise. Instead, you'll be using your flexing *back foot to push your body forward.* Then, when your foot relaxes and your heel lowers, your body will return to where it began.

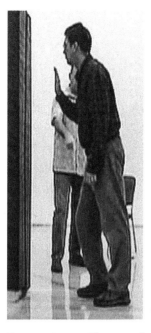

1. Pushing increased pressure into the ball area and toes of the back foot, the relaxed foot flexes and the heel moves upward. This action of the foot, the lifting heel, pushes the body forward.

   The knees can be straight or flexed this time, but having them flexed will help some people apply the required stabilizing pressure down into their feet.

   When the knees are *not* flexed, or do not continue to flex slightly down as the flexing pushing foot pushes the body forward, tipping forward from the front of the forward foot often happens. There are two common reasons for this. One, with the more upright posture, the shoulders easily move too far forward beyond the knee and toe. Two, the downward pressure in the forward foot is weak.

FIGURE 21.11: The toe of Mike's front foot is too far away from the wall. Also note that his feet are very close together. This contributes to the difficulty and instability he is experiencing.

2. When the knees are straightened in the setup, they will most likely remain straightened during the movement. The person is then very upright in the stance, and if their posture is even mildly guarded, their stability is often easily compromised.

   With a guarded posture, movement-impaired people often lose control of the movement and easily tip forward. Why? They must force the foot to flex, and then it often flexes too quickly and/or too much for them to control.

   Then there is the opposite. Many will tip backward because their upright posture often leads them to withdraw their shoulders when attempting to flex the foot. This happens to those who habitually use shoulder movement to help start their movements. The backward tipping tendency also happens when they quickly release the pushing foot when it is flexed. Why? Their posture is too upright with withdrawn shoulders and straightened knees, so when the heel of the pushing foot abruptly descends, the backward movement of the body is often exaggerated. The other factor is that the downward pressure into their feet is often too weak to properly support the movement, so the body moves back.

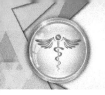

When the person is *relaxed* in an upright stance with knees straightened, they will easily control the movement with the flexing foot, their posture, and the movement of their body, and they will remain stable while adding the appropriate downward pressure into their feet.

Do not forget. Very importantly: After the flexing foot has pushed the body onto the forward foot, *you must continue to hold the push from the back foot, and keep the foot flexed, even after your body's forward movement has stopped.* This is to ensure that your body remains in position where you stopped the movement and does not move farther forward or move backward. Experiment with this. While standing in this "finished" posture, feel how your body moves as you only move the pushing foot's heel slowly up and down.

Bob stops his body's forward movement in picture 4 of Figure 21.12. He holds the push and keeps his back foot slightly flexed, but his posture is mildly tensed, with slight body sway. He is stable in the other parts of the movement, so why is he mildly tensed and swaying at the end of it? In picture 4, the centered red line in the zone of stability shows he still has mildly increased pressure in the heel area of the forward foot, and that is lightly pushing him back to the pushing foot. Therefore, when he releases any of the forward push from the pushing foot, his body immediately moves backward off the forward foot. Also note that in picture 4 his chest and shoulders are back from the front edge of the zone of stability, and his forward knee is close to it. Thus, the shoulder, knee, and toe are not in vertical alignment. This is further evidence of the pressure in the forward foot being toward the heel.

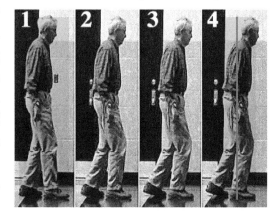

FIGURE 21.12: Relax both knees to relax your feet. Push from the ball area of the foot, and the heel will rise and your body will move forward. Bob does this, but his mildly guarded posture holds his shoulders back, and he is unnecessarily flexing his back knee. Because of this, in picture 4, he has mildly increased pressure in the heel area of the front foot.

How should he correct this situation? With the pushing foot he could add a small amount of heel lift, to move and hold his body forward onto a flattened forward foot; or he could simply move his shoulders slightly forward.

But wait, and take note of a complicating factor. Bob again is flexing his back knee forward to "help" the flexing foot. In this foot-flexing exercise, when the back knee flexes forward, it negates much of the pushing effect of the flexing foot. This is also evidence that Bob is confusing flexing and pushing the back knee forward, rather than using the flexing foot to push his body forward.

3. Done correctly, only a small and gentle push from the flexing foot is all that's needed. This is a caution to those of you with some guarding or stiffening in your posture. When the push from the foot is too strong, it is very easy to push yourself into a forward tip, especially when your posture and knees are not as relaxed as they should be. Therefore, do not force the foot to flex. Instead relax it, to allow it to gently flex.

When you feel you must use a heavy push to move and keep your body forward, the most common reason is that your postural alignment is applying increased pressure into both heels. Stop and correct your stance and posture. When the movement seems to be forced, you are doing something wrong.

4. To move back onto a flattened back foot, simply relax the push from the pushing foot and allow the heel to lower to the floor. Nothing else!

    NOTE: *I did not say stop pushing* from the pushing foot. The controlled relaxing of some of the pressure controls the body's backward movement with the lowering of the heel. The heel moves up and the body moves forward. The heel lowers and that moves the body backward.

5. When you're practicing this movement and have moved onto the forward foot, check to ensure that the heel of the pushing foot has lifted off the floor. If it is still on the floor with your feet on the floor as shown above, you are still using your knee for the movement.

Take it slowly. Feel the movements through the pressure changes in your flexing feet. If you are having difficulties, go back and practice this same heel-lift exercise in a sideward movement to remind yourself how it works and feels. Then simply change your stance by moving one foot forward and use the exact same flexing foot to push your body into a forward movement. If you feel any instability in your feet, relax and flex your knees into a lower ready stance before you begin the forward movement. Because many people with a restrictive posture are not used to keeping their knees flexed, it will feel odd for them. They will say it feels like too much of a squat, but it will most always be not as much as they think it is. For this and many other reasons, use a mirror when possible to see what you're doing, and what you're not doing.

As Bob practiced relaxing into the push from the flexing back foot, and kept the pressure stable in both feet during the movement, he did much better (Figure 21.13). Here, his body is moving only according to the push of the flexing back foot. Follow the sequence of the movement to see what your relaxed forward and backward movement in this

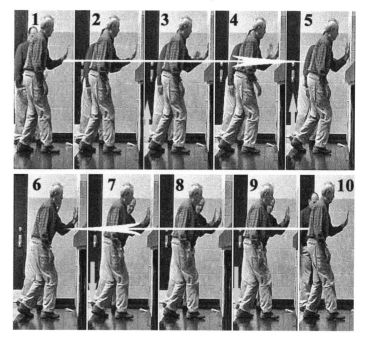

FIGURE 21.13: Top panel: As Bob pushes from the ball area and toes of his back foot, his relaxed body begins to move forward. As the pressure increases into a smaller area, the foot flexes and lifts the heel higher. The lifting heel pushes his body forward.

Bottom panel: As he relaxes the pushing pressure in his back foot, the heel lowers, and his relaxed body moves backward.

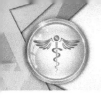

exercise should be. Pictures 1 through 5 show his smooth body movement forward, and note that the heel is lifted higher by the flexing foot in each picture. The heel goes up, indicated by the vertical arrows, and the body moves forward.

Pictures 6 through 10 show the return backward movement of the body. As the heel lowers, indicated by the vertical arrows, the body moves backward onto the back foot.

The vertical green arrows indicate the movement of the heels. The horizontal long yellow arrows indicate the direction of movement of the body. The knees are flexed at the start of the movement and easily flex during the movement. This example shows relaxed postural control and stabilization. It also shows natural movement ability reclaimed.

THE PUSH

"The push" may sometimes sound complicated and seem to be different with various movements, but physically it is always the same force created in the exact same way by the foot. In review: The push is a combination of setting, holding, and using the increased pressure in the correct area of the foot. How do we know where the correct area is? The correct area is created by the relaxed setup posture—the posture that is required for the movement we're intending to do. This is the simplicity of natural movement. The relaxed body sets the required pressure in the feet. Then, when we hold that posture and do nothing more than transfer our body weight to stand on one foot, the pressure is substantially increased in the one foot we're standing on.

Then, because of two factors, the push and movement of the body happen automatically. First, the off-center location of the pressure in the foot causes that pressure to be transmitted into the floor at an angle. This forms the initial push and movement for the body, when the other foot is lifted from the floor. Second, the foot's structure allows the body to be supported by a small and stationary portion of the foot and toes, while the lifting movement of the heel area of the foot continues to move the body.

KNEE DIFFICULTIES

People with a moderate or more significant movement impairment sometimes seem to experience a "disconnect" between knowing what they want to do and actually being able to do it. Within the medical community, practitioners often deem this disconnect to be a direct effect of the disorder. So, the person is instructed to do their best to cope with it. However, when observed in practical application, this apparent disconnect actually more often manifests itself as confusion. There is a direct correlation between the person's level of psychological fear and their postural guarding, and both are indirect effects of the disorder. This statement is based on personal experience, and the observed experiences of many others as I worked with them. Where there was a supposed disconnect, clarity came when the levels of both fear and guarding postures were reduced.

However, it's not just those with a neurodegenerative disorder who are affected. The reality is, virtually everyone has an intellectual disconnect from their natural ability. What does this mean? Because virtually no one knows how their natural movements physically happen, everyone has this same disconnect. The only difference is, those with natural ability can do what they want because their bodies are

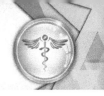

relaxed, functioning cooperatively and doing the movements for them. Those with postural issues and challenging movements are forced to think about how to do their movements more easily or safely. The problem? They don't understand how their movements work, so they also don't know what to change to affect an easier or safer outcome. Thus, in their thoughts they are searching for an answer they do not possess. That is the ubiquitous disconnect.

■ ■ ■

CHAPTER 22

FORWARD STRIDE

When the cause of the problem is understood, a corrective solution emerges.

How well are you doing with the exercises in Chapter 21? Have they become easy, or are you still struggling to remain stable throughout the movements? Are you able to relax to feel the movement and the changing pressure in your feet? Are your knees and feet flexing? And what are the important points to remember to ensure that you're completing the transfer of body weight in each stride?

1. When you push your body onto the flattened advanced foot, your forward knee and shoulder will be in line with the toes of that foot. Look for it. Feel it. The pressure should be equal in the ball and heel areas of that foot.

2. At the same time, your toes, knee, and nipple area on that side of your chest should also be in vertical alignment. Look for it. In this postural alignment, the pressure is centered from side to side in the foot.

3. With these reference alignments, your body will be centered from front to back and side to side over the flattened advanced foot.

When *any* intimidation or instability lingers, remember to practice forward strides by moving from one heavy flat foot to the other heavy flat foot in *baby steps*. A baby step is a very small stride that is approximately one-half of the length of your foot. Why baby steps? They make it easier to remain on flattened feet, even when your knees and feet are not as flexible as they need to be. Staying on flattened feet provides you with the full support and stability of the entire surface of each foot during the movement. Many people with impaired movements and a restrictive-posture have to do this before transitioning to the foot flexing in longer strides. So, very importantly, begin walking using small strides when your posture is not relaxed, and when you feel unstable. And continue with baby steps until your body tells you it's okay to take longer strides. What does that mean? When you begin to relax, the longer strides will simply happen on their own. So do not force a stride or movement your body isn't prepared for.

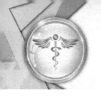

What do I mean by making the foot heavy? Well, imagine that each of your shoes weighs twenty-five pounds. With your legs, push and hold that amount of pressure into the foot you're moving from, and then push that much pressure down into the foot you're moving onto. The added downward pressure and the flattened feet will improve your stability. This will allow you to relax a bit more to work on flexing your knees, and your strides will become easier. What do you need to do otherwise? Stay within your personal limits, according to what your feet and body are telling you.

With each heavy-flattened-foot short stride, you need to trust that you can momentarily stand balanced on just that one foot, *if you want or need to.* When you feel this, then your difficulty with the movement will begin to ease. You must practice becoming and feeling stable standing on one foot, even if it's only for a few seconds. This is vitally important to all your movements. Just a couple of seconds as you move safely back onto both flattened feet. So, practice creating and completely understanding this feeling with *every* advancing stride.

You will note that I've been writing "*flattened*" foot and not "flat" foot. With this, I am not saying that you should try to keep the foot flat on the floor when you have the ability to move beyond baby steps. What I am referring to here regarding shorter strides is only consistently reproducing the temporary feeling of the foot being completely and comfortably flat and stable on the floor, *as you continue through the stride without stopping.* The importance of knowing this flat-foot feeling is simply that it becomes your trust in the movement that allows you to relax into a more cooperative posture. This more relaxed posture allows the foot to begin relaxing, which then allows it to begin flexing. This is required for improving abilities, because a relaxed, flexing foot provides the foundation, support, and push that produce improved abilities.

So, when does this flattened-foot feeling occur in every stride? It occurs in the middle of the stride. It happens when the body is centered over the one foot on the floor, and as the lifted foot is passing by the foot on the floor (picture 3 of Figure 22.1). Importantly, the flattened-foot concept in the walking stride means the foot is permitted to flex naturally during the movement as the person's ability allows it.

This is the *only* feeling in the advanced foot that is of concern or importance, until the advanced foot becomes the pushing foot. Why? Two reasons. First, it signals the stability of the advanced foot. Second, until this pressure happens, the back (pushing) foot is the one important foot for the movement. But some people will say, "It is important to feel the 'rolling' of the foot from heel to toe." *No!* It is not, and for the movement impaired, that arbitrary concept can be very confusing.

Remember, as the advanced foot makes contact with the floor, the pressure in its heel is character-istically a rather light, passive pressure, because the pushing foot is still supporting the body and push-

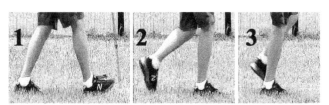

FIGURE 21.1: Pushing forward onto and balancing momen-tarily on a functionally flat foot during a stride (picture 3).

ing the body forward. If the advanced foot's heel pressure is higher when it contacts the floor, it means two not-so-good things are happening. First, when the knees are not relaxed, the higher heel pressure in the advanced foot is pushing the body backward. Second, the higher heel pressure in the advanced foot means the pressure in the back, pushing foot is weaker and is not supporting or propelling the body forward as it should be.

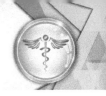

As a side note, some of you may comment that the forward knee is not flexing very much in Figure 22.1, and you are correct. In this example, the forward knee is flexed the amount that is required for the person to feel and be stable in the controlled walking movement. This person's posture is relaxed. With a relaxed posture, the muscles in the legs are working efficiently and providing exactly the correct amount of downward pressure. What is the important message here? The amount your knee needs to flex depends on what is needed to move onto and stabilize your body on the advanced foot. The amount of required flexing always depends on the feeling of what is right for you in that movement and at that moment, and *not on a thought of some arbitrary amount.* You are only searching to find and build trust in **your** correct feeling while doing the movement to the best of your ability. Keep things as simple as you can, to allow yourself to recognize what's right for you according to what your body needs when it happens.

Use Both Feet and Both Knees—Always

All movements begin, continue, and end with pushing stabilizing pressure down into both feet. Remember this. Do not release the pressure and support from the pushing foot even after the advanced foot becomes the pushing foot. In fact, in continuous movements, the pressure in the pushing foot is not "released." Instead, it is transferred to the other foot during the movement of the body and the transfer of body weight. Therefore, the back foot comes off the floor as all the pressure and body weight is transferred to the advanced foot, the new pushing foot. Do not think about when it's time for this to happen. It will happen naturally on its own. Simply use the pressure in both feet when both feet are in contact with the floor, and then just the one foot when it is on the floor by itself. This will ensure that your body is fully supported and stabilized, and your relaxing body will then be able to produce the movement more naturally. There will be much more on this in later chapters.

Lift the Heel, Push the Body, Revisited

Louise's movement impairment was mild, and she stated that she did not feel fearful in any of her movements. In support of that, the pictures in Figure 22.2 show her relaxed posture. However, this example shows that she has developed a reluctance to complete her forward movements. This is a reason why she stops well short of completing the forward movement onto a flattened advanced foot in picture 5.

To better see what is and what is not happening in this example, compare the movements and posture of the person (me) in the background with Louise's. In picture 5, I have completed the forward movement onto a functionally flat foot, with the toe of the shoe, knee, and shoulder very close to vertical alignment. In contrast, Louise does not complete the movement onto her forward foot. Her toe, knee, and shoulder are not in vertical alignment, as the green reference line shows. What's causing this?

In pictures 1 through 3, Louise begins the forward stride with a weak push from a flattened and slightly flexing back foot (red arrow). This push, and the fact that her heel lifts only slightly in picture 5, is inadequate to move her body completely through the movement, and this posture leaves increased pressure in the advanced foot's heel area. This is a common cause of the forward-movement instability problems many movement-impaired people begin to struggle with.

The push from my flexing back foot is strong in Figure 22.2. The lifting heel pushes my body forward beyond the *light and passive pressure in the heel area* of the flattening advanced foot. Very importantly, when the heel of my advancing foot contacts the floor, *the only weight (pressure) going into it is the weight of the advancing leg.*

In contrast, when the heel of Louise's advancing foot contacts the floor, she immediately begins to transfer body weight into it. The increased pressure in the advanced foot's heel then resists and slows the forward movement of her knee and body, because it is pushing against and negating the weak forward push from the pushing foot.

This causes instability, but in this example, Louise is relaxed enough to remain stable. She overcomes the backward pushing pressure from her heel by flexing both knees (picture 5). This pushes increased downward pressure into both feet. It also moves some of the pressure forward out of the heel area of the advanced foot. After this, she increased the pushing pressure in the back foot to flex the foot to continue pushing her body forward with the lifting heel to complete the movement.

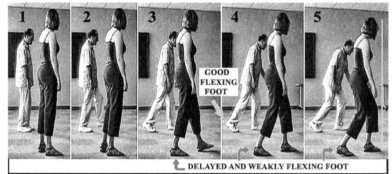

FIGURE 22.2: This shows an unrecognized reluctance to move forward onto the flattened advanced foot. This creates instability from the increased heel pressure in the forward foot pushing the body backward, as well as the inadequate downward stabilizing pressure in the forward foot.

Caution: Louise's mild instability situation shown in pictures 1 through 4 is a very common mistake many people with a mild impairment are not aware they're making. Yes, they do feel the instability, but it is not yet an alarming situation. However, they are reacting to it, and it is becoming more of a conscious reaction. With the mild instability, they begin adding very subtle postural guarding in their movements, with detrimental effects. The forward push weakens while the heel pressure in the advanced foot increases in midstride. This heel pressure frequently causes the body's forward movement to pause, and all too often pushes the body backward.

Minutes after the example in Figure 22.2, Louise stood in the same posture as shown in picture 4. I asked if she felt stable, and she responded, "I think so." I then asked her, "Where is the increased pressure in your forward foot?" "All over. It's flat," she said.

"Okay. I'd like you to test it to make sure," I replied. "To do that, don't change anything about your posture and slowly squat straight down to touch your fingers to the floor." What would you, the reader, expect to happen?

Without changing her posture, as she began to squat, the increasing pressure in the heel of her forward foot pushed her body backward, up and out of the squat. This is exactly what happens to many of you during your movements. This issue has been the cause of a great many of your movement problems and accidents. To eliminate the problem, you must focus on continuing to push your body forward from the ball area and toes of the back foot—the pushing *and flexing* one. This will also help you use the ball area and toes of the pushing foot to support your body better during the advancing movement, and keep the pressure off the advanced foot's heel.

USING, STRENGTHENING, AND BALANCING
ON THE BALL AREA AND TOES

Natural movements require the strength and ability to support your body with only the ball area and toes of the pushing foot. This is necessary to allow the pushing foot to flex and lift its heel to move your body. It also keeps pressure out of the heel area of the advancing foot when it contacts the floor. To have confidence in this ability, you must be able to stand and walk on just that area of both feet without the need for support. Doing this may sound impossible to some, but many of you doubters do have the physical ability to do it. You simply don't trust yourselves to do it.

So, getting up onto the forward area of the feet is the next exercise in our path to improved walking. For support during the practice, you can use a smooth wall, a high countertop, a grab bar or railing, or any other stable object.

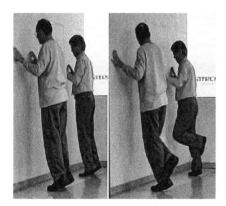

FIGURE 22.3: A slight forward lean of the body moves the pressure in the feet to the ball areas and toes. With fingertips on the wall to steady you, balance on the ball areas and toes, then push into them to move your body upward. Then relax the pressure to lower yourself. The up-and-down movement of your heels raises and lowers your body.

The first objective is to stand and find your balance on only the ball areas and toes of your feet. Then you are to repeatedly raise and lower both heels (at the same time) while keeping the pressure in the ball areas and toes. This exercises your calf muscles. In this exercise, pay very close attention to where the pressure is in your feet and how a small movement of your posture changes it.

Stand facing a smooth wall with your feet about shoulder width apart, and your toes slightly more than one length of your foot away from the wall. For support and to help you stay focused on the exercise, place the *fingertips* of both hands on the wall at approximately shoulder height, as shown in Figure 22.3. Now, slowly lean forward to move increased pressure onto the ball areas and toes of your feet, while remembering to relax and flex your elbows. Pay attention to how this forward-leaning posture removes pressure from your heels.

Initially in this setup, many movement-impaired people will lean too far forward, to rest on the palms of their hands. They do this because of leg and foot weakness, postural stiffness, or simple lack of trust in being on and using just the forward part of the feet. Also, because of these same issues, other people will not lean forward enough, and will then move their fingers to the wall with outstretched arms.

Holding the pressure and balancing on the ball areas and toes of the feet is required in natural movements. Therefore, becoming comfortable with this posture and pressure is key to more complex movement abilities. So, standing at the wall in the leaning-forward setup posture, feel and become comfortable with the increased pressure in the ball areas and toes of your feet. Also feel for a light pressure in your fingertips, and not a heavy pressure from too much of a forward lean. Support your body with your feet, not your hands. Hint: Pushing added pressure into your feet and carefully adjusting your body lean so the pressure feels stable in the ball areas and toes is the way to adjust the pressure in your fingertips.

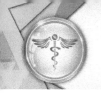

Next, to push your body upward, hold this posture, and push extra pressure into the ball areas and toes of both feet. This will lift both your heels, as shown in the first picture, and push your body upward. Helpful tips:

1. With or without straightened knees, the key is to have a relaxed posture. Re-relax your hands, elbows, shoulders, and knees frequently to help you relax your feet. Then do the movement by slowly increasing the downward push into the ball areas and toes. Feel the pressure and the heel movement. Adjust your posture and correct any mistakes to remain on the ball areas and toes.

2. This movement will feel odd to some. When you do it correctly, you'll feel your upper body and head move slightly forward as your heels lift. This is because *your body is moving upward at the same angle at which it began in the setup posture.* The key to the upward movement is twofold: First, stay focused on holding the pressure stable in the ball areas and toes. Second, increase the pressure to *push* your heels up, to move your body and remain balanced in the movement. Learn to trust that feeling and stability.

3. What about the coming back down? Hold the forward-leaning posture to hold the pressure in the ball areas and toes, and then simply begin to relax the pressure. As the pressure pushing you up is slowly relaxed, your heels and body will slowly move back down. Keep your shoulders in the same forward position. Moving them backward will quickly set you back on your heels and pull your hands off the wall as you tip and possibly fall backward.

4. If you begin to wobble or teeter, increase the downward pressure in your feet and relax your heels to the floor, while also slightly bending your knees. Now restabilize and go back through your relaxation and setup routine. Feel and find where you made a mistake.

    If your toes are too close to the wall, you will easily tip backward.

    If your toes are too far away from the wall, you will lean too much into your fingers, and/or your elbows will be extended to hold your fingers against the wall.

5. Some of you will shrug your shoulders upward to help the movement. Remember, you are practicing postural control and heel lifts, *not* shoulder and head lifts.

No Support

In Figure 22.4, Karey is practicing heel lifts as if he were reaching for something high up on a shelf. In picture 1, he increases the pressure in the ball areas and toes of his feet. Then, in pictures 2 through 5, his heels are moving upward and pushing his body upward. Note that his hand moves closer to the mark on the ceiling, and this upward movement is the exact same amount as the upward movement of his heels.

As his body is pushed upward, it also angles slightly forward, as you can see by comparing the position of his hand, arm, and head with the line on the ceiling in pictures 1 through 5. Also, note that his body has moved slightly forward with respect to the red reference line in picture 5. There are two reasons for this. First, the pressure in his feet moves slightly forward during the movement. Second, his postural

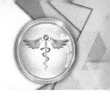

alignment is angled forward in the setup and doesn't change. Therefore, the angled forward movement of his body is the effect of his heels pushing his already angled body upward.

Now set yourself a goal. To gain the strength and confidence required for improved movement ability, gain the ability to do this movement correctly on both feet for twenty-five repetitions without stopping. Next, keep working to gain the strength to do it twenty-five times with all of your body weight on only one foot by itself, and then the other foot, as shown in the second picture of Figure 22.3.

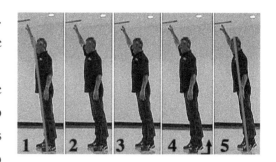

FIGURE 22.4: Karey pushes increased pressure down into the ball areas and toes of his feet to lift his heels, to push his body upward.

This ability provides you with the strength, coordination, and stability your movements demand, especially in forward movements such as walking.

Pushing from and Flexing the Foot

In most of our natural movements, the pressure in the ball area and toes of our pushing foot is by far the most important pressure involved. Why? *The relaxed use of this pressure determines the stability and direction of most of our movements, and controls them.*

With the pressure in the ball area and toes of the flexing foot, *and* with the lifting heel, we push our body through forward and sideward movements. In natural movement, these two forces from the foot combine to provide one continuous pushing force ensuring that the distance the body travels is exactly what is required for the intended movement.

Practicing the Push

Developing, feeling, using, and trusting the support of the push produced from the ball area and toes of one flexing foot is a must. In the top panel of Figure 22.5, I am using the treadmill's handlebar for support. I lean forward on the ball area and toes of my right foot while flexing the elbow of the hand that's holding the bar. With my relaxed body stabilized, I push into the ball area and toes of the foot to flex the foot and lift the heel to move my body forward—which my relaxed, flexing elbow allows. Note the shortening of the distance between my right shoulder and my left hand on the bar. It is the same distance the heel moves upward (green arrows).

In the bottom panel, Jack is doing the same pushing exercise with one heel while standing on both feet without external support. The increased pressure in the ball area and toes stabilizes and holds the pushing foot firmly in place. The foot flexes and lifts the heel to push his body forward. You can see Jack's forward movement by checking the positions of his head with respect to the equipment in the background. In picture 3, his front foot is flattened, and his shoulder, knee, and toe are in good vertical alignment. The continued pushing pressure from his back foot and the pressure in his flattened front foot stabilize his body.

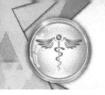

Problems Starting a Forward Stride: Review

The following are typical transfer-of-body-weight mistakes and problems:

1. By far, the most common problem a movement-impaired person has when *beginning* a forward movement is transferring their body weight completely onto the ball area and toes of just one foot, and then holding it there and using it.

2. Another very common problem people with a restrictive posture experience, is straightening of the knees during the transfer of body weight onto one foot. This is most often a result of the shoulders moving up and backward, and the instability of the one foot on the floor. With the changing positions of the knees and shoulders, the location of the pressure in the foot moves toward the heel. This alters everything about the movement. The intended forward movement now begins with instability as a slowed movement, an angled movement, a non-movement, or a backward movement.

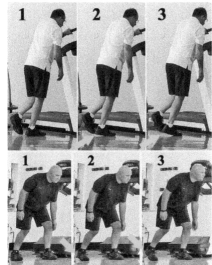

FIGURE 22.5: The combination of the force of the push from the ball area and toes, and the lifting back foot's heel, pushes the body forward.

3. When *only the shoulders* move backward during the weight shift to one foot, the most common result is that the pushing pressure in the foot moves back and creates a flat foot. Then there is no forward push to speak of.

4. When the *shoulders move backward and the knees straighten*, the increased pressure migrates into the heel area. Then the push of the body is backward at an angle. Frequently, the weight shift was incomplete so the push is from the inside of the heel. When the transfer of body weight to the advanced foot is excessive the push is from the outside of the heel.

5. When the transfer of body weight is incomplete and the pressure stays forward in the foot, the increased pressure located in the forward inside of the foot pushes the body forward at an angle. This happens frequently to mildly and moderately movement-impaired people and produces a widened gait.

Reminders and Common Issues

1. The upper body sets and controls the *location* of the pressure in the foot for the movement to begin. Then, during most movements, only small adjustments to upper-body position are needed to hold the pressure stable in that same location in each repetitive pushing foot.

2. The function of the legs is to transfer body weight between the feet, and to apply the required additional pressure into the feet to keep the body supported and stable.

3. The function of the feet is to use the pressure to power and complete the movement.

   When the posture is **not** relaxed, the push is frequently weakened. This creates instability in two ways:

4. The guarded or stiffened pushing foot has decreased ability to fully support the body's weight.

5. The flexing of the pushing foot is restricted, giving it less ability to push the body through and control the movement.
   The most common result: The pressure moving into the advanced foot stops in the heel area and begins pushing the body backward. This unexpected backward pressure triggers additional postural guarding and stiffening, which further increases instability and disruption of the movement.

   A common question is, "If the push was too weak to move the body forward to complete the weight transfer onto the advanced foot, how can body weight continue to move onto the forward foot?" This happens in two ways:

1. The additional body weight moving forward comes from excessive upper-body movement.

2. When the weak push from the back foot slows or stops moving the body forward, the advanced foot immediately begins to be used for support.

STIFFNESS

When your knees are stiff, your feet will be stiffer. This is the difficulty Rhoda is having in Figure 22.6. This sequence of pictures shows her taking one stride forward onto her right foot in pictures 1 through 6, and shows the stiffening of her forward knee (red arrow in picture 7). Also note in pictures 4 through 7 that her upper body is moving forward (indicated by the long red arrow), while her feet are essentially stuck on the floor. She tips forward on the toes of both stiffened feet in pictures 7 and 8, as indicated by the red arrow in picture 8. As her body continues moving forward in the tip, in pictures 9 and 10 she finds the ability to slightly lift her right knee, and then reset the advancing right foot with a flexing knee (green arrows in picture 10). Then, in pictures 10 through 12, she adds another correction to the forward tipping movement: by moving her upper body backward into better alignment. This moves the pressure rearward

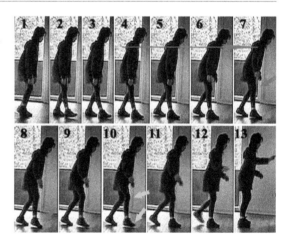

FIGURE 22.6: We control the movement of our upper body with our legs and feet. In this example, Rhoda puts her body in motion with a weak push from her left foot, but then loses control of the movement because of heel pressure in the advanced right foot.

in the right foot and helps to slow the forward movement of her body. Finally, in pictures 11 and 12, she stabilizes on the flattened right foot and moves back to both feet in picture 13.

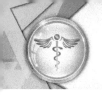

Many people with a restrictive-posture movement impairment frequently experience forward tipping like this. What caused this to happen to Rhoda? She begins the stride with a weak push from her poorly flexing left foot that does not move her body forward enough onto her right foot. This leaves pressure in the heel of the advanced right foot that resists the body moving farther forward, and also begins pushing it backward. She attempts to remedy the incorrect pressures in her feet, and the straightening knee, with forward upper-body movement. In Rhoda's example, fortunately her forward knee did not straighten and hyperextend, but her continuing forward body movement beyond the toes of the advanced foot still caused her to tip forward.

What allowed Rhoda's recovery ability? Note that in pictures 9 and 10 she begins flexing her knees. This strongly suggests that she is beginning to add additional downward stabilizing pressure into her feet. This helps to counteract the horizontal component of the pushing force, and converts some of it to the vertical component pushing force that is required for stabilization. Without doing these two things, she would not have been able to regain control of her forward body lean and tipping movement.

There is another error Rhoda corrects in her recovery. This involves transfer of body weight. She achieves a good transfer of body weight onto her left foot in picture 1. But she fares poorly in transferring weight onto her right foot until pictures 11 and 12. This transfer onto the right foot should have happened in picture 5, but it is completed as she enters recovery mode.

Tipping forward from the increased pressure in the forward areas of both feet temporarily prevents her from lifting either foot. This is an *extremely* difficult situation to correct. To stop the forward tip of the body, we naturally use our calf muscles to quickly add downward pressure into the ball area and toes of the foot, or feet. Thus, she had two components of added pressure pressing the front of her foot on the floor. One, the excessive forward lean of her body moved the increased pressure forward in the foot, and into a smaller area. This concentrated the pressure and increased the forward push. Two, she added extra pressure to that area of the foot with overactive calf muscles. This is why it is difficult to move the foot, or feet, from the floor in a forward tipping situation.

When this happens to a person with natural ability, their recovery is usually not this dramatic, because they remain more relaxed. But when it happens to the movement-impaired with a guarding posture, both legs and knees guard and stiffen more, and typically straighten. Then, as they teeter on the ball areas and toes of their feet, frequently their knees become "locked" in position. This leaves them powerless to transfer any body weight off the front of either foot, or lift a foot to reposition it, in an effort to restabilize their body.

This example serves as another reminder for those with a restrictive-posture movement impairment to keep their strides short until they have worked through the guarding and stiffness in their posture. To help keep your strides shorter, focus on beginning the movement with heavy (pressurized) baby steps, and then slowly allow the strides to lengthen as your relaxing posture allows them to. Your strides will be better controlled, with added stability. The point: You should not be attempting to take longer strides simply because you think you need to, to keep up with others as you walk. Instead, take more strides that are smaller and better controlled, to have the same effect of "keeping up" the pace.

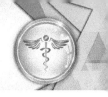

CAN YOU?

You plead to have more natural movement ability, but there seem to be so many obstacles that complicate the learning process. Plus, the process of undoing so many bad habits and challenging issues is frustratingly long, and often difficult. This is a valid reality.

However, the challenges and difficulties you face can also be viewed in a more positive perspective. For example, they repeatedly show why you must uncomplicate and simplify things as much as you possibly can. Yes, they constantly remind you of your mistakes, but you must be careful not to be overly influenced by the negativity that too often comes with them. Instead, focus on the corrections for the mistakes, because that turns the negative into a positive. Consider another positive. Focusing on learning and applying the correction reduces how often the mistake happens. Then, some of your mistakes may likely stop happening altogether.

In mind and action, be productive—not destructive.

What feels right. What feels wrong. When you know the difference between the two, ask the next questions: "What am I doing to cause this feeling?" "Why is this pressure the right pressure?" "Why is it the wrong pressure?" You must come to recognize these things in a way that makes sense to you.

With natural movement ability, you knew the feelings of your movements extremely well, and you trusted them without question. Then everything changed. Your doubting and overthinking mind convinced you that what you did before no longer applied, even though your mind had no idea what was happening. This has been your (everyone's) biggest mistake, *just as it was mine.* Therefore, your greatest challenge is working to change your misunderstanding and misconception of yourself. Only you can do that. If you don't, your life and movement abilities will continue as they are.

The choices are yours to make, and they are yours to act on.

■ ■ ■

CHAPTER 23

Sixth Stance:
Forward Stride Squats and Jumping

To correct movement problems, you must first correct postural mistakes.

The forward stride squat described here is a *modification* of that used in exercise and fitness routines by people with natural ability. Panel A of Figure 23.1 shows a forward *lunge* squat. The body is centered between the feet, with the body weight evenly distributed between the feet. This requires more strength, skill, flexibility, and balance than most movement-impaired people have. For movement-impaired individuals with limited ability, the easier and more stable way to do this movement is shown in panel B. The body is pushed onto the flattened forward foot. This puts approximately 75 percent of the body weight on the advanced foot and 25 percent on the back foot.

People with natural ability routinely do a forward lunge squat in one movement. But many people with a movement impairment, especially those with a restrictive-posture movement impairment, must do

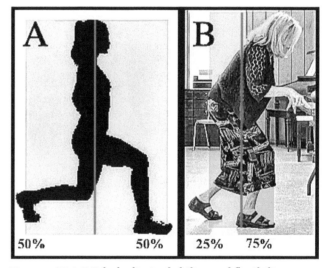

FIGURE 23.1: With the limited ability and flexibility many movement-impaired people have, moving the body forward over the flattened front foot before squatting provides the added stability they need.

This improved support allows them a better opportunity to keep their posture relaxed, which the flexing of the knees and hips requires for lower squatting.

their version in two movements. The first is taking a forward stride and centering the body over the flattened advanced foot, with the flexing back foot holding the body in position. The second movement is squatting straight down onto the flat advanced foot, and the ball area and toes of the flexed back foot, *using both knees.*

In panel B, Kathi does not push quite far enough forward onto her advanced foot. The red line is centered within her zone of stability and shows she has increased pressure in the heel. This is also seen by her

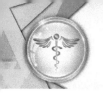

shoulder's position, not yet in vertical alignment with her knee and toes. This is why she is mildly unstable in this position. The effect: the heel of the advanced foot is pushing her body backward. Consequently, she could not lower herself any farther into the squat. Test question: What would happen if she did?

In addition, note her tensed hand and fingers. This reveals her postural guarding and stiffening. However, the strong push from the ball area and toes of the back foot is holding her in this position. The answer to the test question: If Kathi were to squat lower in this stance, the pressure in the advanced heel would increase, and increase the backward push. Is that all? The rest of the answer comes later in this chapter.

A forward stride squat is a more difficult movement than a forward stride, but only because of the added squat. However, it does not include anything new, because the individual parts of this movement have been discussed and shown in previous chapters. For example, recall the exercise of standing facing a wall while pushing your body forward with your flexing back foot and forward knee.

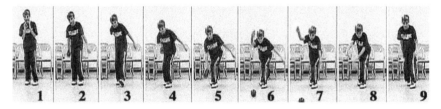

FIGURE 23.2: Jake uses the proper setup, a continued strong push, and a stable squatting posture to do a forward stride squat. For a person with a restrictive-posture movement impairment, centering the body over the front foot before squatting with both knees is the preferred forward-stride-squat method.

The good news: When you can do a forward stride squat with ease and confidence, you will have the ability to do pretty much any other basic movement you want to do. The added qualification to this statement is, *your abilities are always limited by your physical capabilities.*

The squat in this movement needs to happen more easily with a more relaxed posture, and the push into the forward stride must be stronger. This also means the push down into both feet must be stronger to hold the body stable, using both flexing knees as the body is moving forward and downward, as Jake is demonstrating in Figure 23.2.

PRESSURE DISTRIBUTION

There are three different squatting postures in Figure 23.3. In picture 1, Jia and Min are squatting centered over both flattened feet. In picture 2, Wei is in a forward stride squat over a flattened front foot. In picture 3, Jon is in a squat to the side over a flattened left foot. Study these pictures to answer this question: For each person, which foot increases in pressure as the person lowers into the squat?

If you don't know the answer, don't sit and try to guess what you think it should be. Stand up. Experiment. Get in the same postures. Squat and feel what the correct answer is as you do them yourself. Know the answer by feeling it.

Feel the results. Which foot increases in pressure when you squat straight down on both flat feet, as in picture 1? The pressure increases in both feet.

Now pictures 2 and 3. When you take a stride forward or to the side, and then squat with your body centered over the advanced foot, which foot increases in pressure? By far, the most common response is, "The one I'm standing over. The pressure increases in the flat foot that my body is centered over, the

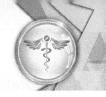

one I'm squatting down onto." But this is **not** the correct answer.

My reply: "Is that what you are physically feeling, or is that what you think you *should* be feeling? Repeat the movement, and this time only feel what you feel and ignore what you think."

Most people give me a puzzled look before repeating the movement. Then, thinking they must have been wrong the first time, on this second attempt their answer most often is, "Okay, now I think my other foot became heavier with pressure."

"Good!" I tell them. "You're finally paying some

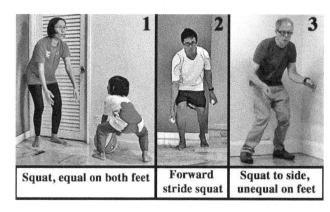

| Squat, equal on both feet | Forward stride squat | Squat to side, unequal on feet |

FIGURE 23.3: Whether we're centered over both feet or one foot, the continued use of both feet is critical to the movement.

attention to your other foot. But no, that still is not the correct answer. To feel the correct answer, stop thinking about what you think the correct answer should or must be. Just *feel* the answer as you do it again. Focus only on *what you are feeling* **in both feet**. Remember to relax your hands and elbows to relax your knees. This will allow you to go lower in the squat to feel the increasing pressure."

Admittedly, on this third try, most people have become so confused that they respond, "I don't know." Many of you will have this same experience. Your mind will be confused because it thought it knew the easy answer, and that is where you repeatedly went for the answer. So, you need to feel what your mama is telling you the correct answer is, and before you start, you need to simplify things. Start by squatting over both flat feet and remind yourself by feeling the pressure increasing equally in both feet, as Jia is demonstrating in Figure 23.4. The pressure is equally

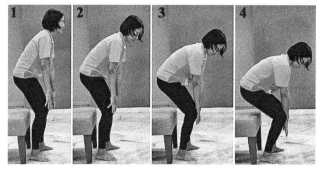

FIGURE 23.4: In this squatting movement, Jia remains very close to being centered over both feet. This means the pressure in both feet is equal throughout her feet in every picture, as the pressure increases in both feet.

distributed in both feet in the beginning and increases equally in both feet in each picture because her body is centered on her feet. Take this piece of information and pay close attention to the other two squats, because where the body is centered is causing an irrational hiccup in your mind.

Now take a sideward or forward stride and center your body over the advanced foot. Feel the pressure in both feet. Now slowly squat straight down over the flattened advanced foot and feel what happens to the pressure in both feet. Next, feel the pressure in both feet as you slowly stand straight up, and then slowly squat down low again.

The difference between the two feet is the percentage of the total pressure being applied to each foot. The flattened foot your body is centered over begins with more pressure, and the pressure increases a great deal during the squat. That is the reason your focus goes to it.

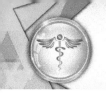

Now focus on the smaller amount of pressure in the ball area and toes of the other foot before you squat, and feel this next part very carefully. As you slowly squat with your body centered over the flattened foot, the pressure in this foot also increases in pressure. Why? You are still using it for support.

This is *always* the case when both feet are in contact with the floor and providing support for the body. The very important point to remember is, when you are using both feet for support, they will both have increasing pressure moving into them during your movements.

This explains the numbers under the picture in panel B of Figure 23.1. Kathi's back foot has approximately 25 percent of the total pressure, and her front foot has approximately 75 percent. Now consider what the percentage of the pressure in each foot will be when she stands straight up while staying in this same position on her feet. The pressure in her feet will still be the same 25 percent and 75 percent of the total pressure. The distribution stays the same. Only the amount of the pressure will change as she moves from the squatting posture to the upright posture.

Both pressures are equally important. In this example, the pressure in the flattened foot is supporting the majority of the body weight. The pressure in the ball area and toes of the other foot is supporting less of the body weight but is stabilizing the movement of the body. Therefore, the pressures in both feet are equally important to the body's stability and movement.

Overuse of the Upper Body

Eric was struggling to remain stable while practicing forward stride squats. Figure 23.5 shows what is and what is not correct in his movement, and why he was unhappy with the results.

Leading up to the throw in pictures 1 through 4, Eric's setup looks okay. However, when you pay attention to his legs and feet, you'll see that it is not.

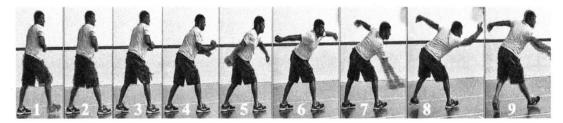

FIGURE 23.5: In this example, Eric's upper- and lower-body movement is unmatched and unco-ordinated. Overdependency on his stronger upper body forces instability on his feet, which is worsened by weaker legs. Having increased upper-body strength to "muscle" the movement will never replace the function and purpose of the legs. Our movements require the coordinated functioning and use of the entire body.

1. He begins with an inadequate push from a flattened and stiffened back foot.

2. The weak push causes him to come down heavily on the heel area of the advancing foot (picture 1). Now the significantly increasing heel pressure in the advanced foot leads to instability that causes the forward knee to straighten in picture 2. With this heel pressure forcefully held in place throughout all

the pictures, the flexing ability of the forward knee is greatly restricted and stops his body's forward movement. His legs, knees, and feet are uncontrollably held in place.

3. On unstable feet, he continues to throw the one-kilogram ball using only his arms with forced upper-body movement, causing his upper body to come uncontrollably forward in pictures 7 and 8. This creates additional instability and pulls his back foot off the floor (picture 8)—and then he fell immediately after picture 9.

This is a *very, very common* problem for many people with a moderate restrictive-posture movement impairment. When their knees and feet become the least bit guarded or stiffened, their upper- and lower-body movements rapidly become uncoordinated and unsynchronized. This greatly reduces their ability to support, stabilize, and control their posture to complete the intended movement.

Eric's series of mistakes begins before the movement does. It begins in his setup posture, which he did not pay attention to. Instead, he was focused on throwing the ball. Because it "automatically" happens without thought for most people with natural ability, there typically is no need to focus on having the proper setup posture for most of their activities. However, when unnatural restrictions hinder our natural ability, our focus must be directed toward making the best possible postural adjustments in the setup, and then toward the activity. Without the stability and cooperative functioning of the body in the movement, the results of the activity will always be less than desired.

Eric worked on relaxing, flexing his knees, and pushing from the ball area and toes of his foot. When he was patient and focused, he did much better and managed coordinated movements. However, when he lost focus and patience, his old habits and bodybuilding routines quickly led him into another upper-body-induced uncoordinated movement. This overuse of the upper body happens frequently with restrictive postures.

So, everyone with impaired movements and a restrictive-posture, any time we are experiencing *any* stiffening or straightening of our knees, we must be very patient with ourselves. We must take the time to focus on the proper setup posture, taking the time time to relax and stay relaxed, and then doing better in smaller movements.

There is another issue that must be remembered with regard to exercising to strengthen the body. Include stretching in your strengthening workouts for overall better results.

STIFF KNEES

Stiffening and straightening knees are a primary source of problems for many people with a restrictive-posture movement impairment. In panel A of Figure 23.6, Mike is trying his best to move onto a flattened advanced foot and then squat to roll the ball on the floor. But his knees and feet are too stiff to allow it. Then, in panel B, he does manage it.

In panel A, he begins with straightened knees. In panel B, his setup posture is much better, with flexed knees, but still it lacks the same important thing that is missing in panel A.

In picture 2 of both panels, the push from his left foot is weak. Now look at the pushing foot from start to finish. In both panels, it stays flat on the floor. A flattened, non-flexing, stiffened foot produces a very weak push.

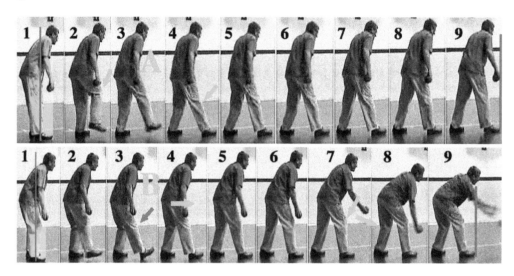

FIGURE 23.6: A common cause of a poor outcome is a poor setup. In both panels, Mike's weight shift onto his left foot in picture 1 is good, but the push from his back foot is too weak to propel his body forward. The left, pushing foot remains stiffly flat on the floor in every picture. The weak push results in the increased heel pressure in the advanced foot that stops his body's forward movement (picture 4 in panel A; pictures 3 and 4 in panel B). This, combined with his stiff right knee, creates instability at the beginning of both movements.

In panel A, Mike is so intent on moving the knee forward that he forgets about where the pressure needs to be in the pushing foot. In panel B, he begins with a focus on having increased pressure in the ball areas of both feet, with knees flexed in picture 1. But the inserted green zone of stability shows that he begins with flat feet in both panels, as shown by the centered red line in the zone.

In picture 2 of panel A, he flexes his right knee forward, but then, in picture 3, he extends it to push the advancing foot forward. In picture 2 of panel B, he extends the knee, and in picture 3, again pushes the advancing foot forward. Then, in picture 5 in both panels, he is centered over both feet with mildly flexed knees. What happens next in picture 6 in both panels determines the outcome.

The movement is compromised. In panel A, his knees remain stiffened. He is unstable, cannot squat, and cannot roll the ball. In panel B, his knees flex. He is stable and does roll the ball.

Your knees will be one of your most troublesome and most difficult things to control in your postures, stances, and movements. When your knees don't flex easily, everything you try to do will be harder. As you try harder, frequently the result is the knees stiffen even more. Stiff knees create stiffer feet, and stiffened feet create stiffer knees and postures. So remember, your feet will not begin to relax until your knees are more relaxed, and the push will always be weaker from a stiffened, non-flexing foot. The solution to work toward is relaxing into the posture and movement to create a cooperative posture, rather than trying harder with an uncooperative posture.

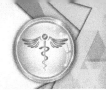

JUMPING

Kids lower themselves into a squat and then easily jump up into the air, which is what Ken and Keri are practicing in Figure 23.7. Jumping requires the sudden and vigorous use of the calf muscles. They forcefully push a great deal of pressure into the ball areas and toes of the feet, and then very quickly flex the feet to push the body upward.

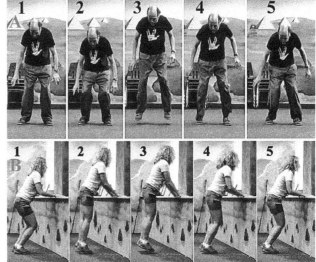

Can you jump like this? Many of you can, but rightfully do not trust doing it. The very beginning of the jumping process is knowing how to squat and stabilize on flattened feet. The next part is having the ability to squat with your body forward and balanced on the ball areas and toes of both feet, and hold it there during the going-up and coming-down movements. The rest of it is a matter of strength, coordination, and relaxed postural control.

The midball areas and toes of the feet quickly push the body up. And, very importantly, this is also where your posture and the pressure need to be when you come down from the jump, to provide you with stability, control, and a softer landing on the floor. Squat to go up, and squat when you come down. You must have a relaxed and coordinated posture to stay forward and to flex your knees and feet—especially when landing.

FIGURE 23.7: Jumping uses the powerful calf muscles and easily flexing feet. A relaxed, cooperative posture keeps the location of the pressure in the ball areas and toes, and allows the hips, knees, and ankles to flex freely.

Think of this in terms of sitting in a speeding car as it goes over a bump in the road. The bump forces the car up, and then it comes down hard on the road. If the shock absorbers are good, then the force of the car coming back down to the road is softened. Your body also has "shock absorbers" for this same purpose. *Your knees, hips, and ankles work as the shock absorbers* of your body. These joints must be flexible as your feet contact the floor to soften your landing, as shown in Figure 23.8.

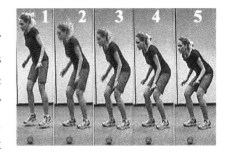

This takes practice for the movement-impaired person. Many of us need to remind ourselves constantly to keep our shoulders forward and flex our knees, so we start and end on the ball areas of our feet.

This movement requires dedicated practice to learn how to hold the correct posture throughout. *This is especially true when coming back down*, to end in the posture in which you began. Keeping shoulders forward and knees flexed will be the most difficult parts for the restrictive-posture movement impaired. Many will come down with a stiff and upright posture, causing instability and tipping back on their heels. To help avoid this, when coming down, think and say the reminder, "Shoulders forward. Knees down. Squat!" (Figure23.8).

FIGURE 23.8: Many movement-impaired people need to force themselves to hold their shoulders forward. If they don't, their knees will be too straight, and flexing their knees will be difficult in the hard and jolting landing. Stay forward on the ball areas of your feet.

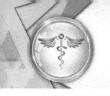

For those who need it, use something solid and stable for support, as Keri is doing in panel B of Figure 23.7. But when you use a support, another factor comes into play. Now you must also remind yourself to keep your elbows flexible while limiting the pressure pushing into your hands. Another option is to have someone with good balance and strength standing in front of you and firmly holding your hands during the practice. But that person must also keep their elbows flexible so they don't unknowingly restrict your movement. Remember, though, even with the support of something or someone, you are still responsible for your stability and movements.

Be patient as you experiment with this. Start with small, jump-like movements much like children's "bunny hopping" if you need to, and many of you will need to do this. Also, try not to be so embarrassed or intimidated that you refuse to try it. Start with small hops to feel and experiment with what is happening in the fronts of your feet.

HOOPS

In Figure 23.9, Joe is practicing shooting hoops. What else is he working on? While playing the game, he is also working on squatting, jumping, postural control, and coordinated movement. He is practicing keeping his posture relaxed, staying forward over the ball areas and toes of his feet, flexing his knees, doing heel lifts, and coming down from a small "jump." In this example, he is doing very well with the going-up part of it, but the coming down still needs some work. As he descends, his posture stiffens and knees straighten. He ends the movement standing upright with increased pressure still toward the ball areas of his feet.

What's happening? As he pushes the ball up toward the hoop, he appears to be relaxed in pictures 1 through 5. But in picture 6, this begins to change.

In pictures 1 through 6, he is up on the balls and toes of his flexing feet with good postural alignment. In picture 7, he still has increased pressure in the ball areas of his feet as he is recovering from the upward

movement. In picture 8, his upper body has moved backward. Then, in picture 9, he is stiffly holding his arms in a guarded posture with straightened knees. What happens in pictures 2 through 5 to yield this result?

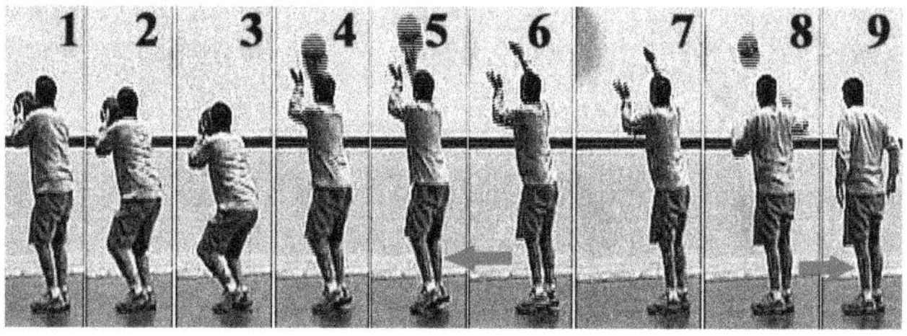

Going up, Joe uses his calf muscles correctly, but he doesn't relax them afterward. Holding them tensed in pictures 6 through 9 is the main cause of his knees not flexing, his upper body moving backward, and the postural stiffness that ensues. So, why did he keep these muscles tensed?

When a person is standing on the ball areas and toes of their feet and feeling unstable tipping forward, the natural response is to use the calf muscles to push added downward pressure into the ball areas to stabilize the body to prevent the forward tip. Thanks to years of frequent instability with increased pressure toward the front of their feet, many people with a restrictive-posture movement impairment learn to overuse these muscles, even at the hint of tipping

FIGURE 23.9: Shooting the ball toward the hoop is the same movement as jumping, with added arm involvement: squatting, pushing down from the ball areas and toes of both feet to push the body up, and then coming back down with a relaxed posture on the ball areas and toes. Coming down relaxed and flexing is often the most challenging part of the movement for those with a restrictive posture.

forward. In time, using the calf muscles becomes an immediate overreaction. This is very difficult for them to stop doing.

Joe was again exhibiting this response even though he was *not* unstable on the ball areas and toes of his feet. He held his calf muscles tight. This caused his feet and knees to stiffen. Then the rest of him stiffened, which intensified when his upper body moved backward in picture 8. This shoulder movement induced another *sub*conscious fear of tipping backward, even though he was not, which created additional stiffening.

POWER, CONTROL, AND MORE FUN

The power in a basketball shot comes in large part from the legs and feet, with the sudden push from the ball areas and toes of the feet. The same is true of rolling (throwing) the weighted ball across the floor, as Eric and Mike were doing in the previous examples. In walking movements, and other similar movements and activities, the push from the ball area and toes is the power.

Yes, you are also using your arms in many activities. But your legs and feet are supplying the power to control the movement and stabilize your body. Consider it this way. The proper use of the legs and feet allows the relaxed upper body and arms to do their parts of the movement.

Even as an adult, "play time" shows and teaches you many things. Playing and enjoying different activities brings things into a better perspective with much more clarity than just "walking practice." Yes, walking practice is important, but it is only a very small part of what you must do in order to reclaim your lost movement skills and abilities. Play to find and re-create them, just as you did to learn them the first time as a child.

Enjoying the activity allows you to release your mind from overfocusing on what you think you should be doing with your movements. Through play, you learn to relax your mind and body, and allow your body's improved cooperative ability to happen. Through play, you set challenges for yourself that you otherwise wouldn't experience, and these give you additional learning opportunities.

Those who practice a great deal in play will improve their movements more quickly than those who do not play. This is nature's way and nature's rules. Not mine.

Which games should you play? You decide. There are no hard-and-fast rules. Try some of the examples you see in this book. Definitely try some of your own, and also try some from any other source. Experiment. There is an abundance of choices. Use your imagination. Give yourself permission.

WATCH THE YOUNG PEOPLE

Young people tend to stay active and are very resilient. The movement-impaired young people I have worked with have had far less guarding, less stiffness, and less fear than the adults. This remains true even when the youths have the same level of physical impairment and the same disorder as the adults. Jake was one of these young people (Figure 23.10).

Jake's posture and movements were not "perfect." He simply was able to use what he had more freely than most adults do. Because of that, on the days we worked, his immediate concerns were not so much about his movement impairment. Instead, they were more directed toward the challenge of the activity. With this focus, his mistakes only caused him to try to do better the next time, especially with his brother lobbing challenging comments from the sidelines. That brotherly competition and encouragement was helpful and gave him another outlet to take his mind off his disorder. In all of it, Jake did what he could

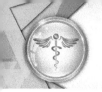

because he wanted to be as normal as he could be. Because of this, he tried his best without complaints of what his disorder would or would not let him do. He allowed himself to play and learn with the challenges in the room, and then he did better and enjoyed the outdoor games and challenges even more.

This is a valuable point for adults. *Be the kid.* Allow yourself to play and do it your way, using the younger-person mind-set. Accept the challenge of playing with friends and family. Allow yourself to make mistakes and learn from them. Make an effort to stop being so apologetic for everything you do. Stop apologizing for the mistakes you "know" you're going to make, and those you do make. Stop apologizing for living and having the issues your disorder or condition has brought upon you. Stop complaining, and give your mouth a rest. Get off your bottom. Learn what you can do to improve your situation. Find the things you *do* have the ability to do. Stop saying and thinking, "I can't!"

◼ ◼ ◼

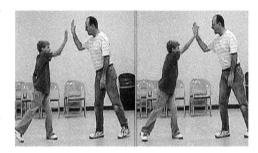

FIGURE 23.10: When doing a high five, move into it with a forward stride, and hold it. The power and control of your hand comes from the push of your back foot.

A younger person's focus is on the game and having fun. This takes their attention away from their difficulties and allows them to have fun despite their problems. So very many adults need to relearn this.

CHAPTER 24

PUTTING IT TOGETHER

With fear in my belly I stand, staring at the problems before me.
So many people. So many steps. So many things scattered on the floor.
These things prevent me from going where I would like to go.

My *phone buzzes with her name appearing* on the small screen. "Hey, Julie. How are you doing up there?"

"I'm doing great, but Oscar is having problems with his walking again. He's having difficulty going up and down the steps and crossing the room, even with someone helping him. He is lifting and pointing his knee when he walks, and he's holding his back foot with pressure just as you told him to do when you were here. We can't figure out why he's not walking better than he is. He walks super slowly and says he feels like he can't move. Tom, his walking ability is going downhill again. Sadly, it's probably due to the progression of his Parkinson's. Can you give us some suggestions that we could use to try to help him do better?"

Oscar's movements are significantly impaired, which means he moves with the typical Parkinson's narrow gait in a very slow, shuffling walk. A year before this call, I had worked with him and his personal trainer, Julie, for a couple of weeks. During those sessions, he had achieved notably good results. His movements and walking ability had improved, and he was walking with more stability and independence. Still, the report I just heard from Julie didn't surprise me, because Oscar leads a very sedentary lifestyle. He seldom leaves the house, and he spends the vast majority of his time sitting until someone forces him to do something. This makes it very easy for him to slip back into lazy, maladaptive movement behaviors and patterns.

From this small bit of information about Oscar, do your best to visualize what he is doing or not doing. Try to see and feel his posture and movements using all the information we have covered about basic movement. Combine that with what you know from your own problems and experiences, and take your mind off his diagnosis. Why? It's because the issues Oscar is having with his movements are the very same that many of you are also experiencing with a different diagnosis. Whether your diagnosis is multiple sclerosis, traumatic brain injury, viral encephalopathy, Parkinson's, SCA, MSA, DJD, HSP, or any other term, word, condition, or unknown reason, separate that and stay focused on the movement.

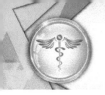

Direct your thoughts and focus toward only the basics of natural movement and the common problems people with a restrictive-posture movement impairment share in their unnatural movements. Focus purely on Oscar's present complaint: walking very slowly.

See the movement and ask, "Why do people sometimes feel they are stuck in the mud with small and slow strides? What causes them to shuffle forward instead of taking a stride?" Make it personal and ask yourself, "What is my posture when I am doing that? Why do I sometimes do this same thing?" Use the KISS principle—keep it simple.

See and feel it. Julie said Oscar is holding down pressure in his back foot, the pushing foot, when he lifts and points his advancing knee, *and* he is moving forward very slowly. What is his posture? Stand up and do what she's described. Feel it for yourself to better understand it.

From Julie's description, you know Oscar is doing a good transfer of weight onto one foot, which also means his posture is stable and relatively relaxed. This information tells you the issue with his slow movement is likely a problem with the pushing foot.

The good weight transfer to one foot strongly implies that Oscar *is not* on the forward part of his pushing foot. This also tells you he *has not* returned to his "Parkinson's shuffle." If he had, he would likely be tipping forward and not lifting the knee. The question then is, "Where is the pressure in his feet when he transfers body weight to one foot?"

The feet are FLATTENED, and the pushing foot is staying flattened and providing a very weak push. This is why he's moving slowly. He is nearly walking in place, but this actually reveals a good thing for Oscar. How? It tells us that he is doing many things correctly.

"Julie, from what you've told me, Oscar needs just one little reminder," I reply. "I will bet you he is on his flat feet, transferring from flat foot to flat foot with each attempted stride. This is why he feels stuck and is moving so slowly.

"Have him continue doing exactly what he is doing and add just one small thing. While he's standing on both feet, and before he shifts his weight to lift a knee, have him shift his shoulders slightly forward to move the pressure slightly forward toward the ball areas of his feet.

"Next, tell him to hold that pressure where it is when he transfers to one foot, and to keep doing everything else exactly as he is already doing it. I'll wait while you tell him."

Through the phone, I hear her explaining to Oscar what I said. Then, seconds later, she exclaims, "You're right! There he goes. Oh my God! Oscar, you're doing it. I missed the obvious by looking at all the other stuff. Oh my God! I can't believe it. I thought it was just his Parkinson's making him that way."

Often it is that simple. *It is so very easy to miss the obvious.*

CATHERINE

Another true story, this time from a woman with a mild movement impairment due to spinocerebellar atrophy.

Catherine called and said, "I fell again, as in the third time in as many weeks. We had been bowling. My game wasn't great, but at least I was out there doing it. I actually had some fun for a change. Well, it *was* fun until I went to return the shoes. One second I was on my feet, and the next second I hit the floor."

"What happened to make you fall?" I asked.

"I don't have a clue. I was fine, and then *wham!* I'm on the floor holding my arm. Now my shoulder hurts again, just like it did when I tore my rotator cuff. I hate this!" she replied.

"How many games did you bowl?" I asked.

"Three. And I never fell once," she said with pride.

"When you left the bowling area and headed to the counter to return your shoes, what was on the floor?"

"Not a damn thing. I just lost my footing, and *bam*, down I went," she said.

"But what was on the floor? What were you walking *on*?" I asked again.

"It was just that thin carpet like any business office has," she replied.

"That thin carpet is why you fell, kiddo," I said.

"No, it wasn't the carpet. It was just me losing my footing again," she insisted.

"Yes, it was you with your 'footing,' and yes, it *was* the carpet. Now listen while I tell you the likely reason this happened. While you were bowling, you were on a very smooth wooden floor. The bowling shoes you were wearing are designed to allow your foot to slide a little on that smooth wooden floor. Now, think back to when you were bowling. Sometimes I'm sure those shoes seemed a little too slippery, right?"

"Yes, they were," she said.

"During the three games you bowled, you gradually became more comfortable wearing them. You were able to relax more as you adjusted to your feet moving so easily on the floor. But still, sometimes you also had to be very careful not to take bigger strides because they easily slipped when you did. These things set the stage for the fall.

"Now the other issues that led to your fall: You had not done this type of activity for a long time. So, by the time you finished, your legs were feeling a little tired. The slippery bowling shoes combined with tired legs set you up for the problem with the carpet. Now think about what else you did at the end of the game.

"When you changed back to your regular shoes [she was wearing athletic-type shoes], two things suddenly changed. But one very important thing did not: The soles of your own shoes are not as smooth and slippery as the bowling-shoe soles. And the carpet wasn't as smooth as the wooden floor. What does this mean? Your shoes didn't slide on the carpet like the bowling shoes were sliding on the wooden floor.

"Now, what did not change? You were still walking on the carpet just as you had been on the wooden floor while wearing the bowling shoes. You were subconsciously expecting your shoes to slide easily on the floor. But on the carpet, your regular shoes did not.

"While you were bowling, it didn't take as much effort to walk, and you didn't need to lift your knee as high to raise the foot off the floor. This allowed you to get lazy in your movements. You became lazy shifting from foot to foot and not lifting your knees as much because your shoes were sliding readily. Then, when you put your regular shoes back on and continued walking this same way on the carpet, that lazy movement mistake and the shoe catching on the carpet is the reason you fell.

"Think back to what happened one second before you fell. You felt the bottom of the *front* of your shoe catch the carpet. Think farther back. This wasn't the first time that foot contacted the floor like this. Especially in the last game you bowled, the bottom front part of your bowling shoes often scuffed the floor. Now go back in your mind and feel again what you felt as you were walking on the carpet just before the fall. So, Catherine, what did you feel just before you fell? What did you hear?" I asked her.

"Well, because it happened so quickly, I really don't remember," she said.

"Yes, I understand that. Just pause and take a moment to think back and relive what happened. You sat down on a chair in the bowling area to change your shoes, and that's when you actually felt how tired you had become. Then you stood up, and it took a little extra effort to stabilize yourself before you started to walk. Then, when you stepped up on the carpeted area, you most likely had to pause again to steady yourself. Is that pretty close to how things went?" I asked.

"Yes, that's actually very close to what happened," she said. "My legs felt the workout from the bowling. But I don't remember feeling clumsier because of it. My legs felt a little heavy. But I thought I was still walking okay."

"Okay. Now take those feelings and think back to when you first walked on the carpet. What were your feet doing? What did you feel and hear?" I asked.

"Well, now as we are talking it through, one foot was scuffing on the floor some of the time," she admitted. "It was the bottom toward the front of the shoe. Not the tip of my shoe, but closer to under the ball of my foot. I have noticed this at other times when I'm walking but haven't paid much attention to it. But you're right. It mostly happens when I'm feeling a little worn out."

"This is why it's so important for you to understand what you feel happening in your feet. You were a little tired and a little lazy picking up your knees. Because of that, you were not completely transferring your body weight from foot to foot. This is what caused your slightly drooping front foot to come in contact with the floor too soon as it moved forward in the stride.

"When you scuffed the ball of your foot on the floor, the forward movement of your foot slowed, but your body did not. That means you tripped yourself. The slowing of the advancing foot prevented it from moving to where your body needed it to be to stop the fall. This is what caused your nose to go on that spectacularly wild, zooming-through-the-air adventure. Then your arm and shoulder tried to save your nose."

"I am so sick and tired of those kinds of thrill rides," Catherine said.

SCUFFING FOOT

In Figure 24.1, Tom is tipping out of control off the toes of his stiffened left foot for the very same reason that caused Catherine's forward fall. In picture 1, his left foot scuffs firmly on the floor and momentarily stops the foot's forward movement. This sudden stop forces an immediate and exaggerated upper-body forward lean that applies backward pressure to his straightening left knee. His left knee hyperextends, and his posture stiffens as his body continues moving forward. These events shift

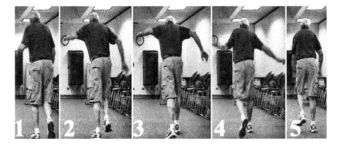

FIGURE 24.1: Tom's left foot scuffs firmly on the floor in picture 1. His legs and feet momentarily stop, but his upper body lurches forward.

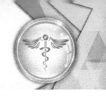

increased pressure into the toes of his left foot, causing an uncontrollable forward push from the tip of his left shoe. Suddenly, he has created an exaggerated, mismatched movement in which his upper body is ahead of and moving much faster than his legs and feet.

Fortunately, Tom *was* able to avoid falling to the floor. But his feet did not catch up with the uncontrolled forward momentum of his upper body. Luckily, he was able to stay on his feet until the far wall stopped him (Figure 24.2).

This is often a difficult, out-of-control situation for people with natural ability to correct. So, it's no surprise that it is extremely difficult to correct for most movement-impaired people. The problem is that they

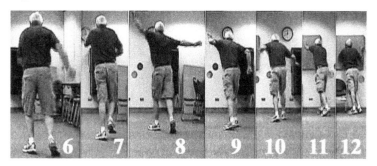

FIGURE 24.2: Uncontrolled upper-body forward momentum mixes with postural stiffness, creating an out-of-control forward movement our legs can't catch up with.

can't remove the continuing push from the increased pressure in the forward ball area and toes of their feet. Uncorrected, this pushes the person forward faster with each stride, making it more difficult to move the legs and feet fast enough to catch up with and stop the upper body's out-of-control forward movement.

KATHRYN

In her walk, Kathryn has this same shoe-scuffing problem (Figure 24.3). The red arrows in pictures 2 and 3 point to the shoe as it lightly scuffs the carpet. Tom, Catherine, and Kathryn have impaired movements. For the same reason, they all scuff the same area of the shoe as they walk. But the reason Kathryn developed a movement impairment is very different from Tom's and Catherine's reasons.

For all of them, an incomplete weight shift is the reason their shoe scuffs the floor. Because of this, the knee doesn't lift the foot high enough to keep it above the floor. Why? As Kathryn shows here, the pressure on the inside of her right foot is pushing her left foot back down to the floor. *Her left foot is at its lowest point as it passes her right foot in midstride.*

Of note, in natural movement, when the ankle and muscles controlling the foot are relaxed, the ball area of the foot is the lowest part of the foot in the midstride arc of the advancing foot.

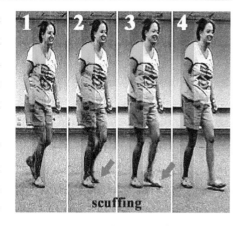

FIGURE 24.3: Kathryn scuffing the bottom of her shoe under the ball of her foot. The scuffing of the shoe interrupts the synchronized forward movement of the foot and body.

You can also see the evidence of an incomplete weight transfer in the pictures when you look at the position of Kathryn's upper body. She is leaning to the left while using her right foot. This adds body weight to her left side that is not removed when she shifts onto her right foot. This adds to the force that holds her left knee and foot lower as they move forward, and holds the pressure to the outside of the foot.

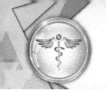

In this example, Kathryn's scuff was light and she was walking slowly. But this light scuff did have an effect, and that is her upper body moves forward out of the green zone of stability in pictures 3 and 4. The push in picture 1 sets her body in motion, and then it continues at the same rate when the scuff of her left shoe slows the rate of her left leg and foot. In this example, she easily corrects the sudden mismatched rates of movement between her upper body and lower body.

To compensate for the slowing of the scuffed foot, Kathryn lifts her left knee and moves the foot forward just a little bit faster from picture 3 to picture 4 to catch up with the movement of her upper body. This positions her left foot on the floor where her body needs it to be for the next stride. When this correction isn't completed in time, the advancing foot comes down to the floor short of where it needs to be, and the result is an unexpected shortened stride that causes the person to stumble forward into the next stride.

These four examples highlight the importance of paying attention to and understanding what you feel and hear from your feet, because this tells you immediately what is right or wrong. When you pay attention, the information allows you to recognize mistakes early, apply the corrections, and avoid bigger problems. These examples highlight very common correctable and *avoidable* mistakes.

MOVEMENT MYSTERIES—NOT!

To understand how to correct a movement problem, first you have to understand the mechanics of the natural movement. Only then can you understand the mechanics of the correction.

In this quest to understand both sides of the issue, take the time to watch and study people as they walk. For example, pay attention to their posture while you observe the movement and placement of the advancing foot in each stride. See how everyone does basically the same thing, meaning the same movement, even though many will be doing something slightly different in the way they are doing the movement. Discern these subtle differences. Study and compare. Ask yourself questions while trying to work out the reasons for the differences you see, and by working through the same movement yourself.

Working through a critical analysis of other people's movement examples will help you to better understand your own posture and movement issues. Study how everyone is using the same basics and then practice to feel the same basics in yours. Try to do their movements as you imitate their postures to help you feel what they're feeling, to come to a better understanding of your own. The following is a summary of some very basic details to focus on:

1. The flexing and pushing action of our feet directs and controls our movements.

    In naturally relaxed movements, our foot swings on a hinge, the knee joint, and the thigh moves the foot.

    In natural movement, when our posture and knee remain relaxed, and we do not attempt to control the foot, the advancing foot always comes down on the floor *exactly* where the body requires it to be. The flexing knee takes care of this.

2. The position of the upper body (shoulders) determines the distribution (location) of the pressure on the feet.

   A problem in the brain is **not** *directly* responsible for the increased width of our gait, *or the length or inconsistency of our stride.*

   For example, the well-documented irregular stride length and wide-based gait seen in people with cerebellar pathology **is directly due** to uncontrolled upper-body positioning and an incomplete transfer of body weight.

   Therefore, uncontrolled upper-body positioning and movement create the erratic placement of pressure within the feet *and force irregular strides and wide-based gait patterns.*

3. To begin an intended movement, the correct pressure is set in the pushing foot. Then, to stay in that intended movement, the upper body must make subtle adjustments during the movement to hold the pressure in that same location in each pushing foot. Thus, movements of the upper body are always relative and coordinated to the movements of the lower part of the body.

   When the changing upper-body position is not coordinated and is not counterbalancing the lower body's movement, the location of the pressure in the pushing foot changes. This always alters the intended movement.

   To see this cause and effect, watch people's postures as they walk. And, most importantly, experiment with this yourself to feel and firmly understand it.

4. The leg and foot power the movement. So, other than ensuring that the pressure in the foot remains constant, no help to produce the movement from the upper body is needed. This is because the upper body's basic function is to adjust and hold the location of the pressure in the foot for the movement to proceed as intended. Therefore, when the upper body is used to further help the leg and foot move the body, its natural basic function is compromised, and the intended movement is altered.

5. *The length of our stride* is how far one foot moves forward away from the other foot during the movement. Basically, the length of our stride is determined by the location and amount of pushing pressure in the flexing pushing foot moving the body.

   Since the upper body adjusts the location of the pressure, *stride length is, in large part, determined by the position of the upper body.*

6. The knee and leg control and/or modify the foot's direction and movement. However, since the upper body sets and adjusts the location of the pushing pressure in the foot, and since the location of the pressure in the foot determines and controls the direction of movement of the body, *in large part, the position of the upper body determines the direction and movement of the foot.*

7. Therefore, in natural movements, *the placement of the advancing foot on the floor is primarily determined and controlled by the positioning of the upper body and modified by the leg and knee.*

8. The pushing pressure we create and use in our feet is a combination of body weight and the added pressure produced by muscles in our legs.

9. The cooperative counterbalancing movements of the relaxed body create and control how the flexing feet function.

TOES AND MOVEMENT

Our toes are vitally important in all our movements. They are an extension of the foot and are used for pushing and supporting the body. They may be small, but the function they serve is enormous. When the foot "flexes," actually the joints where the toes attach to the foot extend. These joints and the movement of the toes allow the calf muscles to pull the heel up, as seen in Figure 24.4.

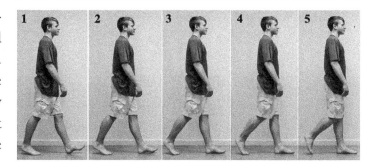

FIGURE 24.4: Toward the end of each natural stride, the flexing foot moves the pushing pressure onto only the toes.

The sequence in these pictures proves this. In picture 1, Lucas is on the toes and forward ball area of his back foot and the heel of his forward foot, with his body centered between his feet. Then, in picture 4, his body is close to being centered over his forward foot, and the toes of his back foot are lifting off the floor.

1. Pressure stays in the toes of the back foot until it is completely transferred into the advanced foot.

2. Then the new pushing foot essentially lifts the toes of the back foot from the floor as all of the pressure and body weight is removed from the back foot. The quadriceps muscles in the thigh lift the foot by lifting the knee, as the pressure that was holding that foot down is removed.

UNDERSTANDING HOW IT FEELS

Steve has a degenerative neurological disorder, and his movements were moderately impaired when I worked with him. Kerry is Steve's sister. She has natural movement ability and wants to help Steve.

On this particular day, Kerry entered the room and exclaimed, "Wow, Steve. You're standing pretty steady" (Figure 24.5).

"You bet he is," I answered Kerry. "And the intent is to get him even better. Want to join in?"

"Sure," she said.

In this picture, he is standing very stable. However, to put Kerry's reaction in perspective, it's important to know where Steve began just two weeks prior. My first introduction to Steve was by the sound he made coming down the hall long before he entered the room. It was his walker making the noise. He was leaning on it so heavily that he was "plowing" through the carpet, as shown in Figure 24.6. This caused the walker to vibrate and groan.

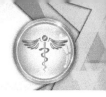

"Good," I said. "First, let me tell you what we're working on. We've been practicing staying on flat feet while making posture adjustments. Now, beginning today, we'll be working on small movements where often the feet are not flat.

"We began this way for this simple reason: Before Steve will ever feel stable and confident in any movement, he must first know how to be stable while standing. To be stable while standing or in movement, he must trust that he can easily control his posture, to control the pressure in his feet. Importantly, he must know and trust this by feeling it, just as he always did before, when his movements were good. This helps him create the needed confidence to relax his body, to then work on improving his movement ability.

"Gradually, due to his instability, he lost his trust in standing on his feet. This led to the postural stiffness you've seen in him. Living the effects of instability adds postural stiffness, and the added stiffness creates more instability. A product of this process is fear. More specifically, it is a fear of falling and injury.

"Many people with impaired movements cannot make themselves stable when standing on their feet. The reason for this is most often a postural problem. Due to stiffness and misuse, their upper body *pulls* them away from stability, and Steve is one such person. What does this mean? Before he can improve his movement ability, he first needs to correct the standing instability that his posture problems create. Once he understands how to gain better control of his pos-

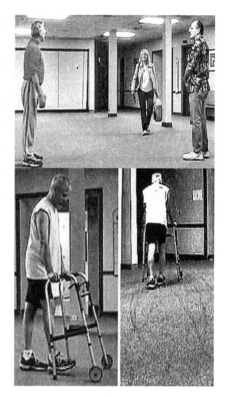

FIGURE 24.6: Steve's arms are stiffly pushing body weight onto the walker, and the plowed lines in the carpet show how forceful that push is. In addition, the walker is much too low for him to use properly and encourages this abuse.

ture to stabilize his body on his feet when standing, then he must relearn how to use his feet to remain stabilized in movement. That brings us to today."

Kerry offered, "I can see a big difference in his stability while he is standing there. What do we do to help him with that and with his walking after you've finished working with him and leave our area?"

"Tell you what, Kerry," I said. "I'm going to let you answer those questions yourself by feeling and understanding what you naturally do when *you* move and walk. Are you up for that challenge?"

"Yes, I think so," she said.

"Okay. As virtually everyone with natural movement ability does, you use your body in your movements without ever knowing what it is you're doing. You know whether what you're doing feels right or wrong, without knowing what the right or wrong actually is. So, basically, the only thing you do know, or care to know, is that your movements work when you need them. That is how it used to be for Steve until his problems developed, and now he is stuck. Without knowing how he did his movements when everything worked, and without knowing how he created the right and wrong feelings in those movements, now he is completely lost in how to cope with and correct the problems he can't identify within himself.

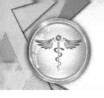

"So, Kerry, to help Steve, you must first understand the right and wrong feelings about your own posture and movements. This will give you a personal reference to understand why he feels the things he does. This also means that today you will be putting yourself in some of the same postures you often see Steve using. Then, to a limited degree, you will be feeling some of what he feels every day. You will gain a better understanding of what he experiences when you begin to understand how the wrong feelings cause a similar instability for you. And you will better understand how this instability also negatively affects your posture and movements. From these experiences, you will then begin to understand the fear he has developed in response to his constant instability that he has had great difficulty correcting. This is the first part.

"The second part is understanding how you are creating these feelings, and then learning to understand how you naturally turn the wrong (bad, unstable) feelings into the right (good, stable) feelings. When you make sense of your mistakes and corrections, understanding his mistakes and corrections will be relatively easy. This is because they will be so very close to the same. They will only be close because of your naturally relaxed posture compared with Steve's unnaturally restrictive posture, when you are attempting to mimic his mistakes.

"During this process, you will be learning your feelings in varying postures and movements. You will be learning *your* natural (right way of doing things) and some unnatural (wrong way of doing things) movement feelings. Understanding yours to better understand his is key. This learning process will be the one best thing you can do to help him after I'm gone.

"In all these things, your reference always comes back to the pressure in your feet. This is because the location and amount of the pressure in your feet are where most of the right and wrong feelings of your posture and movements come from.

"This brings up a very important point about your helping Steve. You must understand how your posture adjusts the pressure in your feet and know the feeling of it. You must also gain the ability to very quickly identify the pressure in your feet with your posture changes. When you do, you'll have the ability to know where the pressure is in his feet by just looking at his posture, because you'll know where it is in yours when you stand like that.

"This is very important and deserves repeating. Our posture adjusts the location of the pressure in our feet. Therefore, in our basic postures, when we know where the pressure is in our feet, we also know what our posture is without looking at it. Then, knowing where the pressure is located in the feet or foot of the person you're watching as they are about to do a movement, you'll also know which way their body will initially move when that pressure is used.

"In natural movements, we set the pressure where it needs to be in our feet and then relax our body (posture) into that pressure. Then we completely transfer our body weight onto one foot, and the movement happens. In this natural process, *our natural movements are not controlled by our brains.* What do I mean by this?

"We do not control our natural movements with thought. A thought only has the ability to help guide you into a posture according to your perception of what you think that movement is. But most people have a misconception about their posture and the mechanism of their movements. With natural movement ability, we seldom think about how we do or should do a movement. And those times when we do, our relaxed body still does what is required to complete the movement, despite what we think it should or should not be.

"For many people with a restrictive-posture movement impairment, extensive thoughts are an active component of the preparation, and of the movement. Like Steve's, their thoughts are frequently combined with fear. This forces them to change their posture to brace for the fear they expect in the movement. This changes the pressure in their feet and the outcome of the movement. The results are unnatural movements and instability, which create more thoughts, misconceptions, and fear.

"Steve has been unstable on his feet because of difficulty controlling his posture, which means he cannot control the pressure in his feet. When he can't control the pressure in his feet, he can't control the movements of his body. This circular problem is the ultimate reason for the fear he's been living with. But today you see him with a more stable posture. This shows you he is learning to control his posture, to control the pressure in his feet. This is the foundation that allows him to begin relaxing his body and mind. This standing stability you're seeing is the first requirement he must meet before he can move on to anything else."

PRESSURE AND MOVEMENT

"Okay, Kerry," I said, "I'd like you to experiment with something. Stand slightly on your heels and walk sideways along that straight line in the carpet. But do it without looking at your feet. Just feel and hold a small amount of heel pressure in your feet as you take four strides to the side." (Figure 24.7)

"Good," I said. Now look at the line the toes of your shoes were lined up with when you started. Look how far you moved backward away from that line on the carpet. Why did that happen?"

"Because I'm putting pressure on my heels?" she asked.

"Yes, and that is the reason Steve tips and moves backward in his movements. He has been asking, 'Why am I always moving and falling backward?' And it is very likely that he has claimed it was never his fault. It was the floor, or the fault of his neurologi-

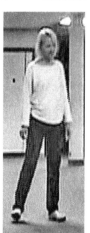

FIGURE 24.7:
On heels.

cal disorder destroying his life. However, for the most part, the floor and his disorder have not been *directly* responsible for this. The **direct cause** of that mistake has always been the pressure he's been incorrectly holding in his heels, just like the pressure you are now holding in yours.

"Many people stand on their heels, and there is absolutely nothing wrong with that, provided they are stable, comfortable, and doing what they want to do. However, what happens if they start walking with that pressure in their heels? Try it. Kerry, stay standing on your heels and take one stride forward." (Figure 24.8)

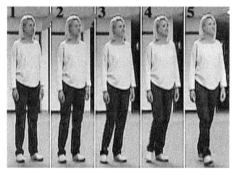
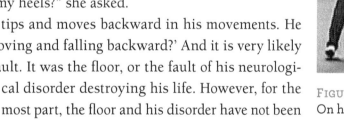
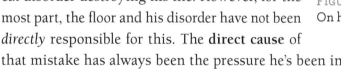

FIGURE 24.8: Naturally, to walk forward we move the increased pressure to the forward part of the foot, to the ball area, and then begin the movement.

"No," I said. "You just changed your posture before taking that stride. As you began, you naturally adjusted your posture forward. That moved the increased pressure forward out of your heels and into the ball area of the foot, and then you took the stride."

This is shown in the pictures. The reference point is the corner of the door frame behind her, indicated by the red arrows in pictures 1 and 2. While transferring body weight to her left foot, Kerry moved her shoulders forward before beginning the forward stride in picture 4.

"Many movement-impaired people like Steve do not do what you just did. In fact, Steve stopped doing that years ago. Since then, he routinely stays on his heels when he begins to move forward. Why would he do that? Through postural stiffening and fear, he lost the natural ability to easily adjust his posture to where the movement requires it to be. The other reason has to do with his non-flexing, stiffening feet. When the pressure is forward in them, he typically tips forward.

"Now try it again. This time, force your 'normal self' to stay back on your heels, and also hold your arms and shoulders stiffened like Steve does. When you do that, you will feel some of what he feels every day." (Figure 24.9)

"Good. Now feel your instability," I said. "Feel what's happening in your body, how your upper body is beginning to sway. Now feel how you are guarding against the swaying, and then stiffening because you can't stop the swaying. Also feel how the pressure in your feet changes with the swaying."

"Wow! This is more than I expected," she replied.

"What you're feeling is coming closer to what Steve frequently feels, with one huge exception. You do not question your ability, nor do you feel the fear he lives with when he feels like this on his feet. The big reason: Your body is still flexible all the way down into your feet, so you can stop and correct this erratic movement anytime you want. But when Steve feels what you are now feeling, his posture is very stiffened, from the fear that he'll fall—*again*. This makes it very difficult for him to stop and correct the problem.

"Okay, Kerry, as you're walking in this posture, what feels the most *unnatural* about what you're doing?"

"My upper body," she said.

"Stay with that and tell me, *when* does it feel the most unnatural?"

"When my foot is going forward. I feel like I'm using more pressure on my torso to hold me up. Yes, it's like my abdomen is pulling me."

"That is what it seems to be, only because you are putting some tension into your body that you're not familiar with in your natural movements. So, feel it again. Feel where that most uncomfortable sensation really is.

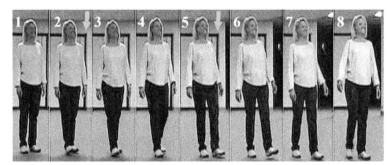

FIGURE 24.9: A person with natural ability consciously holding postural guarding while walking on her heels. In picture 2, Kerry's posture begins to guard, and then increasingly guards throughout the stride. The small amount of guarding quickly turns into more, due to instability in her feet. When she purposefully holds this heel-heavy posture, the additional changes to her posture and movement are much the same as the response a movement-impaired person experiences when they move with increased pressure in their heels.

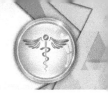

"*There!*" I said. "Right there [Figure 24.10]. You feel it the most when your advancing foot contacts the floor in front of you. Now what do you feel on that forward foot?"

"Pressure in my heel," Kerry said.

"Yes, there is pressure in your heel, and this brings up a very important point. I hope you're paying attention over there, Steve, because this is all for you. Now let's shift gears.

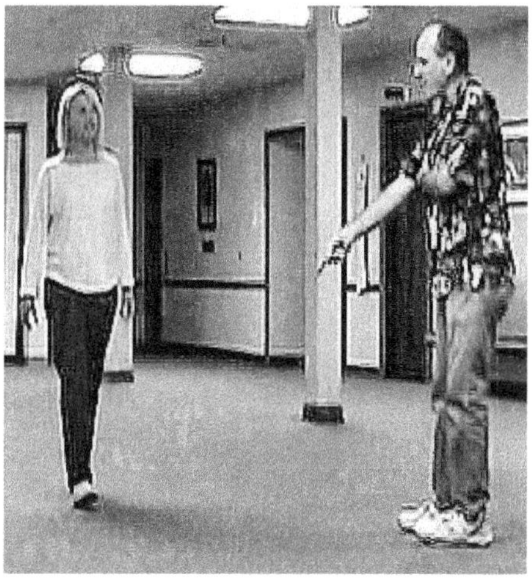

"Today Steve says to you, 'I want to walk again like I did before, like you still do. Tell me how you walk. Help me remember how. Tell me how you move so easily. Please tell me, to help me understand what I'm supposed to do.' So, Kerry, how do you walk so easily?"

"Okay, so I am starting from this point," she said.

"Point? What point?" I prodded. "I don't understand what 'this point' is. I'm confused."

"I balance?"

"Okay, Kerry. Remember that I am playing Steve. Here I am standing balanced just as you said, but I'm not moving."

"I rock forward."

"Oops," I said. "When I rock forward, I go onto my toes and then tip onto my nose." (Figure 24.11)

"My knees are bent."

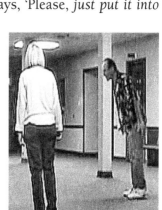

FIGURE 24.10: Stiffened foot contacting the floor with increased pressure in the heel.

"How do I do that? I can't bend my knees, because I'm too stiff. Steve says, 'Please, *just put it into words I can understand and use.*'

"Kerry, can you make it simple for Steve? Can you simplify into one sentence the explanation of what you do to walk? Can you summarize in one sentence the basic part of what you do to begin the movement and continue moving? Okay, why do you need to keep it short and simple for Steve? It's because anything more adds more confusion by causing more thought, and thought is not a part of natural movement.

"Here's a clue," I said. "I can tell you what you do to begin walking with one word."

"Okay, tell me that one word," she replied.

"No, not yet. I would rather you find it by feeling *in your feet* what that word is. I will also add that you already know the answer. Find that word in yourself by walking like you normally do. Feel it so you truly understand it and will never overlook it again.

"Oh, Kerry. Now you're walking too slowly and thinking way too much about what you think you are possibly doing in that slow walk. Let it go, girl! Just walk as you normally do. A little faster, please."

"Yes, you're right," she said. "I am thinking about it."

FIGURE 24.11: With stiffened knees and feet, rocking or leaning forward causes tipping.

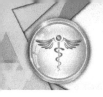

"You won't feel it by overthinking what you're thinking about. You won't find it by thinking about feeling something you think you'll discover hidden in your thoughts. Stop thinking. Only feel. Walk a little faster and simply feel what you're feeling *without* trying to imagine what you think you should be feeling. Only feel what's happening as you are physically doing it. Nothing more."

"I'm rolling on my feet from my heels to my toes."

"You're on the right track. Keep going with it. One word. Simplify it to one word."

"I want to say wave, but I know that's not it. No, I'm definitely not waving."

"You are correct. That is not the word and not what you are doing."

"Rock?" she guessed.

"Really? Remember, Steve does not like any rocking feeling on his stiffened feet. Kerry, take a moment to again *stop thinking. Stop guessing with thinking.* Get out of your head to put a focus down into your feet. Feel only what is happening in your feet, and tell your mind to shut up. Why? Because the answer is in your feet and not in your mind.

"You were closer to the right track when you said, 'I roll from my heel to my toes.' That very vaguely describes your foot flexing on the floor. But the real question is, what is that flexing foot doing on the floor? What is the purpose of it? One word. Continue walking a little faster. What do you feel?"

"Speed?"

"That is a sensation you feel all over. It's the air in your face. I'm asking you to feel what you feel in your feet, and that requires you to get out of your thinking mind."

"Pressure?"

"Ah, *yes!* The lights are getting brighter. Yes. You are feeling pressure in your feet. Now take that feeling of pressure and keep walking all the way to the wall with it. Feel what your feet are doing with that pressure."

"They are transferring."

"Yes, they are transferring, but what does that mean? How does it apply to the pressure you're feeling? Feel the one-word explanation of how we naturally use the pressure you're now feeling. It is a word that describes what your foot is physically doing with the pressure, with respect to the floor."

"It's pushing."

"**Yes! *The flexing foot pushes.*** That pressure you're feeling and pushing with is in a specific location in the foot for the specific movement you're doing. To walk. In all movement, we push the pressure into the floor to move our body."

Kerry then added, "You push into your heel, which then transfers your weight into the rest of your foot, and then onto your toes, and that pushes you forward."

"You got it, *almost,* **but NO.** The first part of what you just said is *not* correct. To clarify this misstatement, go back to a few minutes ago, when you were trying to walk stiffened like Steve. Remember, I asked you what you felt uncomfortable with when your advancing foot came down on the heel [Figure 24.10]. Let's review that.

"Start with *pushing yourself through a natural walking stride*, but I'd like you to do it this way. Take one step and pause on the flat advanced foot. Then take another step and pause. Continue this way to feel what's happening. As you push onto *and stand* on the next foot, look down at it, feel it, and tell me where your body is relative to that foot you're standing on."

She did this, then said, "It's behind it."

"No. In a natural walk, when you transition onto the flat advanced foot, it is not. Again, you are thinking your way into the movement rather than simply doing it. Here's an experiment to prove it. Stand balanced on one foot. What do you feel?"

Kerry stood on one foot. "It feels flat."

"Okay, now start that slow, interrupted walk again, and reproduce that same standing-on-a-flat-foot feeling. Okay, good. Now, as you walk, where is your body located when your foot feels flat?"

"I'm right over it."

"Correct. Now walk a slow walk without pauses. Feel how each time you come onto that flat-foot feeling, you are also feeling very stable, because your body centers over that foot. Naturally, as you walk, *every time* you push yourself forward onto the next foot, you momentarily reproduce that same flat-foot feeling. This is a feeling of 'I am balanced. I can stand on this. I can trust this feeling. I can trust this foot.' This is something Steve has not felt for a *very* long time."

"So," Kerry said, "I don't give way in my other foot until I'm balanced on this foot."

"Exactly. You do not stop the push from the pushing foot until you are fully supported by the foot you're moving onto. This is especially true when going up stairs, down stairs, up or down hills, running, walking, you name it. Every movement. Naturally, we always hold the push until the next foot completely takes over the job of supporting and pushing.

"Now, let's go back to correct something you said earlier in your answer about pushing. Remember when you walked on your heels, and the pressure in the heel of the foot you were moving onto didn't feel good [Figure 24.9]? Slowly repeat that again."

She complied.

"Okay, Kerry, what just happened to your walk when you moved onto the heel of the forward foot? This time you're feeling something different in the forward foot than you did when you were walking to feel the push, and when you were pausing over a flattened foot. This time you're feeling increased pressure in the heel, and some of it is going back up into the leg. This is important to feel and to know, because that pressure coming back into the leg is causing your knee to stiffen and your forward movement to slow."

"Yes, my forward knee is very stiff."

"Steve's knees are even stiffer when he walks like that. This means his knees are stiff almost all the time, as in all day. Now, take that same stride and feel the effect that pressure and stiffness are creating. Are you feeling stable doing that?"

"No."

"Feel how the pressure in that heel is moving up through the stiffened knee and pushing you backward. Many movement-impaired people feel that sensation with every stride, and they have learned to accept it. But remember, just as this heel pressure is not there when you walk naturally, this heel pressure is also not supposed to be there for Steve, or anyone else.

"Now, it's your turn to feel that sensation just as Steve frequently feels it. Holding your forward knee and foot as stiff as you can while taking a stride, try to continue pushing your body forward. Feel what's happening. Can you keep moving forward onto a flat front foot, Kerry?"

"Not really, at least not easily."

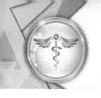

"That's right. It's because that pressure in the heel of the forward foot is pushing you backward, while the weakened push from the back foot is trying to push your body forward. The push from the back foot is weak because it is not forward enough in the foot, because you began with shoulders back and pressure toward the heel. The backward push from the heel of the forward foot is stronger because it's now being used to prematurely support some of your body weight. Both create instability, increase postural stiffness, and promote additional dysfunctional movements.

"Here's another thing to experience. Stand with increased pressure toward the heel of your *back* foot, but relax back into your normal-person mode. Also, keep your knees straight and then walk forward. With this posture and foot pressure, can you push yourself onto your front foot to stand and balance on it?"

"No."

"That's correct. You need that back foot to flex so you can move your body forward onto the next foot. To do that, the pressure in the back foot needs to be in the forward part of the foot.

"Now, what about the straight knee in the front leg with the weak push from the back foot? This time force the forward push from the back foot. Feel what's happening in the forward foot. Do you feel the increasing pressure pushing you backward?" (See Figure 24.12.)

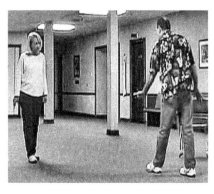

FIGURE 24.12: **A straightened forward knee allows back pressure from the heel of the front foot to move upward into the forward leg, and pushes the body backward.**

"Yes. This is hard to do."

"And now do you feel what's happening with your upper body?"

"It's kind of all over the place."

"Yes. Now feel more of what's happening as you continue to forcefully push yourself forward."

"I'm going backward."

"That's correct. What you are now feeling frequently causes a movement-impaired person with stiffened posture to stop their forward movement and stutter-step backward. Because of the added instability, they stop pushing from both feet to stop the backward movement and instability. But this causes them to lose the little stability they did have. But what happens if they keep trying to go forward?

"To find out, hold a stiffened straight-knee posture again and push yourself forward *through* the pressure coming from the heel, to move onto a flattened forward foot. But first, before you do that, allow me to tell you what to expect. In this stiffened posture, the pressures coming from each foot into each leg are working against each other. The back foot is pushing the body forward, but the forward foot is pushing it backward. Because of this, to move your body forward, you must resort to using your upper body to 'help' overcome the problem.

"As you lean your upper body forward, your straightened front knee will be pushed backward by the increased back pressure your upper body is forcing onto it. Then it is held in that position. With this situation, your upper body forcefully moves forward but your lower body does not, and suddenly you have only two *not-so-good* choices.

"One, you stop moving your upper body forward before the knee locks straight. This leaves you in a very unstable situation with increased pressure in both heels. You're forced to release the push in both feet so you don't push yourself any farther backward. This creates the next problem: This choice removes

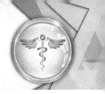

much of the downward stabilizing pressure in both feet and causes additional instability, and you fall in some other direction.

"Choice two is to continue moving your upper body forward. This often *does* move the pressure forward in the forward foot, and into a flattening foot. However, the problem is that the pressure frequently continues moving forward into the ball area of the foot, because you have no way of controlling the movement of your upper body. The combination of the locked-straight advanced knee and the pressure now in the ball area and toes of the advanced foot forces a forward-tipping, pushing fall that is very difficult to stop.

"Added to the other things that cause him to fear his movements, Steve frequently is forced to deal with these problems you're feeling when he is on his feet every day. So, now that you've felt a small bit of what he feels, do you have a different understanding of your movements and his movements than you had an hour ago?"

"Yes," Kerry said. "It doesn't feel good to me, either, and I don't have any of the fear and stiffness that he does."

"Right you are. The combination of the stiffened foot and knee, especially when that knee is locked straight, creates an out-of-control and frightening feeling of utter helplessness, and often terror. Now consider these same issues from a 'what if' perspective.

"Imagine what it would be like for Steve if he could undo just some of this bad stuff. What would it be like if he had the ability to bend that advanced knee? If he could do that, then he could stop many of these problems from happening, and the problems that did happen would be easier to manage and correct. Imagine what his life would be like if he knew how to do that. His standing movements and walking abilities would improve beyond his and your imagination.

"Think about it. If he is not creating these problems, what is there to hold him back? If he is not creating the problems, the things that create and perpetuate the fear are gone. This will allow his fear of the movement to begin to fade as his growing trust moves in. So, very importantly, *to remove fear, you must first physically remove the conditions and situations that create the fear.*

"Think back to when I started working with Steve. First, he had to know how to stand and begin to relax on two stabilized flat feet. That's what he was doing when you walked in today. The next thing he must learn is to stabilize and relax his body when using just one flat foot. Why? That's because every advancing movement requires it. This is what we are beginning to work on today.

"To walk better, he must learn to trust supporting all his body on just one foot, even if it's only for a second or two. Then, to progress into a more natural walk, he must learn to trust supporting himself on only the front part of one foot during each stride. Feel that when you walk. Walk as you normally do, and feel in each foot how you are supporting and pushing your body forward with *only* the front part of the foot. Do you feel that, Kerry?"

"Yes," she said.

"Now feel the rest of it. As you are pushing from the ball area and toes of the back foot to move onto the forward foot, you are momentarily supporting all your body weight on roughly one-quarter of one foot. That is 12.5 percent or less of the total surface area of the bottom of both feet. That is what you're using as your pushing foot easily flexes during each stride. But Steve's feet don't do that. You are easily

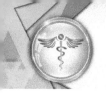
using the forward part of the foot that he doesn't trust using, because his feet are not relaxed like yours. When he moves onto the forward part of his foot or feet, they stiffen more than they already are. So, with that, I have another challenge for you to feel. In your first stride, relax your foot and move onto the front of it as you normally do. But then, in the next stride, do your best to stiffen your foot as you move onto the front of the foot.

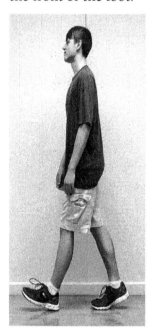

FIGURE 24.13: On the toes of the back foot and lightly on the heel of the front foot. This is a critical balancing act we depend on in each stride.

"Be careful with it. Without a relaxed, flexing foot, your normal movements don't exist. When your foot is held stiff, you will feel yourself tipping forward on your toes. Now try it.

"There. That's good," I said. "Do you now feel and better understand why Steve shuffles and moves awkwardly on his feet?"

"Yes, now that I'm feeling this. It helps me know some of what he's dealing with. That forward tip can be frightening."

"Relaxed, flexing feet can only happen when the rest of the body is relaxed," I said. "This means Steve has much to learn and do before he will achieve that level of total-body relaxation. To remain in a natural walk, we must have the ability to confidently move onto and use just the forward quarter of each foot. This is a *huge thing* for many movement-impaired people to learn how to do again. They must learn how to trust the area of their foot they have come to passionately fear using." (See Figure 24.13.)

"When a person with natural ability walks forward," I said, "there is a quick moment when they are balanced on and supporting all their body weight on the ball area and toes of the back foot. This is just as the heel of the forward foot is coming in contact with the floor. Without the ability to support the body and balance and control the movement with just that area of the back foot, each time the forward heel contacts the floor it would have increased pressure in it. Why? Because the person would be prematurely putting body weight onto it and then creating the problems we just talked about and you felt.

"Yes, there are many people with natural ability who constantly thump their advancing heel onto the floor and lazily put body weight onto it, and otherwise they are doing okay in their walk. They are creating the same potential problems, but they avoid them because their posture remains relaxed.

"Back to Steve and other people with his movement problems. To regain a more natural use of their feet, there are three basic problems people with a restrictive-posture movement impairment must correct: (1) postural instability, (2) stiff feet, and (3) incomplete weight transfers.

"To correct these issues, Steve must learn to understand, control, and use the pressure in his feet. Next, he must learn how to relax his posture. Then he must learn to trust himself using flexing feet again.

"We start this process using two feet, then one foot, and then just a part of one foot. This is the only way to gradually reclaim natural movement. It is the natural way we learn to use it. We have to master the simple basics of posture, foundation, and stability before we're able to do the complex movements.

"Steve, to gradually develop trust in improved walking ability, you need the ability to balance and stand on the front parts of your feet in the middle of the room [Figure 24.14]. This uses your calf muscles, and relaxed postural control provides you with the ability to momentarily use them this way during your movements.

"So, Steve, you must exercise these muscles to get them stronger, because you haven't been using them very much. Your stiffness hasn't allowed it. When these muscles are weak, your ability to use your foot more naturally will always be a problem. When they're weak, your walking ability will *never* be as good as you'd like it to be.

"Every time a person with natural ability walks, they use everything we have talked about. Their posture, knees, and feet are relaxed. Their constantly flexing feet provide them with continuous smooth movement. Their movement is smooth and easy because they have complete control of the pressure in their feet. The comfort of the correct pressure feeling and the stability of the relaxed posture tell us everything we need to know.

"Therefore, everything you want to accomplish in having better movements comes back to the same thing. It comes back to *knowing where the pressure is in your feet, understanding it, and trusting your ability to use it.*"

"This is so wonderful," Kerry said. "But how will Steve be sure of where his foot will come down on the floor when he walks?"

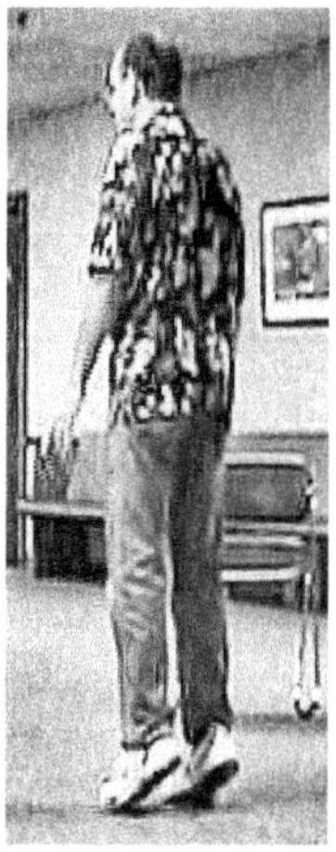

"That, my friend, will be easy. You begin with the proper setup and pressure, do complete weight transfers from one foot to the other, and then hold that pressure in the same location in each pushing foot during the movement. Your advancing foot will always be exactly where it needs to be when it comes back down on the floor. How? It lands according to what your body requires. This means your relaxed body is placing it in the right spot. So, in natural movement, the advancing foot will land *exactly where it is supposed to be when you leave it alone.* Let's briefly go through how this works.

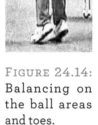

Figure 24.14:
Balancing on the ball areas and toes.

"Okay, Kerry, what determines where your advancing foot comes down on the floor when you walk?"

"My speed?"

"Indirectly."

"How hard I push?" she guessed again.

"You actually just said the same thing."

"Okay. How I flex my knee?"

"You are guessing within a cloud of whirling thoughts. Here it is. The length of our stride is set by the pressure we create and use in our easily flexing pushing foot. So, when you said, 'How hard I push,' well, yes, indirectly that's it. But it isn't the complete answer.

"Go back to this question: What adjusts and sets the pressure in our foot? The position of our shoulders, our upper body, does that. So, according to the *very simplified basics* of our movements, *the position of our shoulders determines the length of our stride.* But yes, we can modify the length of the stride with the additional stabilizing and pushing pressure we produce with our leg muscles during the movement.

"Okay, now consider the concept of the natural push. Our body is pushed into motion as we completely shift our body weight onto the ball and toes of the one foot that stays on the floor. A very light knee lifts the other foot from the floor. *The PUSH is the pressure created by our body weight and the added downward pushing force from working muscles in the leg.* This combined pressure is forced against and directed into

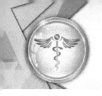

the floor by the forward part of the foot. We push this pressure into the non-moving floor to move our movable body in the opposite direction. The rest of the movement is simply allowing the flexing foot to work, and that requires a relaxed, cooperative posture. In a practical sense, that's essentially all there is to it. This describes the effortless part of our movements.

"Our body weight supplies most of the pushing pressure. So, it's important to do complete transfers of body weight to each foot to maintain the same power and direction of the stride. As the pushing foot moves the body forward, the advancing knee delivers the foot to the precise location on the floor where all the above have determined it is required to be. What does this mean for Steve and your question, and for all of us?

"When you leave it alone, the body and knee will move the advancing foot to the spot on the floor where the advancing body requires it to be, according to the strong push from the pushing and flexing foot. This will always be the exact spot that's needed. The only requirement is staying relaxed to allow it to happen.

"In our basic movements, this is what makes walking feel so easy. The movement 'just happens' and frees our mind to do whatever it wants. Not being relaxed is Steve's problem. It creates his unnatural movements. This is why his advancing foot frequently is not where it needs to be to support his body and the movement.

"Kerry, now it's your turn to feel the answer to your question as you slowly walk. Begin by setting the pressure in the ball areas of your feet. Then completely transfer your body weight onto one foot while keeping the pressure in the ball area. Next, with each stride, focus only on the push from the back foot. Do nothing else. Feel the ease of the movement as that flexing foot pushes your relaxed body forward. Feel how your advancing foot always comes down on the floor exactly where your body needs it to be. *Your body is directing it*, not your thinking mind. You are moving with relaxed dynamic postural control.

"Feel how it all comes together. The simplicity of the seemingly complex movement resides within the postural setup and keeping it. The complexity of how our body works to provide us with natural ability is simplified when we *quiet our mind and allow our relaxed body to cooperate with itself.*

"This natural process falls apart when we alter our posture, transforming natural movements into unnatural movements. Through posture mistakes and modifications (indirect effects), people with a movement impairment make their movements more of a problem than they otherwise would be (owing to the direct effects of their disorder or condition).

"There is a long-standing myth within what I just said. The popular explanation is that the condition or disorder in the brain is directly causing all the changes that are happening in their movements, especially as the disorder progresses. Therefore, *in this theory*, since the brain controls our movements, our movements become a problem because the brain has a problem. Well, as one of my very young grandsons said to me one day when I was teasing him, '*Really*, Pa Pop!' In other words, he was sarcastically saying, 'Do you really expect me to believe that rubbish?!'

"This 'brain causing all the problems' line of thought and theory is simply not true. A good example of it *not being true* is Steve's ability today compared with last week. His posture and balance are better today. But we have not changed anything about the disorder in his brain. So, what did *he* change? He

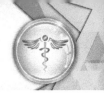

is more stable today only because he learned improved control of his posture and relaxed a bit into his flattened feet, which today are more stable.

"Just like mine, the disorder in his brain will continue to degenerate and cause him added problems. However, he can learn how to better cope with the changes and continue to improve his movements. This will take a great deal of commitment. With much effort and dedication to improving, he will hopefully be able to stay ahead of many of the direct physical effects the disorder in his brain will cause. I have been working through this very same process for many years, and my rewards have been fantastic.

"Steve, does everything make a little more sense to you now?"

Steve nodded. "Yes."

"You'll need to work and play with all these things, and simply use them a great deal before most of it becomes easier for you. Kerry will now be better able to help you with it after I leave the area. But unless you do your part, none of it will make a difference.

"To both of you, when you question what it is you're supposed to be doing or why something isn't working the way it's supposed to, feel what is or is not happening in your feet. Kerry, when Steve is stuck with that sort of thing and you don't have the answer for him in your head, stop thinking about it. Instead, put yourself in the same posture he is in and feel what you feel in your feet. That will be close to what he feels. Then tell him what he needs to be reminded of.

"Feel the mistake he's making when you make it, and then do what you naturally do to move into the correct feeling in your feet. Steve will need to do the same thing. But remember that Steve will almost always have a component of stiffening in his posture that you do not have. This must be undone to allow him to have better movements. You also must take that into consideration when attempting to reproduce what he's doing, to then correctly advise him.

"Always look for guarding and stiffening in his posture. And Steve, always feel for it. Begin in your hands to begin the relaxation of your body, to practice taking that relaxation down to your knees and feet.

"Both of you will forget much of what I've just explained to you, but don't worry about forgetting it. Why? You're not learning my movements. You are learning your movements. Continue learning your movements by being aware of what your feet are telling you, because that is your truth about your movements.

"Keep it personal. The most important words you want to remember need to be *your words* about your feelings, to replace my words, so that you're doing your movements your way while using your present and past experiences.

"*Your movements. Your feelings. Not mine.*

"There is no magic to any of this movement stuff, just as there was nothing magical or special about it when you learned it as a toddler. It is still exactly the same, but now you are a thinking adult. This means you need to intellectually understand the why and the how of it before you will believe and trust it. Without this intellectual understanding to satisfy your mind, you won't allow yourself to use any of it. *This is the permission you must find within you, to give to yourself.* Without giving yourself permission to do this, you will not succeed.

"There is another thing to be aware of, Steve. If you're thinking that maybe if you just understand this in your mind, then you will know how to use it, you are gravely mistaken, and your chances of success will be very low.

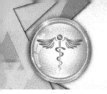

"You must learn how to physically apply and use the intellectual information you're collecting. That only comes through a great deal of work, practice, and play. That is the only way this intellectual information will make any 'how do I use it?' sense.

"*Stay in your head—to stay in your chair. You will never think your way back toward the natural side of the movement world.* You must force yourself to question and be more like the trusting, adventurous toddler you once were. You must find and allow the '**Yes, I can**' to dominate your choices and ambitions."

■ ■ ■

CHAPTER 25

WALKING TO THE PRESSURE IN THE FOOT

*Walking is smooth and easy when the movement of the body
is precisely synchronized with the forward movement of the pressure
through the feet, and the flexing of the pushing foot.*

W*alking is an effortless movement* for people with unchallenged natural ability. It is effortless because the forward movement of the body is precisely synchronized with the forward movement of the pressure through the feet and the flexion of the pushing foot.

SEQUENCE OF MOVEMENT

During each walking stride, the rate of the movement of one foot is different from that of the other. While one foot is quickly moved forward through the air, the other foot "stays in place" working on the floor. See this in the series of pictures in Figure 25.1, which shows the sequence and movements of our feet during one forward stride. In picture 1, as the **right** foot is completing the push of the stride, its toes are still in contact with the floor. The **left** foot is forward and flattening on the floor as the body is moving onto it. In pictures 2 through 5, the right foot is blurred as it quickly moves forward, and then in pictures 6 through 9, it is not blurred while flattening on the floor as the body is pushed forward onto it.

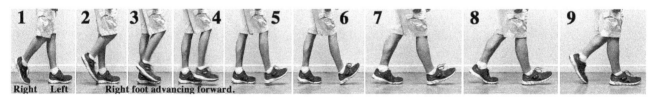

Right   Left   Right foot advancing forward.

FIGURE 25.1: During this stride, the right foot moves forward as the left foot pushes the body forward. Note the changing clarity of the right foot. As it moves forward, its image is slightly blurred. This is due to the speed at which it's being moved forward to be in place to support and push the body in the next stride.

Watch people as they walk, and initially watch only the movement of their body and head. Note that the forward movement of the body and head is steady and uninterrupted. Next watch only the movement of their legs. When one leg is moving quickly, the other leg is moving slowly. And then only the feet. The lifted foot moves forward very fast while the one on the floor is stopped in place, flexing on the floor.

During natural walking strides:

1. The forward movement of the body is continuous, steady, and smooth.

2. The forward movement of the legs is one slow and the other fast.

3. The forward movement of the feet is one very fast and the other stopped.

4. The movement of the legs and feet is interrupted.

How does this work? How does this mismatched rate of movement between the body, legs, and feet make sense? How does a stopped foot on the floor not interrupt the body's steady movement? The answer is rather simple.

In order for the uninterrupted forward movement of the body to be possible, the pressure moving forward through the advanced foot *and* the flexing movement of the pushing foot must also proceed without interruption. This is possible only when the feet remain relaxed. When the pushing foot is not flexible enough to easily push the body through the movement, and/or when the advanced foot is not flexible enough to control the movement of the pressure that the forward-moving body is creating within it, the movement of the body is altered.

In the relaxed advanced foot, the forward-moving pressure stops when it moves into the forward portion of the ball area and toes. The pressure stops as it is being increased to stabilize the flexing foot, to prevent it from moving as the heel is pulled upward. The foot "flexes" at the joints where the toes attach to the foot.

THE PUSH

There are multiple components to the foot pushing the body:

1. The downward (*vertical*) component of the pushing pressure in the flexed foot stabilizes the body.

2. The forward body push is produced by directing the pressure in the flexed foot backward into the floor.

3. The backward moving (*horizontal*) component of the pushing pressure pushes the body partly through the movement.

4. The movement of the flexing foot (lifting heel) produces the remainder of the pushing force.

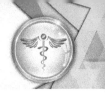

SYNCHRONIZATION

In basic terms:

1. When the downward pressure in the pushing foot is not strong enough to stabilize the body, there will not be an adequate forward pushing force to propel the body into the intended movement.

2. When the downward pressure in the foot is not strong enough to stabilize the body, the foot's ability to flex is compromised and limits the continued push of the body.

3. When the pushing pressure is in the wrong location in the foot, the forward push will be either too strong, too weak, or pushing the body in the wrong direction for the intended movement.

4. The flexibility of the foot is also largely dependent on the condition of the muscles that control the foot. Tightening, guarding, and stiffening of these muscles restrict the flexibility of the foot.

For a person to continue walking at the same rate with **un**interrupted body movement, the pushing pressure in the foot during each stride must be identical. Thus, it must be in the same location and of the same amount and force. Additionally, each foot must be flexing the same amount and at the same rate as the other during each stride.

1. When the forward pushing force increases or decreases, the speed of the walk changes accordingly.

2. The walking stride is altered when the pushing pressure changes location in the foot. In general, moving the pushing pressure forward in the foot produces a longer stride. Moving it backward in the foot produces a shorter stride.

3. When we wish to stop our body's movement, the forward pushing force from the pushing foot and the progression of the pressure in the advanced foot must be stopped.
    Just as it is during continuous movement, the stopping movement of the body must remain synchronized with this stopping process in the feet. This is done with and controlled by the forceful application of increased downward stabilizing pressure into the foot, or feet. The smooth application of this depends on a relaxed, coordinated postural response and flexible feet.

4. To stop the body's movement, the horizontal component of the pushing pressure must be converted to additional stabilizing downward pressure.
    The quickly applied increased downward pressure in the feet must be enough to overcome, convert, and stop the body's forward momentum in a smooth and purposeful movement.

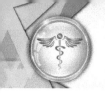
Knee and Hip Involvement

There are critical components to the synchronization of stopping the movement of the body. Primarily this is done by stopping the movement of the pressure in the feet and stopping the flexing of the feet. To accomplish this, flexing hips, knees, and ankles quickly move the body downward to lower the body's center of gravity, by squatting and increasing the pressure in the feet. During forward movement, this is a quick forward stride squat that "forces" the involved muscles to do more work. The result in the feet is the immediate addition of increased downward stabilizing pressure that effectively eliminates the horizontal component of the pushing force in the feet. Thus, the force that was moving the body forward is stopped. This coordinated and controlled grounding of the body is basically how we apply our brakes.

With a relaxed posture, this action is naturally very effective. But with a restrictive posture, often the momentum of the body is only partially eliminated. Commonly this is because the squat is limited and the leg muscles aren't doing enough productive work to produce the downward pressure that is required to stop the body's momentum.

Another limiting factor is that the feet are not relaxed and flexible enough to control the pressure that is being applied into them, and this prevents the complete conversion of the horizontal force component into the downward stabilizing force component. Thus, some of the horizontal pressure force continues moving forward in the feet, and that allows the body to continue moving.

Finally, many times the knees remain straight, and this greatly restricts the movement-impaired person's ability to create the required amount of added downward pressure into the feet. Without the required downward stopping pressure in the feet, the body continues moving in an uncontrolled manner.

These are the reasons many people with a restrictive-posture movement impairment tip or fall forward when they attempt to stop. This is why they are so distrusting and fearful of their ability to stop their movements.

In summary: Naturally, with relaxed postural control, we stop the movement of our body while preserving balance, stability, and control. This requires the synchronization of the horizontal movement of the body and the horizontal pushing force from the foot. They are synchronized when stopping the movement, just as they are during the movement.

*Ultimately, the functioning of the feet determines the quality and outcome of any movement,
be it starting, continuing, or stopping the movement.*

Walking

In a natural walking stride, in the advanced foot, the pressure moves steadily forward from the heel area until it moves into the forward portion of the ball area and the toes. There it becomes the pushing pressure. This pressure applied into the floor begins to push the body forward (see the right foot in pictures 1 and 2 of Figure 25.2), and then the lifting heel continues to push the body forward onto the next advanced foot (pictures 3 through 7). Thus, beginning in picture 5, the increased pressure is moving forward in the advanced left foot as the body is also moving forward.

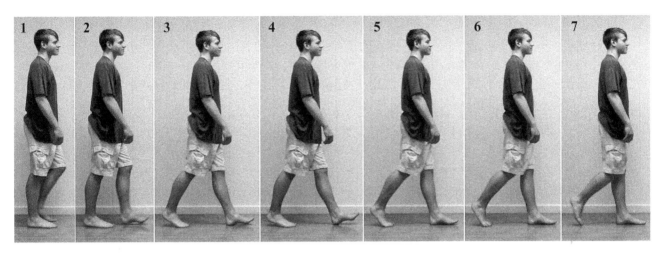

FIGURE 25.2: The pushing pressure is located in the forward ball area and toes of the foot. Early in the stride, the toes of the pushing foot flatten on the floor. This pressure begins to push the body forward, and then the lifting movement of the heel continues the forward push.

The lower portions of the calf muscles form the Achilles tendon, and the tendon attaches to bone at the back of the heel. As these muscles contract, pressure is added to the toes and ball area of the foot. As the muscles continue contracting, the Achilles tendon pulls on and lifts the heel, flexing the foot. This ability and function is vital to natural movement.

Look at this process again in Figure 25.3. In pictures 1 and 4, the red vertical line is at the tip of Bob's forward shoe, and the yellow rectangle in picture 1 is the distance his body has moved forward in picture 4. In picture 1, the pushing pressure is in the forward ball area and toes of the back foot. As the pushing back foot flexes in pictures 2 through 4, the lifting heel and pushing force from the ball area and toes propel the body forward. Of note, the lifting heel moves the body forward because it is adding length to the leg (in this case the left leg).

Near the bottoms of the pictures, the bottom of the inserted red bar marks

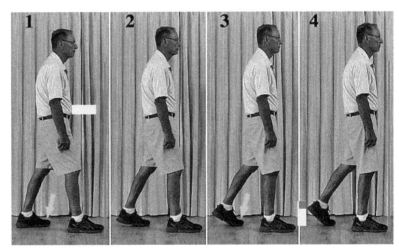

FIGURE 25.3: The function and support of the toes is vital to natural movement. They provide a great deal of support and stability to the foot to allow the heel to be lifted during each stride. They also generate pushing force to move the body.

the bottom of the pushing shoe. The top of the red bar marks the top of the front of the pushing shoe, as indicated by the green arrow in picture 1. Beginning in picture 2, the front tip of the pushing shoe moves under the top of the red bar (the area indicated by the green arrow in picture 3). This shows that the toes of the pushing foot have been pushed down and flattened on the floor by the working calf muscles. This small area of the foot must be compressed onto the floor with increased pressure to stabilize the pushing foot, to prevent it from moving, so it is able to support and move the body.

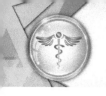
The yellow and red rectangle behind the pushing foot in picture 4 is the same height as the length of the yellow rectangle that is on its side in picture 1. The yellow block in picture 4 has a red insert that shows how much of the movement of the body was produced by the push from the ball area and toes. The remaining yellow block below the red block shows how much of the body's forward movement was produced by the lifting heel.

As the pushing foot flexes and pushes the body forward, the pressure in the advancing foot is also moving forward. When the pressure reaches the forward ball area and toes of the advancing foot, the push from the back foot is ending as the front foot is beginning to take over the pushing process. This is the basis for the smooth and uninterrupted pushing transition in the feet that enables the smooth and uninterrupted movement of the body. These examples show that *our natural movements are totally dependent on the free flexing ability and function of our feet.*

Our feet determine, produce, maintain, and control the movement of our body.
Every other part of the body—including the brain—merely contributes to and supports the feet.

When this ability of the pushing foot is compromised, so is the movement and control of the body. This is exactly what limits the movements of the movement impaired, especially those with a restrictive posture. With a limited ability to flex the foot, to lift the heel to push the body, the movement of the body can only be done using the pushing pressure within the flattened foot. A push from a flattened foot produces a very small stride and is precisely what is seen in many people with restrictive-posture movement impairments.

When the foot is not flexible, the horizontal pushing force and the stabilizing downward pushing force into the floor are much weaker. The result is a shortened movement of the body with interruption, instability, and decreased control of the posture.

Understand What You Need

Keep it simple (and *specific*). Know what you're using, how you're using it, and why. Use your words and thoughts that remind you of exactly what you need to do. Do your movements your way, but always do them using the basics of natural movement.

The basics of natural movement are centered in the functioning of your feet.

1. To begin, I suggest you try using the ten words listed in item 2, below. Then, as you continue, find your own words or very short phrases that work for you. Personalize everything.

   Use focus words to simplify the explanation into a shortened functional reminder of the movement or function. This is much more efficient than trying to recall all the information about your posture and the mechanics of the movement. To avoid becoming lost in confusing thought as best you can, choose words that provoke limited thought.

2. The ten focus words I suggest for you to begin with are **heavy feet, flat foot, stand on a foot, knee,** and **push**. Yes, I still use them when I need a reminder.

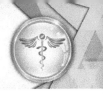

To help eliminate confusion, use only one reminder word or short phrase at a time. This is not to say that you will not or should not use more than one during any movement. The important point is to simplify your thoughts to help simplify your movements.

Another importance of the reminder is to focus on the correct feeling in your feet, to repeatedly convince your mind that this is correct and everything is fine. You need a relaxed mind, to relax your body, to do the movement better. Repeatedly creating and using the correct pressure and feeling also helps rebuild self-confidence and trust in your abilities.

Heavy Feet

To improve your stability when standing or walking, with shorter strides *make and keep your feet heavy* by pushing more pressure into them. People with natural ability do this without realizing it.

This "heavy feet" focus will remind you to continue using your leg muscles, and working leg muscles push increased pressure into the feet. This will also help remind you to flex your knees to lower yourself into a more stable and more relaxed posture (ready stance).

On "clumsy days," this focus is especially helpful. With added pressure going into your flattened feet, you will be and feel more stable and better able to relax. Also, on clumsy days, keep your strides shorter for better control.

The other use for "heavy feet" is working on completely transferring body weight to the foot you're using. For example, pushing more pressure into your right foot on the ground will enable your left knee to lift the left foot higher to step over obstacles or walk on grass, or to simply stop scuffing your feet on the floor.

Flat Foot/Flat Feet

This reminder is helpful on clumsy days and at unsure times when you feel unstable, are leaning, tipping, or "swaying in the wind," and are uncertain how to manage it. The objective is to move from one flattened foot to the other flattened foot using smaller movements.

Remember, you are the most stable when you are standing on a functionally flat foot.

Stand on a Foot

To walk better, you must have the ability to stand balanced on one foot, if only for a second or two. With this "stand on a foot" focus, you are reproducing the feeling of balance and stability with all your weight on one very flat and supporting foot. Remember, you are not to stop on a flat foot as you walk. Simply feel the flatness of the foot *as you pass through the feeling* midstride. In each stride, reproduce the very brief feeling of *I could pause and stay standing on this foot if I needed to.* Allow the foot to continue flexing through the stride and movement without hesitating.

Knee

Direct your walk with your knees. Direct and lead your body into each stride by *pointing and pushing your knee* in the direction you want your body and advancing foot to move. Do **not** think about where your foot is moving. Focus on where the knee is moving. Work on relaxing your posture to develop the

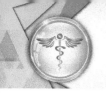

trust that your advancing foot will always be exactly where it needs to be as the relaxed knee and body control and direct it.

Push

Firmly hold the pushing pressure in the ball area and toes of your foot all the way through the stride. Do not, *do not*, **do not** stop the push. Continue the push from the pushing foot until the advancing foot completely takes over. At this point the back foot is easily lifted from the floor because all of the body weight and downward pressure from the leg muscles have been removed. Reminding yourself to keep your knees flexing will be very helpful with this.

When you continue applying a firm push, you'll also be making the forward foot a "heavy foot" and a "flat foot" and a "stand on a foot" as you move onto it midway through the stride.

Trust Mama

Movement-wise, your feet are your mama. Reduce your frustration by learning to pay very, very close attention to what Mama is telling you. Stop the confusion. Stop struggling with your "maybe this is what I should be doing" thinking mind. Keep it simple using the basic facts:

1. With precision, your feet will tell you exactly when it is okay for you to move, and when it is not okay to move. This applies to any movement, at any time.

2. Your feet will tell you exactly when your posture is correct and when it is not.

3. By far, one of the biggest requirements is your mind learning to accept, believe, and trust what your feet are telling you.

4. Without the ability to control the correct pressures in your feet, you will very quickly force unexpected movements that you're unprepared to respond to.

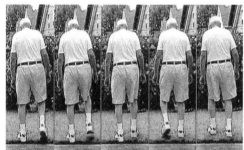

5. **Your successes** in achieving improved movement ability are dependent upon your understanding, use, and trust of the pressures you create and control in your feet.

Do you remember Charlie? In Chapter 16, he was shown taking a very scary backward fall. That fall did not stop him, just as the momentary setbacks will not stop those of you who are determined to work through them. Through persistence and dedicated work, Charlie regained the ability to walk in the thick grass behind his house again, as shown in Figure 25.4.

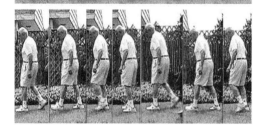

FIGURE 25.4: Charlie walking in the grass again.

Did he do it perfectly? No. And he didn't care, because it's not about being perfect. He was just thrilled to have the ability to be doing it again. For the record, the pictures in this example were taken just three weeks after his fall. His is another example showing that the difficult and frustrating work *does pay off* when you stick with it, *working your program.*

Find your enthusiasm and determination to learn how to reclaim hidden abilities. Use what you already know of yourself and add in the basics of natural movement described throughout this book. This is your responsibility to yourself.

You will never know what is possible until you honestly and repeatedly try.

In fitting form, this chapter ends with the words of another person I worked with, Jeannie: *"Get jazzed."*

■ ■ ■

CHAPTER 26

Movement and Walking Issues

Walking is repeated forward strides done without hesitation.

T*he only person we are working to improve* is the person we are in this single moment in time. We cannot work with who we were in the past, because that person is gone. We cannot work with who we will be, because that person only resides in our imagination. *We live only in the present moment. Our past is a memory and our future, mere thoughts within a projection of possibilities.*

Only in the moment of the present. Only in the here and now. Only in this moment can we do something to prepare for how we hope to enjoy our life in all future moments. For those of us with these problematic movement impairments, every activity, in every moment, is therapy. Everything is our personal therapy in which we are striving to do our best, and learning how to do better in hopes of improving our future moments. Try your best to embrace and further develop this concept.

Going Up

"Why am I struggling so much and not able to do any better?" For years I repeatedly asked myself this question, but then each time I eventually came to the same conclusion. I was simply stuck on another "movement-ability plateau" until I learned the skills that allowed me to push up onto the next-higher one. You can do the same. Consider each improvement in your abilities as one step up on your never-ending, potential-ability staircase (Figure 26.1, for example). When you feel stuck in your ability, you must learn to focus on what is keeping you from doing better. What are you doing or not doing that is preventing you from doing better? From this opening perspective, many things can be realized and simplified.

To move up to the next ability level, you must practice, play, and learn how to improve your present ability. The question then becomes, "How high can you go on your ability staircase?" I don't know—and neither do you! The only way you will ever know the answer is by continuing to work and play, and your answer will eventually be revealed. In the process, you'll also realize that with each higher ability level you achieve, there is another higher ability level to strive for. This means your potential ability is relatively unlimited, and it's up to you to make the best of your potential.

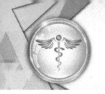
You will never know what your true potential is until you try to the best of your ability. This means that you will only know how high you can go when you get there. It is your responsibility, and your respon-

sibility alone, to push yourself and your abilities until you can honestly say, "This is where I want to be. I am happy here." When that day comes, hopefully you will be very high up on your movement ability staircase, standing with an intense smile on a very high plateau. And better still, I hope that after you say that you are happy there, you then look up at the next plateau and yell back to those below you, "I changed my mind! I'm going up a couple more to see what it's like up there." Big, small, or tiny, there will *always* be another higher plateau. Everything is relative.

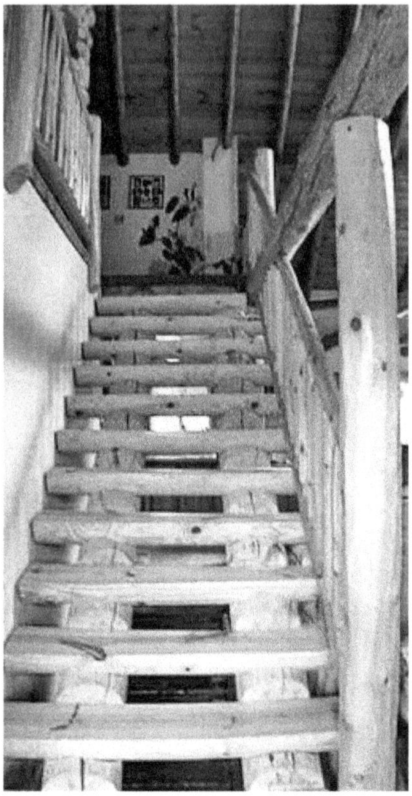

But there is another side to this. You need to understand that *this imaginary staircase works both ways*. For example, if you stop trying and stop doing, you can, and likely will, lose some of the ability you've gained. This means when you get lazy or simply stop doing, you will begin to slide back down to a lower level. Fact: Sliding down is always much easier than climbing up.

Also, on any given day, you may be temporarily on a lower step on the staircase just because of the kind of day you're having. Don't despair when the lower-step days come. One bad day doesn't mean you've lost the ability you have relearned to use. It only means on this day, you're having challenges with your body that make it difficult for you to do better. On those days, just keep doing the best you can with the challenges your situation throws at you, until the higher-step, better days return.

A good example is when we become ill or are injured, and for many, allergies also fit in this category. On those days when we don't feel well and our movements are worse, it too often feels like we've lost a great deal of the ability we had gained. Please don't stress too much over this. When these illness, allergy, injury, or fatigue issues

FIGURE 26.1: In all things, we proceed one step at a time. This is true for reclaiming movement abilities as well. Consider each step up you take as another movement ability achieved. Each step also represents a learning plateau. We remain on each step, or level of functioning, until we learn the required skills that allow us to move up to the next one.

last for a short time, everything we thought we had lost comes back with our returning better health. Try to be realistic. Remember, people *without* movement problems also experience a decline in their function when they're ill. The difference is that our temporary decline is more obvious, and we have more physical challenges than they do.

STUCK

Often, many of you will be disappointed that your successes are not as great as you had anticipated or hoped for. What should you do? Should you throw up your hands and say, "I guess this is as good as I can hope for"? No. Reevaluate. Do an honest evaluation of yourself, refocus, and ask yourself at least these three questions:

1. What have I been doing to help myself improve?

   Or, better yet,

2. What have I *not* been doing?

   Very often, what you have *not* been doing is where the problem lies.

3. What other activities can I try that will challenge me and help improve my chances of reaching my movement ability goals?

The cycle of good days and not-so-good days will continue to churn. So, learning how to functionally deal with the down days without getting overly negative is a big part of helping yourself. You need that, because your improvement process takes patience, practice, play, and a great deal of repetition, and the negative days will turn this process into a burden. The bigger truth you must realize is, you are making a lifelong commitment to yourself. With your condition or disorder, you will always need to pay closer attention to your postures and movements than people with natural abilities do. So, letting go of the negatives, anger, and frustration will allow you to stay focused on more positive attributes.

Stop fighting yourself. Get over the jealousy of what others have, that you have lost.

Put your efforts into the positives you do have, and those you create. Our situation in our brain is what it is. To have a better quality of life, each of us must positively adapt to our personal challenges. So, I encourage you to make peace with yourself, to find and live the better life you dream of.

Stop fighting. There is no battle you wage within yourself that you can win. The "*I have to fight this*" attitude only breeds disappointment. Why? The "fight" is you fighting you. The disorder or condition within you is you. It is impossible to fight with one part of you without fighting with the whole of you. Negativity destroys.

WALKING POSTURE, NATURAL, NO IMPAIRMENT

Dave does not have a movement impairment (Figure 26.2). The pictures in the top and bottom panels are identical, with the bottom panel having the zone of stability superimposed. As a reminder, the green zone of stability is determined by the portion of the feet, or foot, that is in contact with the floor and supporting the body.

In Dave's natural walk, note how closely the center of his body remains within the zone of stability. Also note that the space between his feet varies only slightly.

When his body is centered in the zone, the space between his feet is narrow. When his body is not centered in the zone, as in pictures 1, 3, 7, 11, and 15, the space between his feet is slightly wider. Look closely. What do these pictures have in common?

He is on just one foot in those pictures. Now examine pictures 2, 4, 6, 8, 10, 12, and 14, in which he is on both feet. Do you see a difference? When he is on both feet, his body is closer to being centered in the zone, and his feet are closer together.

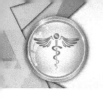

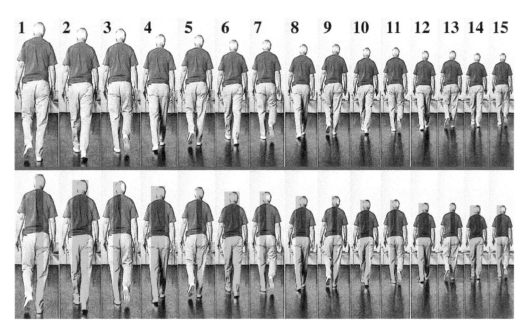

FIGURE 26.2: A functionally normal person in a natural walk.

Now this question: Why does the spacing between his feet change as he walks? His feet are some-times slightly wider apart because he does not fully complete the weight transfer onto the foot he is then supporting his body with. He doesn't center his body over that foot, which means the pressure in the foot is not centered. This incomplete transfer of body weight leaves a small amount of increased pressure toward the inside of the foot. This pressure pushes his body forward at a slight angle to the side, forcing the wider spacing of his feet. This pattern is very common to many.

WALKING POSTURE, MILD IMPAIRMENT

As previously mentioned, I have a movement impairment that is the result of a genetic mutation in my DNA. It is a neurodegenerative disorder called spinocerebellar atrophy (SCA14). Like many other people with spinocerebellar atrophy, I was born with this disorder. Therefore, I have had it all my life, *and not just since 1997* when I received the formal diagnosis, when I was forty-five with mild symptoms.

For the first thirty-plus years of my life, I had no symptoms that I was aware of. Then, by 2003, my movements had deteriorated enough that an examining neurologist recommended that I begin using a walker. But in 2005, at fifty-three years of age, my movement impairment had improved to mildly mod-erate, and that is when I consciously began working to improve my movement ability. That brings us to Figure 26.3. The year was 2012, and my movement impairment had improved to very mild. Look closely at my walk and compare it with Dave's in Figure 26.2. These pictures were recorded on the same day, minutes apart and on the same surface. Look closely for similarities and differences.

I was delighted to see there is only a slight difference between Dave's walking pattern and mine. This is very important to see, especially for those with an impairment. This represents a positive possibility for many. This represents a proof that impaired movements can be improved when you understand how to create that improvement, and when you put forth the required effort to achieve it.

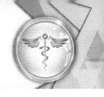

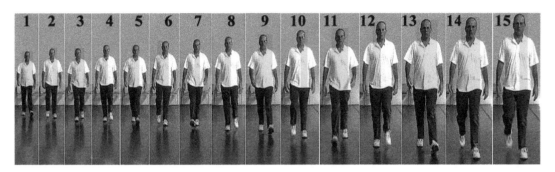

FIGURE 26.3: Typical walking pattern of a person with a very mild movement impairment.

In the walking-pattern comparison, one difference you do see is that when I am on one foot, I tend to move a little more out of the center of the stability zone than Dave does. My transfer of body weight in this example is not as good, and that is why the spacing between my feet is a little wider than his. Personally, this doesn't bother me in the least, because the spacing between my feet *had been* a lot wider years ago, and this shows that my walking ability is much improved. And the important part is, I feel "normal" much of the time when I'm walking.

These pictures show that I have not returned to a completely natural walking pattern. But on an individual basis, how close to a natural walking pattern does anyone need to be before it is acceptable to that person? The only thing that matters is *how comfortable you are* in your movements. It is the feeling, comfort, and control that matters. Not the look of it. This example is the "normal-like" natural movement recovery that I often refer to throughout the book.

I was able to reconnect with the practical use of my natural movements by gaining the knowledge that was totally missing in my intellectual *non*understanding. Learning how to stabilize and relax my posture allowed much of the naturally coordinated use of my body to return. Then, learning how to restore the natural synchronization of my body to my feet became a wonderful and amazing thing to enjoy again. Many others can achieve this very same thing.

WALKING POSTURE, MODERATE AND SIGNIFICANT IMPAIRMENT

In Figure 26.4, Jim has a mildly moderate movement impairment, which is how my movements were in 2005. In Figure 26.5, Charlotte's movements are moderately impaired. They share the same movement problems but have different neurodegenerative disorders.

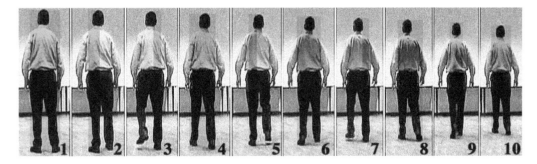

FIGURE 26.4: Typical walking pattern of a person with a mildly moderate movement impairment.

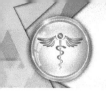

In Jim and Charlotte's examples, compare how far their heads move away from the center of the zone of stability when they move onto one foot. Then go back and compare their movements with the two previous examples. Note how Charlotte moves farther away from the center than Jim does, and Jim moves farther away from the center than I do.

Their postures are guarded and stiffened, with Charlotte having more stiffening than Jim. They both hold their arms out to their sides with stiffened hands. But because she is more unstable, Charlotte's arms are held farther out than Jim's. Because she has more stiffness in her knees, Charlotte is also more upright in her posture than Jim is. These slight differences *cause* Charlotte's movements to be more of a problem, which is exactly what you see happening in the pictures.

Her increased postural stiffness forces increased instability and greater difficulties transferring body weight from foot to foot. For these reasons, the spacing between her feet is wider as she walks. Using pressure on the insides of both feet, she is forced into a wider stance.

Charlotte has more fear of falling than Jim does. This forces her to put more thought and energy into everything she does. Imagine what the difference in her posture and movements would be if she had the ability to release some of that fear and relax some of her stiffness. Could she ever accomplish this? And if so, how long might that process take?

The progressive decline in movement ability seen in these three comparative examples is common with neurodegenerative disorders. As postural guarding and stiffness ratchet up, so does fear. At the same time, movement ability and function diminish.

If Charlotte could reduce her stiffness just a little, her movements would look like Jim's. If Jim learned how to trust himself and relax more, his movements

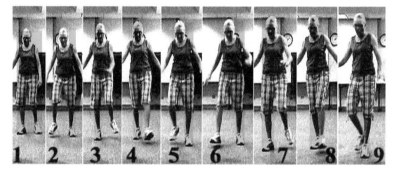

FIGURE 26.5: Typical movement pattern of a person with a moderate movement impairment.

would look and feel very much like mine. If you doubt any of this and it sounds too good to be true, then **please don't take my word for any of what you're reading**. Regardless of what your movement abilities might be, to the best of your ability personally test everything I've written. Prove it to yourself, and learn to trust what you prove. This applies equally to those with natural abilities.

About the Space between Your Feet

The "**good**" of the wide-based stance and gait:

1. The instability of a stiffened and upright posture forces the wider spread of the feet, to use the increased stabilizing force coming from the insides of the feet. This increases the surface area of the supporting foundation, but as the stiffened feet are spread wider apart, the area of the feet in contact with the floor decreases.

   How can that be a good thing? The body weight is being supported by a smaller area of each foot. Therefore, the pressure in that smaller area of each foot is more concentrated. Because of the direction in which the pressure is being applied to the floor, this has a greater stabilizing effect when the person is standing.

2. With feet spread widely, the pressure on the insides of both feet is pushing outward. Thus, the pressure on the inside of each foot pushes the body toward the other foot. Therefore, when standing, the body is naturally pushed and stabilized to the center of the stance by this *cross-bracing force*. The downside is that it only works when standing on a surface where the feet will not slip away outward.

   For example, look at the pictures of Jim and Charlotte when they have both feet on the floor. Note how their bodies are very close to being centered in their stability zones.

3. The widened stance can be corrected. Converting stiffened postures to relaxed postures will naturally create a narrower stance, because the wider stance is no longer needed.

   A stiffened posture relies on body weight to create the downward pressure in the feet. A relaxed posture uses body weight and creates downward pushing pressure from productively working leg muscles.

   For example, toddlers begin walking with their feet held apart because they are in an unstable time in their development. As they mature and their muscles develop, they acquire the ability to apply the downward pressure into their feet, and the spacing between their feet quickly normalizes.

   An adult with a widened stance can learn to do this again by re-creating the exact same thing.

The "**bad**" of the wide-based stance and gait:

1. The increased pressure on the insides of the feet in a stiffened, wide-based stance is stabilizing for standing, but *de*stabilizing for movement.

2. A stiffened posture in a widened stance is stabilized to the sides, but it is *unstable to the front and back*.

   In a straightened upright posture with a widened stance, many people "lock" their knees and then "relax" into a less-stiffened posture. They can do this by using the self-centering pressure from the insides of their feet while supporting their bodies with their leg bones.

   Because it is easier for standing and *very* small, restricted movements, this quickly becomes a habit, and they grow overly dependent on it. Within a short time, this also becomes another reason why they often don't use the natural stabilizing, downward-pushing pressure from their legs. Why? They are using stiffened leg muscles to hold their knees straight. These stiffened muscles are not productively working muscles, so they are not used and exercised as they naturally would be. The result: These muscles then have decreasing ability to apply pressure into the feet, and further limits movement ability.

   Eventually, creating and using downward pressure from the legs becomes unfamiliar to people with this posture and stance. Also, as their postural instability increases, the location of the pressure in their feet frequently and easily changes. Then, when they *do* add downward pressure into their feet, they learn to fear it because they cannot control where that pressure goes in their feet. As

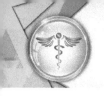
the location of the pressure in the feet changes, the stability and movement of the body also change. So, what is the result? They unexpectedly move, tip, or fall in various directions, and to this sudden movement their posture becomes guarded. As this continues to happen, their posture becomes more guarded due to the growing fear the tipping and falling produces. The combination of this physical and psychological reaction causes them to *stop* pushing added pressure into their feet.

3. A widened stance impairs weight shifting. The farther apart the feet are, the farther the body is away from the center of each foot. The farther apart the feet are, the more pressure there is on the inside of each foot, and this pressure force must be overcome to move the body onto either foot. This forces the person to do more work in each stride.

    Look again at Charlotte as she moves from one foot to the other in Figure 26.5. Then compare that with Dave doing the same thing in Figure 26.2. Charlotte has much farther to go to transfer her body weight, and her stiffened posture makes the transfer more difficult.

4. With a stiffened upright posture, relying on inside foot pressure for stability decreases the need to flex the knees. This allows the person to stand "comfortably" with stiffened, and often locked, knees. Then, when they need to flex their knees, the knees are unprepared and restrictive.

    To flex a knee when it is being held straight, they must first remove the pressure from the joint that is holding it there. But remember, they are using the muscles that support and move the knee to push and hold the knee backward, *and* they are using their leg bones to support their weight.

    Both issues cause major problems. From lack of use, weakening muscles erode the ability to support the body and flex the joints. So, when they are forced to flex their knees, these people experience a high level of instability and sudden lack of standing support.

5. Becoming comfortable in a wide-based stance means you are becoming increasingly *uncomfortable* in a more natural stance, which makes natural movement that much more difficult to return to.

    When *forced or encouraged* to bring their feet closer together, people who rely on this wide stance become increasingly unstable, for the same reasons that force them to have and keep a widened stance. Many well-meaning people need to be aware of this.

6. It's quite all right to stand in a widened stance when you can control it, and when that is what you want to do. However, it is not okay to remain in this posture when attempting to do natural movements.

    For example, people with natural ability often stand in a wide stance. However, just *before or as* they begin the movement, they shift out of it and very quickly assume a narrower stance.

    Because their stiffened posture and weakened muscles won't allow it, the moderately movement-impaired person has difficulty with and often cannot make this adjustment.

Note: Those with natural movement ability will need to force themselves to stay in a stiffened stance *if they wish to honestly feel* what it's like to move and walk feeling like a statue. They need to play with being slightly stiff, and then stiffer still, to come close to feeling the problems they will then create for

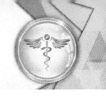

themselves. For those who can hold some postural guarding and stiffening, I guarantee they will experience many of the same problems people with restrictive-posture movement impairments feel every day.

FIRST THREE STRIDES

To those with a movement impairment, especially those with a restrictive posture, have you noticed that when you begin a movement, the first three strides you take are often the most troublesome? When you are stiff, the first three strides are often awkward, clumsy, and filled with panic, fear, and sudden falls. What causes this? You do.

With the improper setup posture for the movement you want to do, you create this recipe for movement problems and failures. It happens when you don't properly prepare yourself for taking the first stride. It happens because you begin the movement with instability, and then things get worse as you conjure up inadequate corrections and overcorrections. It happens because you were impatient. But mostly it happens because you don't know how to prevent or correct it.

The stability of a movement is directly related to the person's posture. Since natural movements depend on a relaxed posture, any posture that is not relaxed will, and does, cause problems. For example, in Figure 26.6, Amy is unprepared to stand up from the chair and then walk forward. Note that

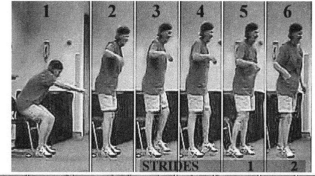

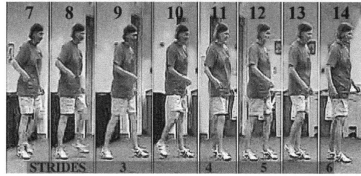

FIGURE 26.6: Amy abruptly stands up from the chair and then very quickly begins "walking." More correctly stated, she tips stiffly forward into a forced forward movement. She was unprepared to stand and very unprepared to begin the forward movement. This is why the first three strides were awkward.

the numbering at the top is the sequence of the pictures, while the numbering at the bottom counts the strides taken.

In picture 2, Amy is standing with a stiffened posture and is unstable with increased pressure in her heels. Her knees are slightly flexed, but stiff and unable to do anything more. Her postural stiffness is evident in her elevated and rigid right arm in most of the pictures, and in her left foot in picture 4, where the front of it is pointing upward. In pictures 2 through 8, her shoulders are slightly forward and elevated, and she is tipping forward. In picture 9, she stops the tip with the advanced left foot and then, in picture 10, begins moving her shoulders back. By picture 11, they've gone too far, so she makes a small adjustment forward in picture 12. What does this shoulder movement mean? This is showing you that she is using her upper body to start and then continue the movement. Moving her upper body forward, she "pulls" her body into the movement, and then slows it by moving her upper body backward.

Now a question to the reader: What was Amy feeling as this was happening?

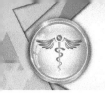

In picture 2, she feels her body tipping forward from the balls and toes of her stiff feet. In pictures 5 through 8, she feels her upper body moving forward faster than her feet and legs are moving. This forces her into the two uncontrolled stutter steps shown in pictures 5 and 6, and then the longer stride in pictures 7 through 9. The longer stride is required for her advancing foot to catch up with the movement of her upper body. This slows her upper body's forward movement and allows her to return to small strides in pictures 10 through 14. These let her begin relaxing some of the postural stiffness.

In picture 9, Amy's straightening left knee forces increased pressure into the heel of her advanced foot. This significantly slows her body's forward motion and replaces it with a backward movement, which is seen happening in picture 10, with the full results in picture 11. In picture 10, her shoulders begin to relax and descend, because at that moment she feels stable. Then increasing pressure moves into her heels as her upper body continues moving back, she becomes unstable, and the stiffening returns in picture 11.

In pictures 12 through 14, she again starts relaxing her posture after finally gaining some control of the movement with stabilization of the pressure in her feet. This allows her to assume a more controlled walk with small strides. The first three strides are awkward and uncontrolled. Then, as predicted and frequently seen, in the fourth stride, control begins returning (picture 11). But what if it does not?

Typically, when control does not begin to return in the fourth stride, the movement has become increasingly uncontrollable and unsustainable. It grows more erratic, with exaggerated overcorrecting and/or noncorrecting postures. Then accidents, falls, and injuries happen. This is the very common pattern that many movement-impaired people with stiffened postures lead themselves into, and typically *repeat multiple times every day*. Much of this is **preventable**. The "how do they do that?" explanations and instructions have been repeatedly given in detail throughout multiple chapters in this book.

UNPREPARED MOVEMENTS AND THE WIDTH OF THE STANCE

Walking with the feet spread widely apart causes problems. For example, the person intends to walk straight forward, but their body moves forward at an angle. This unexpected trajectory causes those with a restricted-posture movement impairment to stiffen and further complicate the movement.

Their body moves forward at an angle because that is where their foot pushed it. In a wide-based stance, the pushing pressure is on the inside forward portion of the pushing foot. Therefore, when they use this pressure, it pushes into the floor at an angle outward and backward. The body responds by moving forward at an angle, exactly opposite to that push.

When this movement surprises the mildly movement-impaired person, they usually can quickly correct the mistake without much mishap. However, those who have a moderate or significant movement impairment will typically go through several overcorrective maneuvers like Amy's in the previous example—when they are having a good day. On the not-so-good days, their movements are more exaggerated and erratic, and they often fall.

The correction begins by first moving into a relaxed ready stance. Then, move the feet closer together, and adjust the posture to a ready stance to create the correct pressure. To begin the movement, the next part is the complete shift of body weight to one foot, and then the use of small strides as the movement continues. Movements work much better when you begin and continue with the proper setup and relaxing posture, and with the correct pressure in the feet that's required for the intended movement.

You can see the results of this advice in Figure 26.7. Compare Charlotte's movements in this example with those in an earlier session with her in Figure 26.5. (In total, we did ten working sessions over 6 weeks, and these pictures come from the video of one of the last sessions.)

This series of pictures shows she has corrected some of her postural mistakes, has better control of the pressure in her feet, and is transferring body weight more effectively. Comparatively, there is a clear contrast between her former reactionary mind-set in dealing with stiffened movements, and this improving, anticipatory mind-set with more relaxed movements.

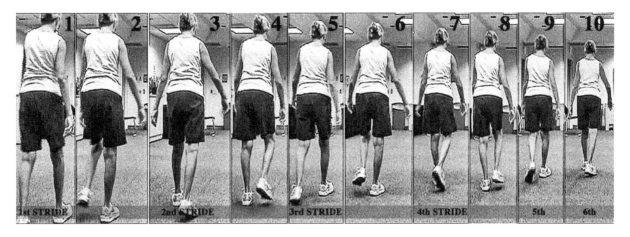

FIGURE 26.7: Finding the ability to create stability and add relaxation to her posture permitted Charlotte's moderate movement impairment to improve to a mildly moderate impairment. This happened within six weeks.

In time, Charlotte realized that what she had believed to be the *only* cause of her movement problems was not the only cause. In her transition to improving movements, she learned that her stiffening posture and fear response were also responsible for making her very real problems even greater problems. In this example, she is not internally fighting herself as she was in the previous example. This allowed her previously moderate impairment to improve to a milder moderate impairment.

This is no miracle cure or quick fix. Yes, Charlotte did very well in a short period of time. However, her real work to continue this trend has just begun. Many people I work with achieve quick improvements while I am working with them, just as she experienced. But everyone also needs to be realistic about what is ahead of them. To keep what they have gained, to rediscover advancing abilities in order to enjoy a better life, every bit of it requires a great deal of steady and dedicated work on nearly a daily basis.

The alternative is straightforward and not so nice. *If you do not continue working and playing*, many of you will quickly lose what you've gained and go back to the way things were before you began.

This is definitely not a "learn it once and then forget it" situation. It is exactly the opposite. To stay ahead of the progressive disorder inside you and keep what you gain, or even maintain your present level of functioning, you must continue to challenge yourself. That is the only way you will come to understand how to apply the knowledge in this book, to then learn how to easily recognize and trust the feelings

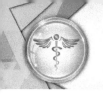

within your feet, posture, and movements. Plain and simple. It requires your strong commitment. Are you worth the effort?

MOVEMENT PREPARATIONS

Learn to use some added patience. Slow down. Take a few seconds to help yourself avoid a preventable disaster by completing the correct setup posture for the movement. Before you begin any movement, you will find it very helpful to do the following:

1. First, stop and feel where the pressure is in your feet.

2. Before you move from the spot where you're standing, practice a few standing-in-place transfer-of-body-weight movements from foot to foot, to "warm up" your legs and knees, and to bring your feet closer together if they're farther apart.

    This *does not* mean scraping, scuffing, or dragging a foot on the floor to bring your feet closer. It means lifting a foot off the floor with your knee, by first properly shifting your weight to and balancing on the other foot.

3. Adjust the pressure in your feet to where it needs to be for the movement you're about to do. If you're confused about where the pressure should be in your feet or how to get it there, **please go back and review** the appropriate chapters.

4. When you are uncomfortable and have any problems beginning the movement, you need to keep your beginning strides small. Keep them very small, as in stomping-on-a-bug small, as in half-the-length-of-your-foot small, as in baby-step small. Why?

    Smaller strides involve smaller movements that are easier to control. They are more stabilizing and safer. This helps you to relax more and eliminate some of your mistakes.

    Stay with small strides until your body naturally begins to relax. It is with that release, and only then, that you will have the ability to safely begin taking longer strides. How will you know? You'll feel it.

5. If you need to move faster when taking small strides, do it by making faster small strides. To do this, simply do quicker weight shifts. This will speed up the number of small strides you can safely make. Remaining stable and in control is the key point.

6. Following this pattern, your relaxing body will tell you when it's okay for you to take longer strides. This will not be something you'll consciously decide. Rather, it will be something you'll feel. Most often, the longer strides will "simply happen" as your body relaxes.

    As an example, after watching a movie in a theater, when the movie is over and the credits are beginning to fill the screen, I don't go anywhere. Unless I need to clear the path for others, I stand up only after

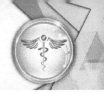

the other people have moved past me. While the others are leaving, I am doing my warm-up of stretching my legs and flexing my knees. I then stand as they're leaving and begin alternating weight shifts from foot to foot while letting my eyes adjust to the dim light. When I need it, I use the back of the seat in front of me for support, and the soft seat is behind me if I need that as well. Whenever possible, I don't start walking out until all the naturally moving people have filtered out of their seats and have mostly moved down the stairs. Now I can move at my speed as my body requires, especially for going down the steps. I *always* do this. I allow myself whatever time I need to make my movements better, even if it takes until the cleanup crew is starting to do their job.

There is another point to be made here. For those of you who cannot let go of the thought "I don't want anyone to see me like this," waiting and preparing by standing in front of your seat will eliminate it. By taking your time, instead of getting lost in the thoughts in your head, you will be better able to focus on your body, feet, and movements.

Feeling even a part of "normal" returning to your movements is a wonderful thing. What's even better is *not* feeling fear that you will make mistakes, because you know you can correct the smaller ones you will continue to make. This is the ultimate goal you are striving to achieve.

*Finding perfection in your movements is **not** what you are seeking.*
*Feeling comfortable doing what you want to do **is**!*
Imagine having that feeling in your life again.

■   ■   ■

CHAPTER 27

ISSUES OF THE SIGNIFICANTLY MOVEMENT IMPAIRED

Walking, relaxed and carefree, gazing into the distance, thinking of nothing.
Life becomes complex when something so simple is lost.

A subset of people with significantly impaired movements still manage to move independently in a very restrictive, shuffling type of walk. Their posture is deceiving. When just standing, these people very often fool the casual observer, because it appears that their impairment is only mild to moderate. Standing still, they often appear to be fairly relaxed and stable. But this changes very quickly as they begin a movement and show how unstable, impaired, and fragile they are in their movements.

Therapists and other helpers: Please pay attention to these details! Not all, but most of the people I have worked with in this category have an impaired voice. This is a tip-off to what you will likely see in their movements. The seemingly relaxed posture they're in when sitting changes to a very stiffened one as soon as they start to move when standing. Because of this posture, their walk is a noisy shuffling of shoes sliding on the floor, and *they are very fragile in their movements.* Frequently, they stutter-step as their shoes hesitate in sliding on the floor. They tip easily, are very prone to falling, and have minimal ability to correct a mistake.

Tom is one of these people (Figure 27.1). To the casual observer, his posture and walk often resemble that of an extremely fatigued indi-

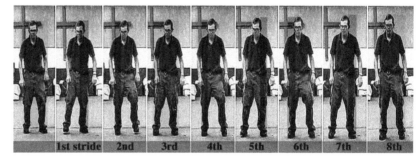

FIGURE 27.1: A very stiffened posture will allow only very small and noisy shuffling foot movements. Tom took eight strides to move a very short distance from the line on the floor.

vidual with natural ability who is moving very carefully. Nothing could be further from the truth. In this example, he moves through eight very small strides. Take note of the black line on the floor behind him. It's a good reference to illustrate how small his shuffling strides physically are.

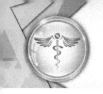

In this example, his arms look somewhat relaxed, and he is slightly flexing his knees. But he is definitely not relaxed. He is very guarded and stiffened, *especially* in his legs and feet. In this very restricted movement, he keeps his arms down at his sides and does not move them as his feet shuffle noisily on the floor. Functionally, he is producing very, very little to no push with his feet. Why? He must remain precariously "balanced" on very stiffened feet using the inside pressure of each foot to push him back onto the other foot. This is shown with reference to the inserted green zones of stability. He "rocks" back and forth from foot to foot, from one side of the zone to the other. Also, remember that the pressure he is using on the inside of his feet is from his body weight, and he is applying very little additional pressure (if any) from working muscles in his legs. He makes very slow forward progress, and all the while, he is very, very close to the edge of disaster. The smallest change in his posture or the position of his arms, or a slight change in the floor, is all that's needed to throw him into an extremely stiff-legged, stuttering, falling mishap.

He is instantly in big trouble when the bottom of his shoe catches on the floor, or he needs to change direction or stop, or a puff of wind forces his body to speed up or slow down, or moves any part of his body. This is the daily experience for this group of people with every movement they do. However, since most of them can stand still very well on their own without assistance, even with these issues and the risks in each movement, many of them proudly insist on continuing to "walk" independently as long as possible.

One day we were discussing and working on his postural and movement issues, but Tom's concern remained centered in this comment. He said, "I think I would walk better if I could take bigger steps." He was referring to his taking longer strides when he uses his walker, but was confused as to why he couldn't do the same without it.

Without the support of the walker, Tom's ability to shift his body weight from foot to foot is very limited. Because of this, he is barely able to lift a knee, to lift the foot off the floor. This is the reason the bottom of the front of his shoe scuffs loudly against the floor as it moves forward. With the very incomplete transfer of weight, the slightly lifted foot is quickly forced back down to the floor, further limiting the length of the stride. As his shoe scuffs the floor, it slows the movement of the foot while his body's slow forward movement continues. Each foot scuffs on the floor, therefore he is constantly tipping slightly forward. But he needs this forward tip. Because there is no push coming from his feet, this is what pulls him into the next shuffling stride. Thus, to continue the "walking" movement, his shuffling, stiffened feet remain slightly behind the slight forward tip of his body. A precarious dilemma. This is why he is always one second away from falling forward.

From one perspective, Tom is correct in saying that he would do better if he could take longer strides. Many movement-impaired people have this same thought, so that is what they focus on.

Yes, if he had the physical ability to take a longer stride, he would be walking better. If he could take longer strides, then he would also have better ability to transfer body weight, and apply pushing pressure with his foot, and lift his knee, and not scuff his feet as much. He would have the ability to catch up with and eliminate his forward tipping—*if* only he took longer strides.

But no! Longer strides are not his or their solution. With that, some of you are saying, "But he does better when taking longer strides with the walker. And since he is, that seems to imply that he does have the ability." No. It does not.

WALKING WITH HIS WALKER

Tom said, "When I'm using a walker, I do better and can take longer strides. *But it keeps pulling me forward, and that messes up my walking.*" Many people who use and abuse a walker feel and say this same thing.

I responded, "So, Tom, if what you say is true, then your binky [the walker] has a secret power source. But you know it does not, and you know it has no ability to move itself. So, tell me, friend, how exactly does your binky pull you forward?

"It does not and cannot," I continued. "Your binky is *not* pulling you forward. The problem is with what *you* are doing. I refer to this as the 'love-hate relationship' people create when they *abuse* their walkers."

This situation is shown in Figure 27.2. The inserted blue line behind Tom in the pictures serves as a reference to show the movement of his *upper* body. When he moves his upper body forward, he pushes the walker away with his stiff arms and takes a forward stride

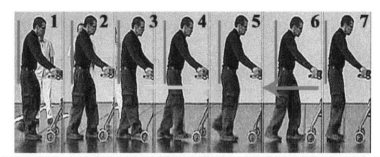

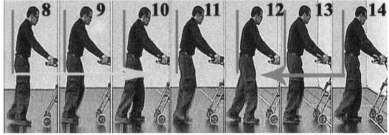

FIGURE 27.2: When your walker "pulls" you forward, you are causing it. Tom leans forward, his stiffened arms push the walker, and his upper-body lean pulls him forward with the walker. He then stops the forward movement of his body using the walker's brakes, and then moves his feet forward as he moves his upper body backward.

with it. Because this also moves pressure forward in his feet and increases the speed of the movement, he squeezes the brake handle more than he already is to slow "the walker's forward movement." This is showing that Tom is controlling his movement by controlling the movement of the walker, which is exactly the opposite of what is meant to be happening. Many people develop this bad habit with walkers.

The arrows in the figure indicate the direction his upper body is moving. Since his strides are very small, this body movement is subtle. The green arrows indicate that his upper body is moving forward, and the red arrows indicate it is moving back.

His stiffness and lack of control of the pressure in his feet are still the problems. For example, if his elbows were flexing, the walker wouldn't move as much when he leans forward.

So, it's not the fault of the walker pulling him forward. The fault is with the person pushing the walker forward with body lean, adding more pressure to the toes of their shoes, and increasing the forward push of the walker. This is what they interpret as the walker pulling them forward.

Many people abuse a walker this way. "Push the walker away so it will pull me forward. Stop the walker by tightly squeezing the brake handle, to pull it back to me."

This is a love-hate relationship. It's as if they hate the walker—partially releasing the brake handles and leaning into it to push it away. But then they realize they love and need it—squeezing the brake handle to stop it and pull it closer.

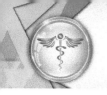
Explaining this to him, I continued, "Tom, you are actually fighting yourself as you are walking with the walker. You are fighting to stop from falling forward, and the walker is *not* causing it. Look at your hands. You have a death grip on the handgrips and brakes. Your fingers and knuckles are white, and the muscles in your forearms are tight. Feel how locked up and tight your elbows are. Are you honestly trying to tell me that your walker is making you do that?

"Now consider something else that has nothing to do with your walker. Where is the pressure in your feet when you're being 'pulled forward' by your walker? Feel the increased pressure you've put in the ball areas and toes of your feet. What does that tell you?

"Test what I'm saying. Try to stand like that without squeezing the brakes on your walker and tell me what you feel."

He hesitated for a few seconds, so I asked, "Are you having a problem with trying to let go of the walker, Tom?"

"I feel like I'm falling forward," he said.

"Imagine that," I replied with a smile.

People with a restrictive-posture movement impairment have another common problem using a walker. As they walk, their feet are spread as wide apart as the wheels and legs of the walker, so the forward-moving foot very frequently hits the wheel or leg. So, how do they remedy this? To avoid kicking the wheel or leg, they push the walker farther away and then must lean forward to grip the handles, creating many of the problems we've just discussed.

With wheels, the walker moves very easily, but their feet *do not*. With their hands, arms, and body pushing the walker away, they must tighten their hold on the handgrips and brakes to keep it close. For most, this alone causes increased postural stiffening and moves increased pressure to the forward ball areas and toes of their feet. This combination makes it very difficult for them to transfer body weight to move either foot.

Relaxing Frozen Postures

Jerry has a very tight, shuffling walk that is even more restrictive than Tom's. He also has the same deceptively "relatively relaxed" posture and appearance when standing. Yet in reality, his posture is stiffly held in place. For the record, they both have the same type of degenerative neurological disorder.

In Figure 27.3, Jerry is walking very close to the wall. Things to note in the pictures are:

1. He takes eight strides, and his posture and shadow on the wall only change ever so slightly.

2. After eight strides forward, he is still close to the red chair he was sitting on.

3. The space between his feet, and the space between his shoulders and the wall, do not change.

4. During the seventh stride, his head moves slightly forward and then returns in the eighth. The position of his right arm changes very slightly in the seventh stride to counterbalance the slight head movement.

Like Tom, Jerry has only slight movement of his knees and shuffles his feet just as noisily. However, Jerry uses a different method to "power" his movements. He uses a *slight* forward-and-back movement of his head. This is

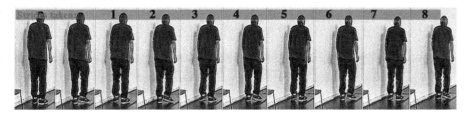

FIGURE 27.3: The numbers at the tops of the pictures count the strides taken. Due to a nearly "frozen" posture, Jerry's movements are extremely restricted.

shown in the pictures with reference to the inserted green zones of stability in Figure 27.4. To begin the stride, he moves his head forward. To stop it, he moves it back. In picture 1, he moves his head forward and then takes two small shuffling strides. In picture 6, he again moves his head forward, but this time only slightly. He completes the third stride in picture 8 and then prepares for the fourth stride by continuing to move his head forward.

In this profile view, you can also see the extremely limited movement of his upper body. His posture is nearly "frozen" in place like a statue.

Both Tom and Jerry have nearly zero trust in their independent movement ability. Surprisingly, though, their observed behavior does not rep-

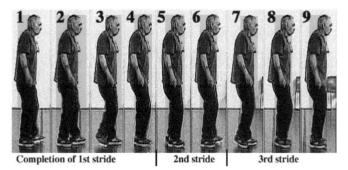

Completion of 1st stride | 2nd stride | 3rd stride

Figure 27.4: With an extremely stiffened posture, Jerry uses small head movements to inch his body forward.

resent that lack of trust. Be very careful of this paradox, because people with these characteristics are constantly on the edge of falling.

FLAT FEET

When people like Tom and Jerry want to move, they are limited to staying within one "moving spot" on the floor until they tip and/or stutter-step into another spot. Standing on their own, their one and only "strength" is also their greatest liability.

When standing, they are *very still* and often look more stable than they actually are. How is that possible? Well, if you patiently watch them, you will see that they're standing on *very flat, stiffened feet*, so everything they do is slow and methodical. Their stability problems begin as soon as anything happens that even slightly moves the pressure in their feet. So be very, very cautious when you see a person like this. Because they have very limited ability to adjust their posture and the pressure in their feet, they very easily become unstable. In an instant, they will quickly become a startling surprise when something forces them out of their stillness. Often all it takes is a bit of wind or the light brush of someone or something against them.

There is another uncommon characteristic they share. Look at Jerry's and Tom's feet as they lift them off the floor to take their ministrides. Note that the front of the foot drops down as if it were relaxed. Well, to do this, it has to be. Lifted in the air, the foot is somewhat relaxed. But on the floor, it functions as if it were as rigid as ice. What does this mean? Again, it means they have hidden ability, naturally working parts, and a better potential for improvement than their overall appearance reveals.

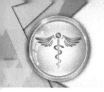

The problematic issue is discovering how to get them to release their potential. The caveat in this is understanding the source of their stiffness. The percentage of physiological stiffening contributing to their total stiffness is unknown, but from my observations it does appear to be very high. By itself, this factor presents the greatest difficulty in helping them gain better ability. When physiological stiffening is the stronger component, releasing the developed psychological postural stiffening is very difficult to do. Why? They are unable to relax enough of the physiological postural stiffening to effect a marked difference in their posture, to flex their joints more, to move into a more stable stance.

What else is deceptive about these two men in the pictures? Both have rounded shoulders with an almost uncaring look about them. This look is even more natural appearing when you see them standing still, and it is a look that conveys relaxed comfort to the casual observer. For example, compared with the other people with neurodegenerative disorders I work with, it's uncanny how this group of people's outward appearance **does not** match their inner restrictions. They are by far the most restricted in their movement ability, yet they display the least amount of outward fear.

■ ■ ■

CHAPTER 28

Changing Directions

When we're walking, a forward stride prepares us for the change-of-direction stride.

At the beginning of our last working session, Howard said to me, "When we're working together here in the room, I'm more stable than when I'm at home or at work. I'm thinking it's because of the mental distractions. When somebody talks to me from over there, or someone calls to me from back down the hall and I turn to look at them, I have problems. I tend to 'corkscrew.' I lose my balance when I turn, especially when I do it quickly. Sometimes I even get that way when I only turn my head. I'll be walking pretty well one second. Then suddenly, the next second I'm a spiraling mess."

"You're correct, Howard," I said. "There are fewer mental distractions and very few physical distractions in this room, and it is large. The floor space is open, with only a few chairs placed against the walls. At the office, there are chairs, tables, lamps, and desks filling the room, and other people walking around. In the real world, there are always obstacles of some kind that you must move around and through. Here, there are none of those obstacles. Out there, you're forced to make adjustments to whatever crosses your path. But here, you aren't. So, with that thought in mind, what is the first thing you feel yourself doing when you walk into a room with things or people in it?"

"I feel like I tense up a little bit," he replied.

"Exactly. You begin by mentally reacting to what you see. Your fear issues flare and throw you back into old, maladaptive reactions. Every time you react that way, you subconsciously remind yourself that you don't trust your movement abilities. You remind yourself that you are expecting to have the problems you will then have. For example, you walk into a restaurant and immediately focus on the tables, chairs, and people crammed into the confining spaces and how little space there is to walk. Or you walk into a busy mall and your focus jumps to the problems *you know you will have* when walking with the crowds of people moving in every direction. Subconsciously and consciously, your mind is on high alert.

"Your first impulse is to immediately withdraw and guard as you remind yourself, 'I shouldn't be here.' This frequently repeating, self-destructive psychological response creates most of the reflexive tensing you still feel happening in your posture today. Your mind is forever primed, awaiting the next bad situation, and is very easily activated. This results in a stronger and quicker response, and it kicks in even when it's totally unnecessary, when there is nothing to fear. We've both experienced it. It is not fun and

305

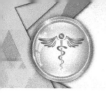

is often very ugly. With your ongoing movement problems, you use it more than you don't. This ensures that all your perceived fears will absolutely come true. So, where does this leave you?

"It leaves you in another disappointing failed attempt. Repeated failures eventually convert your subconscious doubts into conscious doubts. Essentially you have a big neon sign flashing negative images in your mind, prompted by all your scary thoughts and fears. Why do you keep them? You think you're using them to help keep yourself safe. But the reality of it is exactly the opposite. They make you worse. And you'll never be rid of them until you fix the physical problems.

"You use the exact same movements out there as you do right here without . . . without what, Howard? Your negative thoughts. You use the same movements here without the negative thoughts, and most of the time you are showing improvement. In a controlled environment in this open room, you are learning to use a positive focus on improving your movements. This is the very same focus you must learn to use and trust wherever you are, especially in small and confining spaces.

"Here in this large, open, and empty room, your focus can remain on just your movements. Out there, your focus is easily divided and distracted. Here, the environment is stable and unchanging, and everything is simplified. Out there, it becomes complicated. The environment constantly changes, and things happen unexpectedly. This forces you to focus on the distractions, and then you forget the positive focus you need to apply to your movements and posture.

"In short, situations become confusing and scary because of the way you negatively perceive them and yourself. The result: *You become the unstable part of the changing environment.*

"To correct this, you must stop allowing the scary things in your mind to immediately lead you down an imaginary path filled with problems you might need to react to. You must learn to stop becoming obsessed with the 'obstacles' in the space around you—to have the ability to see them as the innocent things they are. You must learn to stop focusing on things you cannot and need not control, and instead focus on the only thing you can control: you. Keep your focus on the same basics that you use during these sessions. They will allow you to walk out there much more like you're walking in here."

SHOULDER WITH HEAD MOVEMENT

When you react as Howard describes—"I feel myself tensing up"—you create a problem where there is very likely no problem. Your subconscious alarm causes your body to physically guard and stiffen. You must learn to pay attention to what you feel when this happens to you. Feel the physical reaction in your head, neck, and shoulders, and then follow that pattern all the way down to your feet. You must learn to recognize this transition from both the mental and the physical perspective, and work to correct both.

As discussed in previous chapters, when movement-impaired people with a restrictive posture guard and stiffen, many of them also hold the muscles in their neck and shoulders tighter. With a stiffening neck, when they turn their head, the head and shoulders move together rather than the head moving independently. This is the cause of Howard's "corkscrew" movements.

Howard was walking across the room when I called out to him in Figure 28.1. He then turned to look toward me and ended up in one of his corkscrew movements.

First, note the stiffness in his hands, arms, and shoulders. In picture 4, he begins to turn his head toward me, but then his shoulders follow the movement of his head in picture 5. Also, in picture 5 his left knee and foot are beginning to move outward to the left. Then, in picture 6, his pelvis is rotating left, lagging behind the movement of his shoulders. His intent was to continue walking forward while glancing to the left. Instead, this sequence of events caused his entire body to turn. This is a self-induced problem.

Howard's postural stiffening includes his neck. With stiffened neck muscles, he must use his shoulders to help turn his head. This shoulder/upper-body rotation precedes and causes the rotational movement of his pelvis, which forces his left knee and foot outward. Also, take note of his left shoulder drooping downward in picture 1. The drooping shoulder quickens the rotation, moving pressure toward the outside portion of his left foot on the floor, and more

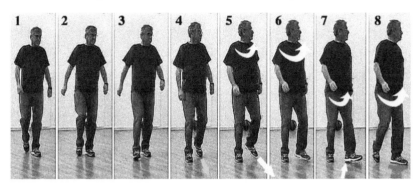

FIGURE 28.1: Howard complains that when standing or walking, he often becomes unstable when he turns his head. Many of you do this, too. Above is an example of why that happens. His head and shoulders turn together when he is wanting to turn only his head.

so in picture 8, as his body is rotating to the left.

He has created three forces in picture 8. His upper body is leaning to the left, his left foot is pushing him to the left, and the upper-body-initiated body rotation is to the left. This creates an uncomfortable, unstable, and uncoordinated rotational movement—his corkscrew feeling.

Food for thought: The weight of a typical adult human head ranges between eight and eleven pounds. When you carry bags in your hands with that much weight in them, what happens to your balance and movements when those bags begin swinging? They pull your body in the direction they're swinging, and the force of the moving weight moves the pressure in your feet.

This same problem often happens when the muscles in our neck are tight, as happens when we have a "stiff neck," for example. With this uncomfortable neck stiffness, we turn our head with our shoulders in an awkward movement. When a person with a restrictive-posture movement impairment has tight or stiffened neck muscles and turns their head, they also use their shoulders. However, with the rest of their body also being guarded (stiffened), their movement is more awkward and uncoordinated because they are not rotating their body with their knees to match the shoulder turn. Thus, there is no counterbalancing, and the weight of the moving head and shoulders moves the pressure in the feet, and alters the intended bodily movement.

This does not happen when your neck is relaxed and turns your head, because your head remains centered, because the movement is coordinated and counterbalanced.

CHANGING DIRECTIONS WHEN WALKING

Naturally, the foot we use for changing the direction of our body movement is always the foot on the side opposite the direction we want to go. If we want to turn or move to the left, we use our right foot to push our body to the left. When we want to turn or move to the right, we use our left foot to push our body to the right. We change the direction of our movement by taking a stride at an angle, which is the second stride.

Every turn begins with a forward stride. When walking, we prepare ourselves to move in a new direction by first completing a forward stride in the same direction we are walking. We then use the advanced foot to push our body in the new direction. Jiyoung demonstrates this in Figure 28.2.

There is nothing new here. The only difference between the first and second stride of the changing-direction movement is the location of the pushing pressure you create in your pushing foot. For moving straight forward, it is centered in the ball area and larger toes of the foot. For the angled movement in the new direction, the pushing pressure is located in the *inside* forward portion of the ball area and in the big toe.

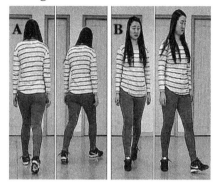

FIGURE 28.2: Changing the direction of your movement when walking always begins with a forward stride. Then the next stride is taken in the new direction.

Many movement-impaired people experience a major problem when they begin moving in a new direction. They create the problem by using the outside of the wrong foot to "push" the body into the movement, when they should be using the inside of the other foot.

An example of this is Kerry in pictures 1 through 6 of Figure 28.3, in which she is changing direction to her left by using her left (wrong) foot to initiate the movement. In pictures 7 through 9, she is using her right (correct) foot for the same movement.

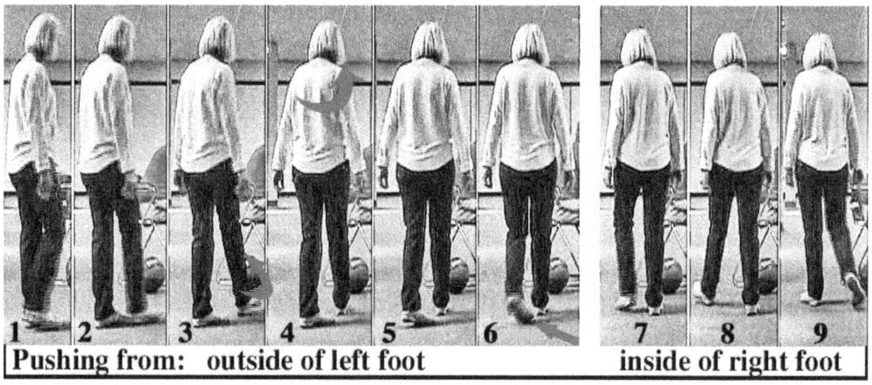

1. In picture 2, Kerry begins the changing-direction movement with her left foot, which is flattened on the floor with all her body weight on it. For this reason, it cannot move or pivot on the carpet.

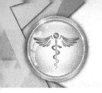

Pushing from: outside of left foot   inside of right foot

FIGURE 28.3: Using the left foot to push the body to the left forces the use of the outside of the foot. This is destabilizing and complicates and restricts the movement (pictures 1 through 6). The natural method is using the right foot to push the body to the left, using the inside of the foot (pictures 7 through 9). This simplifies and stabilizes the movement.

2. To move her right foot into position to support the continuing body movement in the next stride, her right leg must be brought forward and then to the left (pictures 2 through 4), crossing in front of her left leg.

3. To properly position her right foot, she has to rotate her body to the left, *while standing on her left foot, which does not move on the floor* (pictures 3 and 4). This creates an unstable and uncomfortable twisting action in her left knee and ankle.

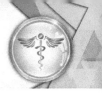

4. As her body rotates and her right leg crosses her left leg, the pushing pressure in her left foot moves to the *outside* forward portion of that foot (pictures 5 and 6).

5. When the ankle and knee are flexible, they will compensate for this mistake. However, with many movement impaired people, that knee is now not flexible in this position, and is often straight.

Think about this situation and see it in this example. Kerry is pushing her body to the left with her left foot, and that means there is no foot on her left side to naturally move onto as her body moves in that direction. In other words, there is no naturally "advancing foot" in this setup, because the foot that is supposed to be the advancing foot is supporting the body and doing the pushing. Therefore, the free right foot, which is unnaturally trailing on the outer side of the turn, must be brought around very quickly to become the advancing foot, to be in place when the body requires it for support.

This further complicates things for a movement-impaired person, especially when their posture is not relaxed. In picture 5, Kerry moves onto the toes and outside forward area of her left foot. This allows the foot to pivot on the carpet. However, the movement-impaired person with a restrictive posture is typically standing on the entire flattened foot while rotating their body, and the location of the increased pressure in the foot is highly variable. This means their foot typically does not rotate as Kerry's does in this example.

1. When the foot remains flat on the floor, the foot is fixed in place and is immovable on the floor. This is how twisting knee injuries, ankle fractures, and spiral fractures of the bones in the leg happen.

2. With increased pressure in the heel area, the foot will often pivot on the heel, but only when the pressure is far enough into the heel to allow the front of the foot to lift partially off the floor. This heel pivot forces a very awkward pushing fall from the outside portion of the heel. This creates a dramatic corkscrew movement with the body rotating to the side at a backward angle.

3. When the increased pressure is in the outside and forward part of the foot, the person typically will not pivot on the foot as Kerry did. This is because of the instability and lack of support they feel in that area of the foot. Therefore, a common outcome is stiffly twisting on the entire length of the foot while falling in the direction of the body turn, while being pushed by the pressure in the outside of the foot. This leaves the foot, ankle, and knee at significant risk of fractures and other injuries.

4. These are *very common AVOIDABLE mistakes that movement-impaired people with restrictive postures frequently create.*

Comparison

In Figure 28.4, Jiyoung, with natural ability, is demonstrating the issues we've just discussed. Panels A and B show the movement of the legs and feet when the outer portion of the wrong foot is used to

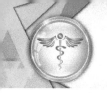

initiate the change of direction. In panel A, the increased pressure is in the ball area and toes. In panel B, she stays on a flattened foot. Then, in panel C, she uses the inner portion of the correct foot to show the naturally correct movement.

Compare these three examples and study the movements of the body, legs, and feet. Which panel of pictures looks to be the easiest, the most stabilizing, and the most natural way of walking through the movement?

In panel A, the direction change is being done with a push from the weakest portion of the right foot, which is the forward outside portion of the foot and the smaller toes. Using the foot in this way requires a very flexible posture and flexing supporting knee to complete the movement in a comfortable manner. It also requires a pivoting movement in the area of the foot in contact with the floor (indicated by the green arrow in picture 4).

Compare Jiyoung's posture in panel A with Kerry's posture in pictures 1 through 6 of Figure 28.3 to note a subtle difference. Kerry was walking on carpet, and her foot could not easily pivot. This restriction caused her to guard slightly in her posture in response to the uncomfortable feeling. For these two reasons, Kerry could not move as far in a new direction as Jiyoung did on the smooth floor.

In panel B, Jiyoung is changing directions while standing and pushing from the outer portion of the right foot, which is initially *flattened* on the floor (indicated by the red arrow in picture 2). Note that her body does not rotate as much as it does in panel A. This is because her body weight is pushing down into the entire foot, and this prevents it from pivoting on the smooth floor. *This non-moving, non-pivoting foot restricts the rotation of the body to only what the hips, knees, and ankle can provide.* This is one reason the next stride is shorter. The other reason is that the outside pressure is

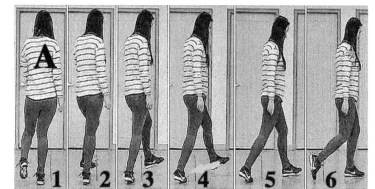

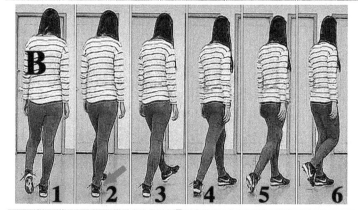

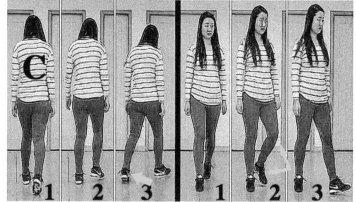

FIGURE 28.4: Comparison of using the inner foot (the one inside the turn) and outer foot (the one outside the turn) to push into the change-of-direction movement. The inner foot: wrong. The outer foot: correct.

A: Using the ball area of the inner foot.

B: Using a flattened inner foot.

C: Using the outer foot.

pushing the body to the side, and the rotation of the upper body makes it a backward push at an angle. Compare the stride lengths in panels A and B to see the result.

This situation causes stress injuries to the leg joints and forces uncontrollable, awkward falls. *This is also a very common mistake people with a restrictive-posture movement impairment make **when beginning a movement from a standing position**.*

In panel C, Jiyoung is demonstrating the correct way to do this movement. Note that there are only three pictures showing the rear view of the natural movement and three showing the front view, while six pictures are needed to show the movement done the complicated way in panels A and B.

Panel C shows the easy, natural, simple, and uncomplicated movement. Relaxed and controlled, using the inside portion of the left foot to push her body in the new direction and stride. One, two—done.

■　■　■

CHAPTER 29

Backward Stride

Before the question appears in your mind, your body is giving you the answer.

n most of our natural forward and side movements, we push our body through the movement using the front part of one foot. We also do this for moving backward. As with the forward stride, the push for a backward stride comes from the ball area and toes of the foot. However, the placement and contact of the foot we advance behind us in a backward stride is very different.

1. In natural forward movements, the heel is the first part of the advancing foot to contact the floor.

2. In natural movements to the side, the inside of the ball area and big toe are the first parts of the foot to contact the floor.

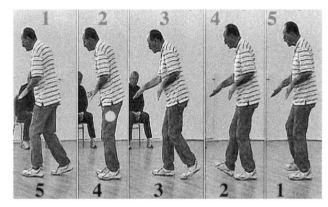

FIGURE 29.1: Which direction am I moving? Two strides. Are the top numbers correct, or are the bottom numbers correct?

3. In natural backward movements, the first parts of the foot to contact the floor are the toes, followed quickly by the forward ball area.

In Figure 29.1, I take **two** strides. Study them to determine in which direction I take them. Are the numbers at the tops of the pictures in the correct order, or are the numbers at the bottoms in the correct order? There is truth in both. Demonstrating the movement for Howard, I begin in the second picture from the left (labeled 2 at the top and 4 at the bottom), where my feet are together on the floor.

1. Using the red numbers, I begin the demonstration standing in picture 2 (with the green dot) with both feet together.

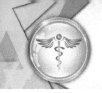

2. With my right foot, I push forward into the posture in picture 1, and pause.

3. Then I return to standing in picture 2 and again pause with both feet together.

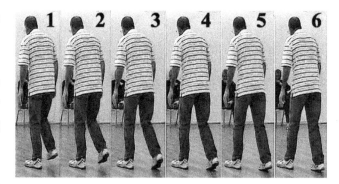

4. I then push with my right foot to move into a backward stride in picture 3, transfer onto my left foot in red picture 4, and then am moving onto both feet in picture 5.

FIGURE 29.2: Foot placement during a backward stride. The push comes from the ball area and toes of the pushing foot. The initial contact point of the foot advancing backward is the toes.

This example shows a very important point. In a forward and backward stride, we *use the exact same posture* with increased pressure in the ball area and toes of the pushing foot.

There are basically only two practical differences between the two movements:

1. The initial contact of the advancing foot to the rear. Figure 29.2 shows the initial contact and placement of the advancing foot during a backward stride, as shown in picture 3.

2. The direction the pressure is being pushed into the floor by the pushing foot. In a forward stride, the push is directed backward. In a backward stride, the push is directed forward.

HEEL PUSH

Many *moderately* movement-impaired people with restrictive postures commonly make two mistakes when taking a backward stride. This is especially true when their posture is guarded or stiffened.

1. Their knees are too straight.

2. Their shoulders are not far enough forward.

With shoulders too far back, the posture is too upright, and the increased pressure in the pushing foot will be toward its heel. This postural mistake commonly happens in one of two ways.

1. They begin the movement with straightened knees and shoulders held back.

2. Their shoulders move back as the movement begins, and then their knees straighten.
   The result is the same. The push comes from the heel area. This causes additional postural straightening and stiffening, leading to increasing instability.

With this rearward-moving postural shift, the placement of the foot advancing to the rear changes drastically. Instead of the toes contacting the floor first, the flatness of the foot with increasing heel pressure is first to contact the floor. This frequently forces the person into an uncontrolled heel-pushing, backward stutter-stepping fall that happens very quickly.

For the *mildly* movement impaired, this dangerous issue has four parts, as shown in Figure 29.3. Initially in this example, the push is from the ball area of the right foot (picture 1). But note how upright the posture is. This contributes to the coming problem.

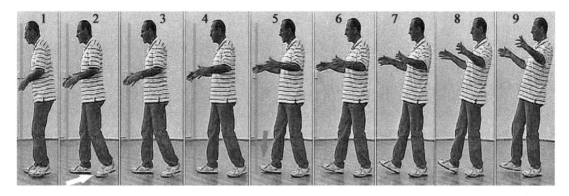

FIGURE 29.3: A common mistake while moving backward is beginning with shoulders too far back, and/or allowing them to go farther back during the movement. In this example, the starting posture is okay, but then the shoulders begin to fade backward. This causes knee straightening, moves the pushing pressure farther into both heels, and forces the body into a backward pushing accident.

1. As the upper body moves backward, away from the inserted blue line in pictures 2 through 5, increased pressure moves to the heel area of the right foot. Now the push is coming from the right foot's heel, and the effect of that is first seen in picture 2. Note that the rearward-moving advancing foot is forced down before the intended backward stride can be completed (yellow arrow). Then, in picture 3, the top of the body begins to move at an angle away from the inserted blue line.

2. The backward tipping of the body continues in the remaining pictures.

3. As the pushing pressure increases in the heel area of the right foot, the front of the foot lifts from the floor (indicated by the red arrow in picture 5).

4. There is another force that has been created and is fueling the coming accident. The rearward-moving body also moves body weight into the heel area of the left foot. Now both heels are pushing the body backward.

5. This is a common and preventable cause of head injuries.

In any stride—forward, to the side, or backward—the pushing foot controls and pushes the body onto the advancing foot. The pushing foot then stabilizes the body over the advanced foot, until the body and foot pressure are moved into position so the advanced foot can support the body by itself. The previously supporting foot is then freed so it can be moved. Note: When a *heel push* is used in a rearward stride, the feet very quickly lose all of these natural functions.

Read it again. In *any* stride in *any* direction, the pushing foot is the controlling, supporting, and stabilizing foot for the movement, until the other foot takes over this very important duty.

BALL AREA OF THE FOOT

When walking **forward**, we move from the ball area and toes of one foot, and the heel of the forward advancing foot contacts the floor with light pressure. As the body continues moving forward, the pressure moves forward through the advanced foot and into its ball area and toes. The pressure is then increased and concentrated into the ball area and toes by the action of the heel lifting, as any pressure in the rest of the foot is removed.

When walking **backward**, we move from the ball area and toes of one foot, directly onto the ball area and toes of the foot advancing to the rear. In continuing backward strides for those with natural ability, often the ball area and toes of both feet are the only areas that are used, but frequently the remainder of the advanced foot does lower to the floor as the body moves rearward. However, the increased pressure remains in the ball area and toes during continuing rearward movement.

An exception to this is when we take short rearward strides, and when the heel area is intentionally being used for support. But still, in the natural movement any pressure in the heel is kept *small* in comparison with the pressure in the ball area and toes.

TAKING A STRIDE VERSUS A STEP

In most of our natural movements, we push. We push our body into the movement to take a stride, and our body moves the other foot to a new location. But sometimes it is necessary to step into a movement, and stepping is a different movement than taking a stride. A common definition of stepping is: *a movement made by lifting the foot and putting it down in a different place, without respect to the movement of the body.* Therefore, when stepping we stand balanced on one foot as we extend the other leg away from our body to place that foot.

Only under certain required circumstances and in certain activities do we lift a foot and then direct it to a different place by itself. In most of our natural movements, we push our body into the movement, and our body places the foot where it needs to be. This is an important distinction, because the two movements are very different.

1. A stride is one movement. It is a controlled pushing action from the supporting foot in which the body and advancing foot are pushed away together as a unit.

2. A stepping movement requires two movements. A stepping movement begins with the supporting foot and body remaining relatively in place as the advancing foot is purposefully extended out in the direction of the next movement, and is then placed on the floor.

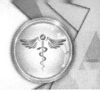

3. In the second part of the stepping movement, the body is moved onto the extended foot as the pressure is transferred from the supporting foot to the advanced foot.

Naturally, we walk backward by taking strides. *However*, in the backward "stride," we often begin with a stepping movement and then follow it with a pushing movement. In a more careful and more deliberate movement, we first extend a foot backward to place the toes and/or ball area of that foot on the floor, *and only then* push our body backward with the forward foot. We do this to ensure that we have a stable supporting foot behind us before committing to the movement.

Many people with a movement impairment have difficulty doing this.

1. Since they can't easily balance on one foot, people with a restrictive-posture movement impairment have difficulty moving backward, even when they are in the correct starting posture.

2. With an excessively upright posture, it's difficult for them to extend a foot backward, usually because they are unstable on the heel area of the pushing foot.

3. Staying on the ball and toes of the pushing foot with a flexed knee, and balancing on that foot, is often a challenge. Consider this: This backward movement is the equivalent of doing a mild, one-legged squat on the ball area and toes of one foot.

STABILITY FIRST

Those having problems with backward movement should practice using a stepping movement, securing the advancing foot, and then pushing the body back onto that foot. This technique *allows the use of both feet when your body is moving*, and it provides improved stability and control.

1. With knees slightly flexed, stand balanced on two flat feet that are side by side. Then, move your shoulders slightly forward to move the pressure forward into the ball areas, *but only lightly into the toes*.

2. Transfer your body weight onto one foot, holding the increased pressure in the ball area and keeping the knee slightly flexed.

3. Using the knee of the other leg, extend the lifted foot behind you approximately one length of your foot or less, and place the toes and ball area of the foot on the floor. Now push pressure into that part of the back foot and *hold* it. What about the pressure in the front foot? *Hold that push too.*

    When you hold your shoulders in a forward position while doing a small backward movement, the toes and ball area of the backward-advancing foot will always contact the floor first. So, when they don't, your posture is too upright, with shoulders too far back.

4. From the ball area of the forward foot, continue to slowly push your body rearward onto the remainder of the back foot, until you are standing balanced over the flattened back foot—**BUT** *with increased pressure still toward the ball area of the back foot.*

   Then, *AND ONLY THEN*, transfer all your body weight to the back foot before moving the *lifted* front foot back and next to the back foot.

5. Practice repeating this sequence of backward stepping until you are confident, and only then practice continuous backward strides.

6. *HINT!* **Before** you begin the movement, during the movement, and at the end of the movement, *remind yourself to keep your shoulders forward.*

7. Also, remind yourself to keep your knees flexed. Stay down.

8. For stability, comfort, and control: Baby steps and small strides.

Helpful Points

I have learned through experience:

1. When your shoulders move up and back enough to put you on **any** part of your heel, *your upper body has moved back much more than you think.*

   This will *always* put you in a tipping-backward posture, regardless of the direction you're intending to move. When this happens during a backward movement, the backward tip of the body is often more aggressive.

2. In the beginning, when you do this backward movement correctly, you will often feel that your shoulders are too far forward. Be very careful. This will cause many of you to change back to your old bad habits without realizing it.

   Listen to "Mama." Feel what your feet are telling you. That is your truth.

   Always. Feel your way through every movement.

■ ■ ■

CHAPTER 30

HILLS, SLOPES, AND INCLINES

When walking on a flat floor is a problem,
the thought of walking on a hill is mind-blowingly scary.

The surface we walk on does not alter the basic principles of our movements. But, because of what we see and think about some of the places we have to go, our minds are quite capable of causing us to alter the basics of our movements. With thoughts of doubts and fears, we create problems where there actually are few to none. Images of unpleasant situations and outcomes force us to misinterpret things. We change our posture accordingly, and create feelings of instability.

HILLS

Walking on a hill, compared with walking on stairs, is often thought to be very different. One is an angled surface, and the other has steps cut into the angled surface (Figure 30.1). However, when we walk on either of them, our movements and posture are actually more alike than they are different.

For the movement-impaired person, the length and steepness of a hill (incline) are often the aspects that frighten them the most. Seeing the hill, they focus on their difficulties and quickly imagine the worst outcome. Their mind prepares their body accordingly. How do they prepare? They guard and stiffen their posture *before* they move onto the hill.

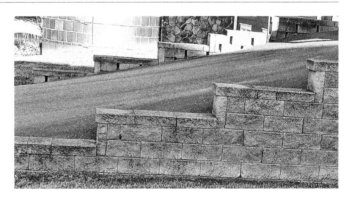

FIGURE 30.1: We walk up or down stairs and hills. The operative word here is walk. This is the reason our movements on them are so very similar. However, with respect to posture and the pressure in our feet, there are some notable differences.

Characteristically, their fear is much greater when going down the hill than when going up. Yes, gravity is a wonderful thing—until it becomes your enemy and pulls you tumbling toward the bottom

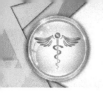

of a hill. But honestly, people with a restrictive-posture movement impairment are nearly as prone to falling *up* a hill as falling *down* it.

The problem with falling on a hill is not gravity per se. The problem is with the person not knowing how to adjust their posture to remain stable, to counter the force of gravity. What must be done is no different from what must be done when walking or standing on any surface, with one basic exception. This exception is one very natural posture rule they need to understand and use.

On a hill, on any slanted or angled surface, always adjust your posture to the surface you are walking on by **leaning your upper body toward the top of the hill**. Always, always **push with your feet into the bottom of the hill**. This stabilizes you to the *relative* flatness of the earth, so the pull of gravity is then straight down with respect to your posture.

As I walk uphill in the top panel of Figure 30.2, I am leaning my upper body forward toward the top of the hill. As I walk downhill in the bottom panel, I am leaning my upper body backward toward the top of the hill. In both examples, my upper-body adjustment places me in the proper posture to be *naturally pushing with my feet toward the bottom of the hill*. On this steep incline, I remained as stable, balanced, in control, and comfortable as if I'd been walking on a flat, horizontal surface.

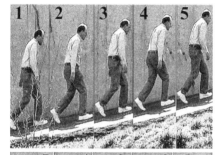
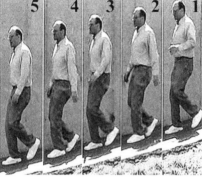

FIGURE 30.2: Push to the bottom. Lean to the top. Relax and go.

1. To walk up a hill, the push from the foot into the bottom of the hill must be greater than the force of gravity.

2. To walk down a hill, the push can be *slightly* less than the force of gravity. However, the force of the push must be enough to ensure a stabilized foundation and posture, because lowering the body down the incline in each stride is done with flexing knees. Also, the advancement of the movement going down is still done with a pushing foot, because it is a stride that is being taken.

Walking Up

Think of this as walking on a flat floor while pushing a shopping cart filled with heavy things. To move the cart and keep it going, you must lean your body into it and continue pushing with each foot as you hold that leaning posture. You do this same thing when walking up a hill, except the cart is your body weight, and the degree to which you lean forward depends on the steepness of the hill.

When pushing the cart across the flat floor, you can stop pushing and it will stay where it stops. But if you are pushing the cart up an incline (angled floor) and then stop pushing it, the cart will roll back down the incline. To prevent it from rolling back down when you stop pushing it up, you must continue to hold enough push with your feet to hold it in place.

This same principle applies to walking up a hill. In each stride, each foot must push with enough force to continue advancing your body farther up the hill. If you stop to rest, you must continue to hold

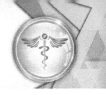

enough push to hold your body in place. The point: When walking or moving on an angled surface (hill, incline), the active pushing with your feet never stops. If it does, gravity will pull you down. This is one reason many people with a restrictive-posture movement impairment have difficulty standing and walking on hills, or on any angled surface. They make mistakes in applying and holding the push.

The problem arises from their learned maladaptive habit of stopping the push from their feet when they are standing or moving on a flat surface. Recall from previous discussions, they learn to stop the push when they are having difficulties controlling where the push is coming from in their feet. This is also saying that they are stopping the push when their body is moving in an unexpected direction. When they are on a sloping surface, these same mistakes happen more quickly and create a much bigger problem.

Naturally, for the best stability and balance when walking and standing on any surface, we adjust our posture to the relative flatness of the earth. This concept is shown in Figure 30.3. When on a surface that is *not* horizontally flat, we tend to hold our body perpendicular (at a ninety-degree angle) to an imaginary surface that is horizontally flat, as if we were walking on a flat floor. This is not a conscious effort. It simply happens when we create and use the correct pressure in our feet for the movement, by doing nothing more than correctly adjusting our posture to the surface we are on.

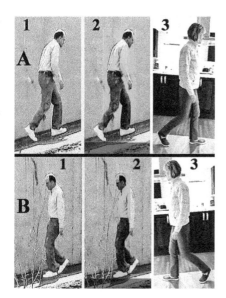

FIGURE 30.3: The red insert in picture 2 represents a flat floor. The inserted green zone of stability shows that my body is perpendicular to the red area as I walk up and down the hill. Now note that the posture for walking on the hill is essentially the same as Eileen's in picture 3 as she walks on a flat floor.

This is shown in the comparison of my postural alignment when walking up the incline in panel A and down the incline in panel B, to Eileen's posture as she walks on a flat floor in picture 3. The inserted red area in picture 2 in both panels represents an imaginary horizontally flat floor. With that reference, note how the postures are essentially the same when going up the incline, going down the incline, or walking on a flat floor.

Walking Down

When walking down an incline, any person struggling with impaired movements and a restrictive-posture should *keep the pushing point of pressure concentrated in or toward their heels*. In this location, the pushing pressure resists gravity, slows the speed of the walk, and provides improved stability. This allows the downward pulling force of gravity to help gradually lower the body down the hill in a slower, better-controlled, and more stable movement. *But* don't allow this to mislead you.

Yes, gravity will assist you down the hill only when you control each stride with the correct pressure in the pushing foot, and use flexing knees. Flexing knees lower the body in each stride, and the pressure in the pushing foot controls the stride and rate of descent. When the feet and knees are stiffened, not flexing, gravity controls the movement.

The knees *must* be flexing going down the hill. With *non*-flexing knees, the posture will typically be too upright with guarding and/or stiffening and will create a top-heavy situation. This means your

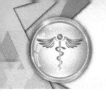

head is starting to lead you down the hill. When the knees are not flexing, each stride will be jarring, relatively uncontrolled, unstable, and shortened. This posture creates instability, so that the smallest added mistake results in an awkward fall, either up or down the hill.

When preparing to walk **down** a hill or incline, any person with impaired movements and a restrictive-posture, who feels stable, should begin by first adjusting their posture to move increased pressure into their heels. How far back in the heels depends on the steepness of the hill, and the person's functional ability to flex their hips, knees, and feet. But there is no need to guess at how much heel pressure is needed. In fact, the one and only thing to use and understand in the setup is the following. Very simply, the upper body (shoulders) is moved back and held in the position that allows the person to stand comfortably and stable on the hill. When they are standing without tipping or moving, that is how much pressure they need on their heels, and that is exactly how far their shoulders need to be held back while they are in the walking-down movement or standing posture.

Then, as the person shifts body weight to one foot, the next part is to let some of the pressure in the heel move *slightly* forward to allow the stride to be taken with a foot that doesn't fully flex. With the pressure moved slightly forward in the heel area, gravity will gently move the body forward, as the person *lightly* allows a soft forward push of the body to happen with the minimally flexing foot.

However, for many of them this is basically not a push. Rather, it is simply allowing the foot to begin flexing. Therefore, those people who have guarding and stiffness in their posture are advised not to focus on pushing with the foot. They should just try to relax enough to allow the foot to begin flexing. Then, later, as they become more comfortable and relaxed, they will begin to naturally add a gentle push on hills with a gently sloping angle, and most often without being aware that they're doing it.

The amount the foot flexes during the stride ultimately determines the length of the downhill stride. Just as it must in any other walking movement, when going downhill the foot flexes to allow the body to move more naturally in a forward stride. However, the difference when walking down a hill is the decreased amount of push that's required to produce the stride. Walking down a hill requires less of a forward push because the pull of gravity is also moving the body forward, using the flexing foot. However, this feeling of the foot flexing while going downhill is uncomfortable for many people with a movement impairment. Initially, they feel out of control when it flexes, and are fearful they will move too fast and won't be able to stop the faster movement. They envision themselves racing and stumbling out of control to a tumbling accident at the bottom. In reaction to the fear, they stiffen and stop the foot from flexing. To avoid the faster movement and tipping off the toe of the shoe, they also hold their shoulders farther back in a more upright posture. Both of these reactions cause instability and jarring during any movement.

With flexing hips, knees, and feet, the correct setup posture and heel (foot) pressure will control how fast or slowly you walk down the hill. But be very careful with any postural change you make while you are standing or walking on an angled surface, because the location of the pressure in your feet will also change, and instability and unwanted body movement too often quickly follow.

For those whose posture is moderately guarded or stiffened, movements of the upper body very often move the pressure in the feet or foot too quickly and too much. Then, too often, a potentially dangerous situation of erratic and/or uncontrolled upper-body movement and further changing of the foot pressure is the outcome—one that stiffened hips, knees, and feet cannot keep up with. Yes, this is a problem on a flat surface as well, but it is a much bigger problem on an angled surface. For example, when the pressure moves forward in the feet, the body will then move faster down the hill. Then the next problem is, too often the restrictive posture cannot flex enough, nor respond quickly enough, to keep up with, support, and stabilize the faster-moving body.

But, for argument's sake, let's assume that the forward-moving leg *does* move fast enough to move the advancing foot down the hill to where the moving body needs it to be. What is the common outcome? It is not so good. With a restrictive posture, the person fears falling down the hill, and with this faster body movement, they react with postural stiffening. Next, as they move onto the advanced leg, the knee is stiff and straightened, and the foot is stiffened and acting like a nonfunctional block of wood. Because of this, *they frequently do tip, with their upper body moving quickly beyond the stiffened knee, and they do fall forward down the hill. In this situation, they are pushing themselves forward down the hill from the toes and ball area of the forward foot.*

So, especially when they are fearful and having difficulty flexing their knees, anyone with a restrictive posture is well advised to maintain increased heel pressure while slowly moving down the hill with a controlled posture and controlled foot pressure, taking small strides. This allows them to remain more stable and provides them with more opportunity to remind themselves to add some postural relaxation.

When *walking* down a hill, especially a steeper one, it is difficult to flex your feet when your fear reaction is causing panic. And when your feet don't flex, it's very likely that your knees also are not flexing. This causes a very stiff, jarring, awkward, and slow walk that is highly unstable, with frequent backward and forward tipping.

Walking across a Slope

The slope is the angle, or slant, of the hill compared to flat ground. For those with impaired movements and a restrictive-posture, walking across the slope of a hill is often more challenging and scarier than walking down the slope. But it doesn't have to be. By simply using the exact same principles of posture that apply to walking up or down a hill, you can greatly reduce and often eliminate both fear and instability.

1. Whenever you are on any part of a hill, *always lean your upper body toward the top of the hill.*

2. Therefore, when walking across the slope of a hill, lean your head and shoulders to the side that's toward the top of the hill.

3. This posture sets both feet so they are functionally angled to push toward the bottom of the hill, to hold your body in position on the slope.

4. As shown in pictures 2 and 4 of Figure 30.4, the outside part of the uphill foot is used.

5. As shown in pictures 3 and 5, the *inside* part of the downhill foot is used.

Therefore, the push from the foot that is higher up on the hill comes from increased pressure on the *outside portion of the foot*, and the remainder of the foot may or may not be in contact with the ground.

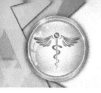

For the foot that is lower on the hill, the push comes from increased pressure on the *inside of the foot*, and the remainder of the foot may or may not be in contact with the ground.

In Figure 30.4, Melinda's posture is held in position as she walks across the steep slope of the hill, in the same position it's in when she is walking on a flat surface. Compare her posture with the slope, and then with the trees in the background. What do you see? She is standing in the same line as the trees are growing out of the ground.

When you're balanced and stable standing on the angled surface, the increased pressure in your feet will be exactly where it needs to be. Holding this posture to keep the pressure in this location gives you the ability to comfortably stand or move on that angled surface. Therefore, the only new task here is learning to be comfortable, and trusting yourself to stand and walk using only the inside or outside part of one foot at a time.

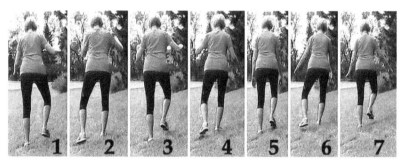

FIGURE 30.4: To walk or stand balanced on a slope, lean your head and uphill shoulder toward the top of the hill.

As Melinda walks across the hill, she is supporting all her body weight on the inside half of her left foot in pictures 3, 5, and 7, and on the outside half of her right foot in pictures 2, 4, and 6. This feels strange, scary, and unstable when you've been dealing with restrictive-posture movement issues. So, practice on small hills with a gentle slope to help you become comfortable and confident with this.

Reminder: There is only one slight change in what you need to be doing when standing, moving, or walking on a hill, or on anything else that is not a flat and open floor. You must be doing the very same things *better*. Not differently. Just better.

1. You must apply and hold the push better, with more authority.

2. If you release or weaken the push, gravity will take control and pull you tumbling and rolling toward the bottom of the hill.

3. When you're standing, if you do not continue pushing toward the bottom of the hill, gravity will take control and pull you tumbling and rolling toward the bottom of the hill.

4. When you're moving or walking and not doing complete transfers of body weight with the pressure where it needs to be in each foot, gravity will take control and pull you tumbling and rolling toward the bottom of the hill.

5. Because they have these same issues on a flat floor, people with restrictive, upright postures will *always* have *more* difficulties on an angled surface. Their same problem issues are simply more noticeable, and the effects more dramatic.

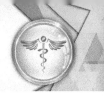

Compare the walking postures of the three people in Figure 30.5. The woman labeled 1 and the man labeled 2 are both in midstride, and their posture is forward because of the hill they are walking on. The posture of the woman labeled 3 is more upright because her left foot is still on flat ground. Her advancing right foot is off the ground and about to contact the ground where the small hill begins. At this moment, she is distracted, looking to the left. The question is, how much of a problem is she about to have when her advancing right foot contacts the upward-sloping ground?

Is she prepared for the incline she is one second away from stepping onto with her right foot? As it happened, yes, she was. With natural ability, she quickly adjusted her posture as soon as the foot touched the ground. She continued without hesitation up the hill, even though she was still looking to the left. How did she know this was coming and what to do? She felt the change in the foot, and that told her everything that was needed to make the perfect adjustment with her relaxed, cooperative posture.

In this very same situation, many movement-impaired people with a restrictive posture will not make the required postural adjustments when they move onto a changed surface.

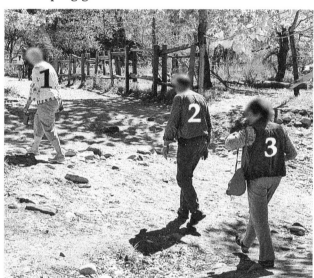

FIGURE 30.5: Transitioning from flat ground to a hill. The woman labeled 3 will adjust her posture forward as her right foot comes in contact with the hill she is about to move onto. She will do this mostly by only feeling the suddenly different pressure in that foot when it contacts the ground.

1. When they see the change coming, a common response is to *react with guarding to the problems they expect they are about to have*. This ensures that they will have problems, because they have reset their posture to one that ensures they will make mistakes.

2. When they are *not looking* to see that the change is coming, the most common response when they move onto the changing surface is a *startle reaction*, which often causes them to very quickly stiffen, straighten, and become more upright.

When the surface they are moving onto is angled *upward*, this often results in a backward push from the advanced foot. Why? With a restrictive, upright posture, typically the shoulders are back, the knee is straightened, and the foot is stiffened. This results in the heel of the advancing foot contacting the ground with increased pressure that does not move forward in the foot. Then a significant amount of the pushing force from this heel pressure moves up into the advanced leg. Frequently this stops the forward movement and pushes the body backward into a stutter step, and pressurizes the heels of both feet.

When the surface they are moving onto is angled **downward**, their chance of falling forward is much greater. This is due to the sudden forward lean of their body, because they have not adjusted their posture

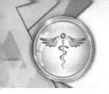
for the changing surface. For example, their posture has been upright for walking on a flat floor with limited flexing of the knees. Then suddenly this upright posture is thrust forward as the advancing foot must move farther downward before it contacts the surface that is angling away. Suddenly their restrictive upright posture becomes an angled-forward, stiffening upright posture. The pressure has moved into the forward-most part of the advanced foot and pushes the body forward, as the forward-leaning upper body is pulling them forward.

Another very common postural mistake happens when they see the angled surface and react with fearful guarding and stiffening. This frequently involves moving their shoulders farther backward in a very upright posture. So, once again, this holds the forward-advancing foot even higher and farther away from the downward-sloping surface. Now, when they attempt to move forward onto the downslope, more of a forward upper-body lean is required to get the advancing foot down to the surface. However, they will not do that. Instead, they will hold or increase the backward upper-body lean—because they are afraid of tipping forward and falling down the slope.

The restrictive upright posture, backward lean, and stiffened, straightened knees prevent them from lowering the foot. What commonly follows is a stumbling, tipping-*backward*-and-to-the-side fall.

Consider this. On a flat and level floor, being too high in your stance raises your center of gravity and leads to instability. This is *a much bigger problem when you are on an angled surface*. Being too upright with a restrictive posture is one of the biggest reasons for the problems and falls movement-impaired people experience on angled surfaces. *Moving down the angled surface is always more difficult*. For many, just the thought of being on an angled surface quickly fills them with dread.

Of note, for a person with impaired movements and a restrictive-posture, there is one thing that is more frightening than being on a hill. Only one thing. It is going up and down steps, but going down is the most difficult and frightening. One, two, or many steps, or even a curb. For the movement-impaired person, all these are full of danger, and reactive guarding and postural stiffening make them more dangerous.

Therefore, anyone with a restrictive posture, and those of you who question your abilities, should pause before moving onto a surface that is different from the one you've been walking on. During this pause, at a minimum you should do the following:

1. Relax and adjust your posture according to the surface you're about to move onto. This is very easy to say but extremely difficult for some to do.

2. Reduce your anxiety by reminding yourself of what is real and what is not, about the changing surface you are about to move onto. This requires a good and rational working understanding of the difference between the imagined challenge and the true reality of the sameness of the required movement and posture, and postural relaxation.

    Of note to those who don't have these movement issues: You need to realize that for those with the frightening movement issues, every single one of their problem issues and fears is very, very real to them. So, what does this mean for many well-meaning people? You might want to stop trying to convince them they need not be frightened, because you are missing the point of why they are frightened. The truth is, the only way they will become convinced there is a difference between what is real and what is imagined is by proving it to themselves with their actions.

The only way they will find the ability to relax and quiet their fears on an angled surface is through the practice of personally doing it correctly. They must practice both indoors and outdoors, moving up, down, and sideways on smooth, firm surfaces that have a very shallow angle, with easy access to a handrail.

3. There is no way of getting around these things. You, the person with the movement issues, must learn to make this difference for yourself. Talking and thinking about it does nothing. Repeatedly fighting it does nothing. To learn how to correct your mistakes and improve your movement ability, you must actively practice the basics of posture to stabilize on your feet. This requires your very dedicated commitment to yourself.

Not-So-Scary Hills

On *any angled surface*, lean your upper body toward the high side of the hill to create the correct pushing pressure in your feet. In Figure 30.6, Melinda has a neurodegenerative disorder, and her movements are mildly affected. In pictures 1 through 8, she is holding her upper body back to keep the pressure in her heels as she walks down the hill. Then, in pictures 9 through 11, she transitions from walking downhill to walking uphill with the pushing pressure in the toes and forward ball areas of her feet.

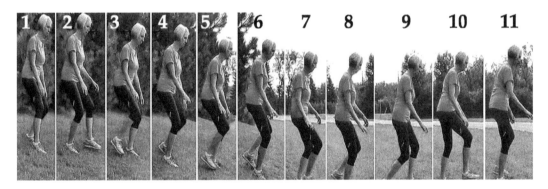

FIGURE 30.6: Whether you're heading down or up, flexing knees and a relaxed posture are critical to stability. Increased pressure in the heels when going down, and then in the forward ball areas and toes when going up. This is your focus.

Look closely at Melinda's posture in all the pictures and pay attention to the angle of the ground she's walking on, and then compare her posture in each picture with the one before and the one after it. In every picture, she makes subtle postural adjustments. This is very good. In each stride, as the ground beneath her feet changes, she adjusts her posture accordingly.

Also note that she is exaggerating lowering into a lower ready stance and is also mildly exaggerating the pressure in her heels. She did this to slow her descent and to add stabilizing pressure into her feet. The important thing is that she remained stable and in control while adjusting her posture to what she needed to feel. Melinda breathed a big sigh of relief when her practice on the hills for this day was complete.

Knees

If you cannot stay down in your stance with flexible knees, you will have problems, especially when you're on an angled surface.

I am walking with Carole on a gently sloping hill covered with short grass in Figure 30.7. Note the differences in our postures. With stiffened knees, she is upright in her stance, with a guarded and sometimes stiffened posture. Because of this, the slight movements of her upper body are relatively uncontrolled, as it is constantly changing position. This means the pressure in her feet is also relatively uncontrolled and constantly changing location. The result is instability and balance problems.

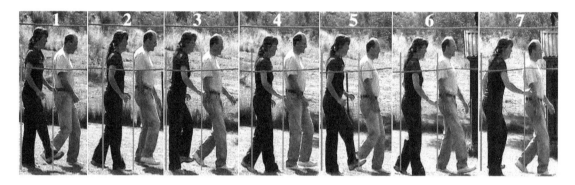

FIGURE 30.7: Having control of your movement is what allows you to keep your posture relaxed. To control your movement, you must remain stable on your feet, and to do that, your posture needs to be relaxed. So, which comes first? The answer is always the same. Adjust your posture to create the correct pressure in your feet, then relax into that pressure to hold your posture stable as you move.

In contrast to Carole's, my posture is relaxed and stable on the unchanging slanted ground beneath our feet. To better show the differences between our postures, I inserted vertical lines behind us. Note that the space between the red line and Carole's back changes in every picture, but the blue line is consistently in the same position on my back. The exception is the subtle change in picture 6, where my upper body moves slightly up and back. Do you see why? I looked up and out toward the horizon, and adjusted my posture accordingly to continue walking at a steady, controlled pace with the same stride length.

What Carole's movements show in this example are typical for those with restrictive-posture movement impairments. From top to bottom, what are the problems?

1. Her posture is guarded. This is why she is holding her shoulders up and has stiffness in her arms and hands.

2. Although she uses a small amount of knee flexing (the left more than the right), mostly her knees are straightened.

3. While advancing forward, she holds the fronts of her feet up, showing how stiffened they are.

When you feel or are told of these same problems in your posture that Carole is showing, STOP and make the needed corrections. Begin with your feet. Where is the increased pressure, and where does it need

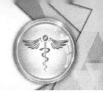

to be? What should you do if you can't relax enough to feel the pressure? You should then pay attention to which way your body is trying to move. This will tell you where the pressure is located in your feet.

The next thing to do is adjust your posture so your body is balanced and stable with respect to the angle of the ground you're standing on. Then relax your hands to begin relaxing your knees. Holding this posture, slightly squat to flex your knees—and then go back and relax your hands and knees again. Now you are ready to adjust your posture for the movement, and then completely transfer your body weight to one foot to begin the movement.

This first stride is the scariest, so be sure you relax to hold the posture and pressure stable. When the scary first stride works, simply keep repeating the transfers of body weight from foot to foot, while holding the pressure in each foot where it needs to be to remain balanced and moving slowly forward with each stride.

When the scary first stride does not go as planned, STOP and repeat the posture setup process from the beginning. *The biggest key to success is having the ability to keep your body relaxed, even partially.* This is necessary if you are to stay in the correct posture. Easily said. Difficult to do.

The pressure in the foot being used must be allowed to move far enough forward to enable the forward stride to be taken. Often this means moving the shoulders slightly forward. Those with a restrictive-posture movement impairment have great doubts about this because they have mistakenly learned to lean their guarded or stiffened body too far backward, because they fear falling down the hill. But this tactic actually does the opposite. This fear-driven stiffening posture reaction holds the pressure too far back in the heel, and the feet and knees are stiffened. Everything about this upright, uncooperative posture prevents movement. It does not allow the body to move forward into a stride. Instead, typically the initial movement is backward as soon as they transfer onto one foot, even on the hill. This is how they fall up the hill.

The truth: This fearful response *only makes their chances of falling on the hill much greater.*

Here is another tidbit of information. Many people with impaired movements and a restrictive-posture do this same thing when going *uphill*. Yes, they pull their shoulders back while transferring to one foot when beginning an uphill stride, and then they often tip and topple back down the hill. Been there, done that, many years ago.

That is the problem you create. Holding your shoulders back puts increased pressure into your heels, regardless of what you're standing on. Then, regardless of the angle of the ground, when you use that pressure, it always pushes you backward. Yes, standing with a restrictive posture and facing toward the downslope of a hill, you want some increased heel pressure, but remember you are using that pressure to slow your forward movement. It is not to stop and prevent movement when your intention is to be walking.

As a reminder, the setup posture for movement and taking forward strides is a ready stance, with your upper body adjusted so the distribution of the pressure in your feet is such that you are balanced and stable when standing and moving. This applies to any surface, flat or angled.

In **natural-ability** walking movements, the increased pressure is typically farther forward in the flexing feet than it is for those with a restrictive posture. Therefore, the necessary correction for **walking more naturally** for both up and down hills is actually shoulders forward, to move the pressure into the proper location in the foot for the surface we are on.

Yes, this includes people with impaired movements, too, but only *when they have the ability to control it*. And yes, many people with natural ability have the pressure in the ball areas of their feet when going down a hill. Think it through. Where else would the pressure be when those with the ability walk faster or run down a hill?

MAKING IT BETTER

When I am walking on any surface and begin to feel clumsy or unbalanced, there are three basic things I immediately remind myself to do to correct the mistake(s) *I allowed* to happen:

1. Relax hands and elbows to relax my shoulders down.

2. Flex and relax my knees down more than they are.

3. Increase the downward pressure into each foot to improve the transfer of body weight, to stabilize each stride and lift the other foot higher.

BACKPACKS

You must compensate with the proper postural adjustments for the things you strap on your body. Otherwise, you will have instability issues.

When you strap on a backpack, how much it weighs and how high you carry it make a difference. This is more of a problem for a person with a movement impairment, and especially for those with a restrictive posture. And, quite honestly, when your movements are impaired, even a relatively light pack can cause unexpected postural changes and problems. As we tire, we are much more likely to straighten too much, and too quickly, because we often do this when we are carrying nothing. As we tire, our knees become more resistant to flexing, and this is exaggerated when we're carrying something that is adding to our posture issues. So, please realize that having just a little extra weight on your upper body easily sets you up for bigger problems when your postural control is already compromised, even on your good days, and especially when you're fatigued.

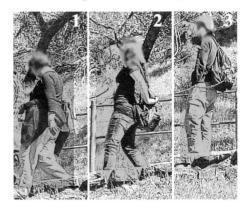

FIGURE 30.8: The things you carry and wear will often alter your posture and affect your movements. With a relaxed posture, you will naturally adapt and stabilize by counterbalancing. When not relaxed, you will struggle with instability caused by difficulties counterbalancing.

Compare the postures of the people walking down the same hill in Figure 30.8. The woman in picture 1 is not wearing a backpack, while the woman and man in pictures 2 and 3 are. The two wearing the backpacks are holding their upper bodies much farther back to counteract the weight of the backpacks. They're doing this to move the pressure in their feet toward the heel areas, to prevent the packs' extra weight from causing them to walk faster down the hill. (Note: The inserted zones of stability are approximated to the locations where the back and front of the shoe are assumed to be.)

The woman and man wearing the backpacks moved down the hill more slowly than the woman in picture 1. This was because the pressure in their feet was farther back toward their heels. The woman in picture 2 had a small amount of jarring in her legs and body with each stride. The man's strides were smooth.

When you're wearing a backpack and your movements become difficult to control, stop fighting it. Take it off. If you are having difficulties with a backpack but need to have something to carry personal items, try wearing a smaller waist pack. These will naturally be more centered on your body, will not pull on your shoulders, and will not cause the postural changes a backpack often does.

BAGS

Anything you carry in your hands will have negative effects when you don't adjust your posture to the added weight. Postural issues become more of a problem when you hold the bags high, especially when they are heavy or bulky. Another irritating problem frequently arises when the bags swing freely, constantly pulling you forward, then backward and to the side. These same things apply to shoulder bags.

For added stability and balance, carry these things *lower* to the ground with relaxed, extended elbows and flexing knees, and hold them in a manner that limits the amount that they swing. Having equal amounts of weight in both hands also helps to provide better stability and balance.

A basic point: Stop allowing or creating a problem where there really need not be one.

THE WIND

When you don't know how to compensate for it, the wind can quickly turn your best day into a terrible day. But realize this: Compensating for the wind and adjusting your posture in response to it is merely another simple concept. Treat the wind as an invisible hill.

Whether you're walking into the wind, with the wind, or with a crosswind blowing you sideways, the postural adjustment that's needed is exactly the same as when walking up, down, or across a hill.

The direction the wind is blowing from equals the top of the hill.
Always lean your upper body and head into the wind to properly adjust the pressure in your feet.

Try to keep your movements and strides smaller when the wind is blowing hard or gusting. Why? When the wind's force suddenly changes, stops, and starts again, you'll be better positioned and prepared to readjust your posture and stance accordingly.

Our goal is simply to do better with what we have.
To that end, everything we do is therapy, working and playing to enjoy life.

■ ■ ■

CHAPTER 31

Uneven and Shifting Ground

Pay attention to where the pressure needs to be in your feet.

The top of a manicured lawn is smooth and even to look at, but often the ground under it is not. The unseen and unexpected ups, downs, and slants of the ground hidden beneath make walking on **grass** much more challenging for the movement impaired. This is especially so for those who react to unexpected changes in footing with exaggerated postural guarding and stiffening.

The nature of grass itself is another issue for them. When a lawn is thick and growing healthy green, it is soft when stepped on and feels rather nice to people with natural abilities. But for many people struggling with impaired movements, that soft carpet of grass is a spongy hazard under their feet, even when the ground below *is* firm and flat.

When standing on thick grass, many people with impaired movements and a restrictive-posture *are not* standing on the flat and solid surface of the ground below. Instead, they are standing on a cushion that allows their feet to move, tip, and wobble. But, interestingly, a person with natural ability standing beside them **is** standing on the stable, solid ground beneath the grass. How can there be this difference between two people standing side by side?

Most all people with natural ability easily push the increased downward pressure into their feet to effectively compress and stabilize themselves on the grass under them, without realizing they're doing it. However, many people with restrictive movement abilities do not add enough downward pressure into their feet to adequately stabilize themselves on the cushion of grass.

For these reasons, many times those with impaired movements and a restrictive-posture are standing on an unstable, movable surface. This leads to oscillating feet and shaking legs, anxiety, and increasing postural guarding and stiffening in a vain attempt to find stability. This same situation often happens when they walk indoors on thick carpet, or on carpet with thick padding under it, or on a spongy, thin carpet like the one Sue was having problems with in chapter 13.

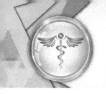

*A small amount of movement in the feet
often creates big movements in the upper body.*

The correct response to this situation is the same as it is for each of the instability examples in previous chapters. To correct the instability caused by the soft surface and the uneven ground, the downward pressure going into their feet must be increased, and that is done as they slightly lower themselves with flexing knees and hips to get the muscles in their legs working more productively.

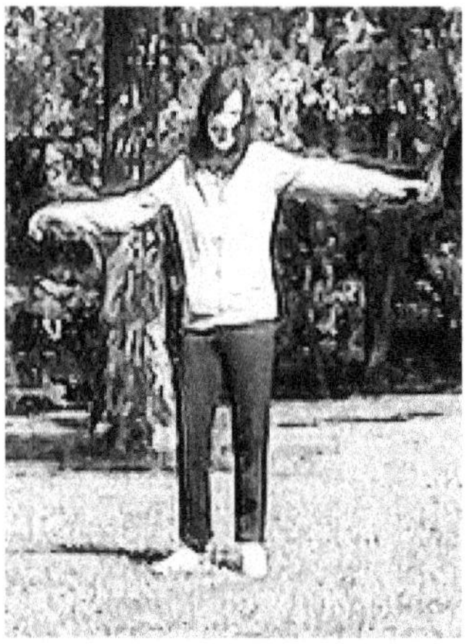

For the person who learns to overcome these physical and psychological obstacles and regains the ability to walk comfortably on grass again, there are no words to adequately describe how it feels. For those of us who have experienced it, it is an absolutely joyful and exuberant adventure. We frolic like children, so happy to be there again, while people who do not know us watch and wonder why we're so excited.

"As I walked and played on the grass today, I did not feel fear or worry. Without hesitation, *I did it*. I proved to myself that it is okay for me to be here, and I love it." This is what Rhoda in Figure 31.1 is signaling to everyone the day she experienced that moment. Caution and fear slipped away into a newfound permission to be, to do, and to feel the independence and freedom of living again. Another piece of life is renewed within another fresh awareness that will no longer be denied.

FIGURE 31.1: For those who had lost the ability, to walk comfortably on grass again IS a big deal.

"MIND" FIELDS

Why are **small stones** in the driveway or in an area of the yard so scary to walk on? They shift under your feet, and the same is true for walking in loose sand. For many people with a movement impairment, this slipping of their feet makes it scary and difficult to remain stable and balanced.

"Why did I ever put rocks between the house and garage? I have to walk on them every working day to get to and from the car," Tom repeatedly said to himself. "And God help me when they're slippery in the winter. That is when I really *do not* like those rocks." This was Tom's personal "mine field" that was filled with constant danger when he had to walk on it. It was also his "*mind* field," creating anxiety and fear. His psychological anticipation of walking on the stones of the driveway altered his physical "preparation" and created additional physical problems beyond those that were already there.

WALKING, ON ANY SURFACE

Pay attention to what's happening. Quiet your mind and listen closely to the sound each foot is making as it moves forward. Do not think or talk about what you're doing. Only listen to the sounds your feet make as they brush against and through things. Hear the sound by itself, listening for only what that sound means when you hear it.

When you have clearly heard the sound, continue the same walk using a different focus. Now pay very close attention to what you feel in your foot when you hear the same sound, to put the sound and the feeling together. Make sense of what is physically happening.

Combined, the sound and the feeling will tell you a great deal about your walking pattern and posture, so you can better understand why the sound and feeling are happening. For example, what do you hear, and why are you hearing it? Is it loud or is it quiet? What do you feel in your foot, especially when the sound is louder? What is your posture, and how relaxed are you when you hear and feel these things? Then, using the sound and feeling as a guide, you can work to improve your walking posture by reducing or eliminating the sound and feeling.

Now try your best to do essentially the opposite. By this I mean for you to pay attention to see if you are feeling the correct sensations (pressure) in each foot as you walk. So, as you walk, what do you *not* feel when your feet are making a lot of noise? Compare this with what you *do not* feel when they are quiet. Many times, you'll be surprised by how much you discover.

When you were young, were you ever told, "Perhaps you'll learn something about what I'm trying to teach you if you'll be quiet and pay attention"? Just as it was then, this statement remains true today. For all of us, it's often difficult to quiet a busy-thinking mind enough to have the ability to simply listen, feel, and learn from an experience. This is especially true when you are having difficulties with your movements.

Example: "Mike, do you feel the fronts of your feet digging into the grass as you walk?" In the first three pictures of Figure 31.2, you can easily see why Mike is having a difficult time walking in the thick grass. As he takes a small stride forward, the front of his right shoe moves through the grass, as indicated by the red arrows. Then, in picture 4, he lifts it slightly to slide it forward on top of the grass, to complete the stride in picture 5, where the front of his shoe is above the grass (green arrow). Look at his posture to see why this is happening.

He begins with increased pressure in the forward portions of his feet in picture 1. Then he uses an upper-body forward lean, seen in picture 2, to begin taking a stride with his right leg, and that moves additional pressure into the toes of his left foot. This pressure buries the front of his left shoe in the grass. But why is he leaning so far forward to take this very small stride?

Mike was mildly unstable on the thick, soft grass. This lush carpet of grass was not firm like the concrete floor we had just been working on. In addition, the grass was approximately two inches high; the concrete floor was flat and smooth. The thick and taller grass created a spongy cushion under his feet.

With the sponginess of the grass, Mike does not feel as stable as he did a few minutes earlier on the hard, flat, and smooth concrete floor. In reaction

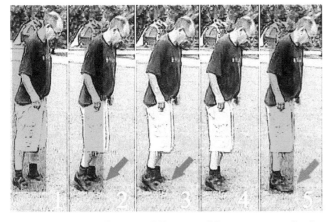

FIGURE 31.2: Mike is mildly unstable. His upper-body forward lean pushes the toes of his shoes into the grass. As a result, the transfer of body weight to his left foot is incomplete, and he drags the toe of his right shoe through the grass.

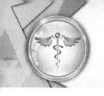

to the mild instability he is feeling while standing on the grass, his feet are mildly stiffened, and he is using his calf muscles to help him stop tipping forward. This is why the toes of his shoes are under the top of the grass in picture 1.

Recall that the calf muscles push pressure into the ball area of the foot and the toes, and then flex the foot (pull the heel upward) to push the body forward. In this example, Mike is using these muscles to stop a forward tip, so all the added pressure going into the foot from these muscles is directed downward. That is why he is unable to use these muscles to flex his foot to make the push to take the stride. This means his only option is to use a forward upper-body movement to tip himself farther forward to pull his body into the stride. This upper-body movement is better illustrated by the green zone-of-stability insert in pictures 1 and 2. Note how he is farther forward out of the zone in picture 2 and then moves his shoulders slightly back beginning in picture 3. This is seen in the toes of his shoes moving up to the top of the grass in pictures 3 through 5.

Mike had a mild-to-moderate movement impairment when I worked with him, and he shows mild postural guarding in these pictures. You can see this in his straightened knees, and in the way he's holding his arms and hands in place away from his body. Again, the reason for this is that he was mildly unstable, wobbling slightly on his feet when standing, and more so when moving. This is also why the transfer of body weight to his left foot in these pictures is incomplete, and when his right knee does flex in picture 2, it does so only slightly.

As previously discussed, to stand stable on the grass, *Mike needed to do more work with his legs than he had been doing* on the concrete, to produce the necessary additional stabilizing pressure to compress the grass. This is a very common mistake many people with a movement impairment repeatedly make. They fail to prepare themselves for the transition when they are moving onto a changing surface. They then have instability reactions and fearful thoughts when they move onto it. Why do they not prepare? Basically, they don't know how.

The height of the grass and other things on the ground cause problems. All of them require the knee to be lifted higher, to raise the foot out of the grass and/or over obstacles during a stride. As covered in earlier chapters, this also requires the transfer of weight from foot to foot to be more deliberate and complete. It requires that a greater downward pushing force be applied into each foot to stabilize the body on the softer surface, to allow the complete transfer of body weight to happen. When body-weight transfer to the supporting foot is not complete, the lifting of the other knee will be compromised, and the advancing foot will often not adequately clear the top of the grass or the obstacle on the ground during the stride. Hence, the same problem Mike has in Figure 31.2.

Simplify things. When your movements become challenging or difficult, stop what you're doing. Stop and go back through the basics of your setup posture. Remind yourself what you're forgetting to apply. Also, listen to the noises made as the foot moves forward, and feel what is happening in both feet. Then deal with what you find, to do a better job in every movement. The changing surfaces and conditions will not adapt to you. *You must adapt* to them.

When you're feeling unstable, create a firm and flattened foundation under your feet by moving into a ready stance, and then push your feet firmly down to find the stabilized bottom. This will likely mean you will need to flex your knees and hips more. Your next challenge will be to hold the downward pressure,

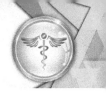

then complete a weight transfer to one foot and apply the push, while keeping your posture as relaxed as you can to enjoy a more natural experience.

Remember the helpful tip: When you feel unstable walking on any surface, focus on moving from and to a "flattened foot" during each stride ("standing on a foot," creating a "heavy foot") to establish a better foundation. Then, to improve the stride, lead it by pushing the advancing knee forward. To accomplish both of these when you are more stable, simply "push" strongly into and from the ball area and toes of the pushing foot.

The overwhelming point is, push downward with more force into the foot you are standing on. That will enable a more complete transfer of body weight onto that foot. Then the advancing foot will be more easily moved to the place where your body needs it to be for the next stride. When you can do these things, each stride will be stronger and more stabilizing, and will allow a more relaxed posture.

Sounds from Your Feet

When your shoes brush and drag against things on or close to the ground, it negatively affects your walking. The louder sound means the resistance to the movement of your feet is greater. This slows the movement of your feet and forces you to do more work. For many people with impaired movements, this extra work typically causes them to guard and stiffen their posture as they attempt to "try harder." Often then, they assume a more upright and straightened stance as they begin using their upper bodies to "help" their legs do the extra work, and the quality of the movement suffers. Commonly, their transfer of body weight onto each foot becomes less complete, and the sound of scuffing shoes grows louder. The result: Every stride becomes more challenging as each foot drags through the grass or kicks stones as it moves forward in a stride.

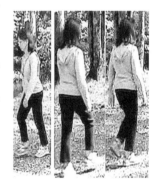

These people frequently experience stumbling, tripping, and falling, and blame the grass or other things on the ground. But what is the actual reason for these problems? It is an incomplete transfer of body weight from foot to foot. Now, honestly, what are very common reasons for this sequence of events? Lazy movements. Misunderstood and poorly done movements. Poor postures. Guarding and stiffening postures. Anxiety. Fear.

FIGURE 31.3: Walking on loose stones requires a relaxed posture, stabilized feet, and complete weight shifts onto each foot.

Because her knee lifts her advancing foot above the stones on the ground, Rhoda is not kicking the stones in Figure 31.3. But a few weeks before this day, she had problems walking and tipping forward on the floor in her house (shown in Chapter 22, Figure 22.6). How this transformation came to be is no great mystery. She only needed to understand what she was doing incorrectly that allowed her neurodegenerative process to appear worse than it was, and then learn how to apply the corrections.

Weakness

Why do some people have problems walking on grass, uneven ground, and stones when their walking ability on a smooth, flat surface appears to be okay? Why do they suddenly have problems as soon as they move onto this different surface? Many times, the answer is related to their level of physical conditioning and anxiety.

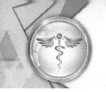

1. The muscles in their legs are weak. The muscles are strong enough to support walking with a rather shuffling type of walking movement on a flat and smooth floor. However, their legs are not strong enough to do the extra work that uneven surfaces call for.

2. When their confidence and trust in their abilities on a smooth, flat surface is low, they have little to no confidence or trust when on anything that is not flat and smooth.

   The reader also needs to realize that people with this issue are not on these other surfaces by choice. It is by necessity. So, when they are on them, they desperately want to get off them.

   When they are forced to be on uneven surfaces, fear dominates and rules their thoughts and movements. Because of this, they typically have little or no mental capacity to recall how to use the basics. They are in survival mode.

When a person doesn't have the physical strength to control their posture, they also do *not* have the ability to control the pressure in their feet. This means they do not have the ability to relax or stand momentarily on one foot to do a complete transfer of body weight. This also means they will have limited ability to lift the other knee, to adequately lift and move the advancing foot. Quite simply, with this weakness, they have very limited ability to do the movement any better than they already are.

Many people with impaired movements have weak calf muscles because they routinely are only partially using them, or are not using them. When a person's calf muscles are skinny and poorly developed, these muscles are very weak, and *the person's movement abilities are very limited*. Their movements are limited because their ability to flex their feet, lift their heels, walk, or do any of the activities that involve moving and supporting their body weight on the ball areas and toes of their feet is greatly restricted. For many, *this weakness issue is correctable, but it does take a good deal of time and committed effort.*

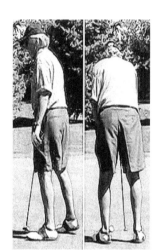

FIGURE 31.4: Weak calf muscles have a profoundly negative impact on your movement potential.

For example, if Tom's calf muscles were better developed (Figure 31.4), his golf swing would be better. How are the calf muscles involved in the golf swing? As it is with all our natural movements, the golf swing depends on staying on and using the ball areas and toes of the flexing feet, as well as easy heel lifts during the body's rotational movement. Now recall that the function of the calf muscles is to stabilize the foot on the ball and toes, and flex the foot to lift the heel. Without this function, the foot doesn't flex, and the movement of the knee is very limited. This was discussed in Chapter 13.

When your calf muscles are weak,
*you will **ALWAYS** have limitations and problems with your walking and other movements.*

How the Movement Looks

People I work with often ask, "Does this look right?"

My most frequent response is, "It really doesn't matter what it looks like to me. What matters is how it feels to you. What matters is that it feels comfortable and stable—to you. What matters is that you are comfortable doing what you want to be doing. *So*, if anything doesn't feel right to you and you are not doing what you want to be doing, then something is most likely not right." That is when it's time to ask, "How does this look? It doesn't feel right to me. Do you see what I am doing, or not doing?"

Stop dwelling on the thought of needing the blessings of others for your movements. Learn to focus on and trust what you feel and know is correct according to your comfort level, because they are *your* movements. Feel and listen to what your body is telling you. Learn the correct and good feelings. Trust them. Trust yourself.

Does it feel right? Does it sound right? Are you doing what you want to be doing? Are you relaxed and stable? If your answer is yes to these questions, then you absolutely *do not* need approval from anyone.

■　■　■

CHAPTER 32

WALKING STICKS

A walking stick will not be of much help if you can't walk comfortably without it.

A *walking stick (or hiking stick) is intended to be used* by someone who ordinarily does not need it. Sadly, many movement-impaired people using a walking stick don't know how to use it properly and as a result are overly dependent on it for support. These issues create additional instability and movement problems for them.

This is also true of many people with impaired movements using **canes**. Far too many people misuse a cane by leaning heavily on it, and the cane, especially when it is relatively short, encourages leaning. By design, the heel of the hand rests on the cane's curved top or handle. This makes it very easy to lean inappropriately into the heel of that hand for additional support and balance. Admittedly, though, it is quite difficult for those with an injury or movement impairment *not* to lean on a cane. This is a major reason I personally do not advocate that people with impaired movements and a restrictive posture use one. But when they do, they simply need to understand how to lean on it less, to remain more dependent on their legs and feet for support, and to avoid moving increased pressure into the outside edge of the foot next to the cane.

In Figure 32.1, Bonnie has a degenerative neurological condition and an unrelated problem with her left leg. After years of dealing with these combined issues, her walking posture has become what is shown in pictures 1 and 2. Stooping forward and leaning to one side, Bonnie became dependent on the walker because she didn't know how not to.

These pictures show Bonnie on the first day we worked together and demonstrate her physical dependency on the walker. However, as she moved around the room, it became apparent to me that she was not physically dependent on it. She was only psychologically dependent on it, because she

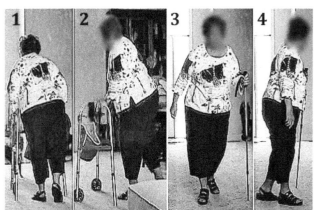

FIGURE 32.1: From leaning on her walker, Bonnie progressed to using a walking stick. She improved her posture by improving the support, stability, and function in her feet. Hidden ability and independence restored.

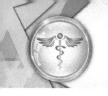

often had the ability *not* to lean on it. This suggested that it had become too easy for her to unnecessarily become dependent on the walker. It had become too easy for her to convince herself that she had to have it. Then, the poor posture shown in pictures 1 and 2 seemed to confirm that she was correct. Bonnie had fallen into a mostly self-made dependency trap, just as many others do. But then, after we worked together a few times, she transitioned from being overly dependent on the walker to becoming more independent while using a walking stick. She was surprised to find that she did have the ability to stay relatively relaxed and stabilized on her feet without the walker.

This enabled her to use the walking stick without being overly dependent on it (pictures 3 and 4. As she became more comfortable with not leaning on the stick, she felt and realized how she had been causing additional movement difficulties for herself, by leaning on the walker. Her challenge then was to make this realization a new adaptive habit, to replace the maladaptive one.

When Bonnie uses the walking stick properly, her posture is more upright and produces increased stability in her feet. Yes, she still has a mild lean to the left because of a left-leg issue, and this is applying some added pressure into the walking stick. However, because she is supporting her body weight much better with her feet and legs, that pressure is minimal compared with the pressure she had been putting into her walker.

Correct Use of a Walking (Hiking) Stick

There is a right and a wrong way to hold and walk with a walking stick. To begin, the correct grip on the walking stick is very similar to the grip you use when casually walking hand in hand with your sweetie.

Both of you walk independently, with your fingers very relaxed and loosely entwined. As you walk and something catches your attention you want to share, you gently tighten your grip on your sweetie's hand to signal, and then relax it again when you have their attention. This is the same way to hold and use a walking stick.

Much of the time, the hand and fingers holding it are not used to control the movement and placement of the walking stick. Instead, the stick is allowed to move *within* the relaxed and lightly gripping fingers. This enables it to remain functional and useful when it is *needed*. Therefore, to make the point clear, most of the time your fingers should be loosely holding the walking stick in place and *not directly controlling it*. Instead, the movement and placement of the walking stick are controlled by the movement of your body, with added adjustments coming from your relaxed elbow and wrist.

A very light grip on the walking stick allows it to move independently with your body's movement. This free and independent movement of the stick allows it to be placed in the position where your body needs it to be, if you want or need to use it.

The pushing foot supports and controls the movement of the body, and the forward-moving knee controls and places the advancing foot.

Your elbow and wrist control the walking stick according to the movement of your body, and your body movement is controlled by the pushing foot. The movement of your body places the walking stick. Therefore, the pushing foot determines the placement of the walking stick.

The correct height of your hand holding the stick is slightly lower than your elbow. With fingers lightly gripping it, the weight of your slightly downward-angled forearm will hold your fingers in place on the walking stick (Figure 32.2). When you're standing in this manner, the stick will rest in your fingers and hand while the weight of your relaxed forearm is gently pressing the stick's tip on the ground, slightly in front and to the outside of the toe of your shoe.

For many movement-impaired people, especially those with restrictive-posture issues, any additional pressure on the grip or pushing the stick to the ground will too easily cause problems. This overcontrol of the walking stick too often results in an under-control situation in the movement of their body. For example, a tighter grip on the stick with the hand and fingers and pushing down with more force from the arm too often induce generalized guarding throughout the body, with the knees and feet guarding and/or stiffening the most. In addition, now the walking stick is unable to move freely in response to the movements of the body, so the stick must then be moved primarily by the hand and arm. In trying to control the walking stick's movement to ensure that they have it for support, the person makes everything about their body movement worse.

A note to able-bodied people with natural ability: Many of you will tighten your grip or push down on the stick and not feel much of anything happening in your knees and feet. Natural ability works that way. Just remember that you do not have the component of psychological or physiological guarding and stiffening that movement-impaired people have.

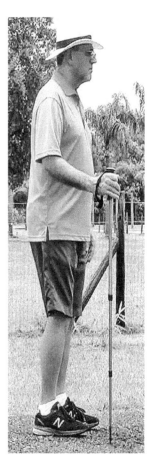

When using a walking stick, the majority of the time the hand holding the stick is relaxed and "just barely" holding it with a couple of fingers. This loose grip is just enough to keep the walking stick from falling from the hand. Then, keeping this loose grip, now *walk as if the walking stick were not there.* For many people with a movement impairment that is beyond mild, keeping a loose grip is difficult. When they are stable while standing their grip is loose, but when

FIGURE 32.2: **A slightly downward-angled forearm and a gentle, loose grip with relaxed fingers.**

they begin to walk they tighten it. When they are unstable while standing their grip is tight, and it gets tighter when they begin to walk. What does this tell you when you are the one doing this? It is you telling you that you are not ready to be walking with a walking stick.

For example, when I walk with a walking stick, I use my thumb and first two fingers to gently hold the stick. This allows it to readily swing with the movement of my body while the relaxed but controlling elbow and wrist easily guide it when needed (Figure 32.3). Another very important observation is the relative *non*-movement of the *upper* arm. From beginning to end in pictures 1 through 9, my upper arm moves very little.

These points are key. A loose finger grip with a relaxed and freely moving elbow and wrist allows the relaxed body's cooperative movement to control most of the movement and placement of the freely movable walking stick. Additional control is done with a gentle movement of the wrist and elbow, and a **gentle** tightening of the fingers on the stick. There is no need or cause to forcefully lift or guide the stick when you're simply wanting to walk with it. Additionally, keep your *relaxed* elbow close to your side in a relaxed position, but *not* hugging or pressed against your side.

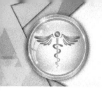
As I walk in Figure 32.3, the rise and fall of my hand and forearm follow with the walking movements of my legs. In this example, in all the pictures, the downward pressure on the stick is only that of my arm's weight. That minimal pressure holds the tip of the stick on the ground and doesn't restrict its movement, and allows it to lift and swing forward with the movement of the body. When you use more pressure than this, you alter the stick's movement, because you're controlling it more deliberately with your hand and arm rather than with your body's motion.

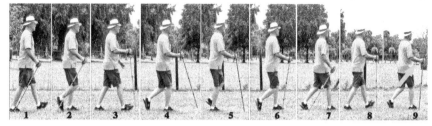

FIGURE 32.3: Walk *with* the stick, not on the stick. Also, do not move the stick where you think it should be. Your cooperative, relaxed body movements will guide the stick to where it needs to be. The walking stick is not to be used to hold you up or to control your postural instability.

Hand Location

Relative to your feet, is there an absolute placement on the ground for the end of the walking stick while you're walking? Yes and no. The stick's placement on the ground will vary somewhat with your movements and strides. During relaxed-posture-controlled movements, the walking stick's movement and placement "just happen" per the body's movements. Therefore, the location of the tip of the stick on the ground will vary as the body's movements vary.

However, when you're standing, the location of the tip's placement on the ground is very consistent and determined by the proper placement and grip of your hand, which correlate to the pressure in your feet, and the width of your feet. So, yes, when you're standing, the tip of the stick will be in the same position with respect to your body, unless the ground you're standing on dictates that the tip must be in another location.

The elbow adjusts the location of the hand on the stick.
*The wrist and **fingers** adjust the angle of the stick to the ground.*

During casual movements, the relaxed wrist and fingers provide the primary control of the walking stick. This is often a problem for many movement-impaired people with a restrictive posture. Too often their wrist is too stiffened, especially when their setup posture is incorrect. This causes them to over-control and be overdependent on the walking stick for support. Examples of this are shown in Figures 32.4 and 32.6.

To help relax your fingers and wrist while holding a walking stick, refer to this same topic discussed in earlier chapters, such as Chapter 8. For example, review dribbling a basketball using a relaxed elbow, wrist, hand, and fingers (Chapter 19). The only actual difference between that activity and holding a walking stick is in the way you are using your fingers. Dribbling the ball, they remain open. Holding the walking stick, they lightly flex to hold the stick. Since many movement-impaired people frequently hold things tighter than they need or want to, learning to keep the fingers and wrist relaxed will take a

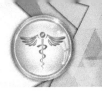

good deal of practice. Therefore, I strongly recommend that you *do not use a walking stick until you have developed the ability to not grip it tightly.*

To properly use a walking stick as a walking aid, first adjust your posture for the movement as it must be *when not using* a walking stick. *Then* adjust your hand position on the stick.

When your **hand is too low** on the walking stick, your elbow will too quickly straighten during movements. This presents another problem for the movement impaired with a restrictive posture. It makes it much easier for them to apply too much downward pressure on the stick. Much of that pressure often comes from their leaning on it for support. *But*, because a walking stick often cannot provide them with the stabilized support they need, additional postural guarding and stiffening typically come with this. Why? They are unstable leaning on the wobbly walking stick, so they tightly grip the stick to stabilize it, so *the walking stick* will stabilize their body. In this example, the stick quickly becomes a useless obstruction. So, what is the moral of the story? This self-induced problem destroys the benefits of having the walking stick.

A **hand too high** removes the light pressure the weight of the forearm pushes into the walking stick. Now the pressure needed to hold it against the ground must be actively pushed downward into the stick with the elbow and wrist. However, it is very easy for a movement-impaired person to overdo this push and create stiffening in their fingers, hand, wrist, and elbow. Problems using the knees and an overdependency on the walking stick quickly follow. Sheryl provides an example of this in Figure 32.4.

People who are overly dependent on a walking stick for support are showing that they do not have the required movement skills to be using it, and causes some very common problems.

1. Leaning forward moves increased pressure forward in the feet and transfers body weight into the stick as if it were a third leg. To compensate for the body tipping forward, the stick must be moved farther forward for support (indicated by the red arrows in picture 1 of Figure 32.4), so the person can carefully take a small stride. However, for fear of creating a fall, it is now very difficult for them to move the stick or their feet to correct their forward-tipping posture in order to transfer body weight to take a stride.

   This is the situation Sheryl puts herself into in picture 1. The walking stick is forward and to the side, and she is leaning on it. Slowly and carefully, she takes two very small strides forward. This creates an additional stability problem (picture 2). During the strides, she is constantly leaning on the stick, making it impossible to move it. This is why the stick is now close to her foot, with the top of the stick pushed forward beyond the bottom of the stick in picture 3. Also take note of her posture in picture 3. Her upper body is leaning farther forward. How did this happen?

   In picture 2, she is pushing into the backward-angled walking stick for support. This pushes her upper body forward (picture 3). Now she stands tipping forward even more, on her toes with straightened knees.

   Fortunately, in picture 4, Sheryl does a very good thing. She stops her body's forward movement by slightly flexing her

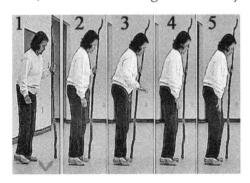

FIGURE 32.4: Sheryl's hand is too high on the walking stick and is holding it tightly. This greatly limits the stick's usefulness, increases her dependence on it, and hinders her movements.

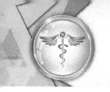

knees to flatten her feet, and moves her upper body back to regain stability. With this adjustment, she is able to move the walking stick slightly forward. In picture 5, she continues to flex her knees and stabilize, transferring more pressure out of the stick and into her feet.

2. Having the hand high on the stick will also coax some people to stand and walk with shoulders too high and too far back, which moves increased pressure toward their heels. In this setup, when the movement-impaired person experiences a tipping-backward movement, their reactive startle response typically straightens their arms and lifts the walking stick from the floor.

When this happens, they try desperately to force the stick back down onto the floor, thinking they need it to stop the backward tipping and prevent the fall. Unfortunately, this "getting the stick down" response is too often a worthless effort. The body is angled backward and the stick held high in the air by a stiffened posture and arm that are unable to move and place the stick.

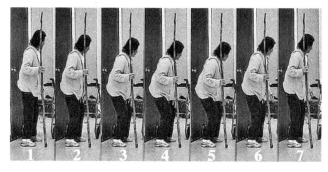

FIGURE 32.5: Stable, supportive feet and a relaxed posture allow for easy hand adjustments and placement of the walking stick.

Occasionally, they do manage to thrust it back down onto the ground, but frequently the result is not pretty. When they are tipping backward on their heels and the stick *is* forcefully thrust back down onto the ground, often the force of this striking push is transmitted up the stiffened arm and holds the shoulders back. This ends in an awkward stance with mixed results. When their hand is high on the stick, often they still have pressure in the heels of their stiffened feet, and a more aggressive backward push sometimes occurs. When the hand is low on the stick when it is thrust back to the ground, the body is leaning and rapidly moving forward in the attempted recovery movement, making a forward fall more likely.

In picture 1-4 of Figure 32.6, Carole is relatively relaxed and stable walking up a very gentle grassy slope. The walking stick in her hand is adjusted to the correct height, and the position of her forearm is good. However, she is firmly grasping the handle in her hand. Now note her posture change in pictures 6-9. Her right arm is now extending outward. This is a postural stiffening reaction. Why does this change happen?

It begins with the guarded stride she takes when moving into picture 5. The push for the stride from her left foot in picture 4 is weak, and that forces her to place too much body weight and pressure in the heel of the advanced right foot. This sudden heel pressure begins pushing her body upward and backward (red arrows in picture 5), and lifts the walking stick off the ground. Her response is increasing postural stiffness, and quickly lowering her left foot backward and onto the ground in 6 and 7 to stop her rearward movement. Beginning in picture 5, the walking stick is useless, and, in fact, detrimental to her recovery efforts.

Carole was able to stop her body's backward movement. In the process she moved her hips backward due to her rapidly forward-moving upper body, and that takes her forward. This allows her right knee to lift, to move her right foot forward in an effort to catch and stop her runaway upper body.

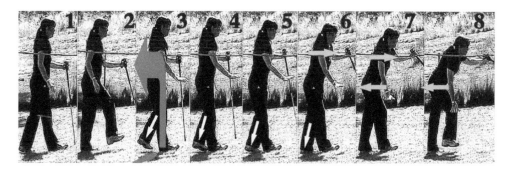

FIGURE 32.6: An example of a stiffening posture forcing the arm and hand to overcontrol the walking stick. The heel pressure in Carole's left foot in picture 3 is pushing her body backward and sets up the bigger problem starting in picture 4. She recovers, but having the walking stick in her hand causes additional difficulties during her startle reaction and recovery effort.

In this example, Carole recovered without falling. But where was the walking stick during her recovery? It was held up in the air with a very stiff left arm. It was useless. It was a problem, and it was a hazard. For example, suppose she had continued in an uncontrolled forward fall with her stiffened arm holding the walking stick in front of her, as seen in the pictures. The tip of the stick was angled down and would have stuck in the ground as her body fell forward. What was the location of the stick? It was directly in front of her. So, what do you think the chances would have been that she would have fallen onto the walking stick that was stuck in the ground like a thrown spear? This presents a very real danger.

As the uncontrolled body falls forward, the person can easily be impaled by the end of the walking stick if its tip lodges in the ground during the fall. This does happen. Several years ago, I came very close to doing this exact same thing.

Improperly used, **anything** can quickly become your worst nightmare. If you are struggling with a guarding and stiffened posture, a walking stick is not the best choice for a walking aid. But if you insist on using one, I suggest you use a long, tall walking stick, as Sheryl is in the above examples. There are safety and use advantages that are covered in the next few paragraphs.

Hills and Walking Sticks

When you're using a longer, **nonadjustable** walking stick on hills, or any place where the height of the ground significantly changes, the placement of your hand on the stick must also change with the change in the ground. Importantly, this is also true when you step up on or down from a curb or step.

When you're using an **adjustable** walking stick, as the ground changes, do not change the placement of your hand on the grip of the stick. Instead, adjust the stick's length to suit the situation.

1. When you're **going up a hill**, your upper body and hand are closer to the ground, because you are leaning your upper body forward toward the top of the hill. Therefore, to use the walking stick properly and remain in the correct posture for the movement, you must *shorten the length of the adjustable stick or lower your hand on the nonadjustable stick.*

2. When you're going **down a hill**, the opposite is true. You are standing more upright, with the ground sloping away from you. This moves your hand and upper body farther away from the ground in front of you.

   This requires you to *lengthen the adjustable walking stick* to maintain the correct posture using the stick while walking down the hill. With a *nonadjustable* walking stick, you'll need to move your hand higher up on the stick to use it properly.

3. Be cautious with adjustable walking sticks. They are also collapsible when you push too much body weight on them.

It happened to me. As I was walking down a forested hill, I did something careless and was suddenly tipping forward. The length of my adjustable walking stick was properly adjusted, and the stick was where it needed to be as I walked. But then the hill suddenly became steeper in the next spot I was moving onto. Feeling confident, I kept going, but then slipped forward a very small amount. That slip was just enough to cause a slow-motion, tipping-forward movement on the balls of my feet that I could not stop. The walking stick was rightfully in front of me, and this slip caused me to lean heavily on the stick with my chest.

Because of the steepness of the hill, I was unavoidably leaning too much on the walking stick. For a few seconds, I was stuck in that position as my upper-body weight slowly collapsed the adjustable walking stick. At the time, I thought I was pushing it into the soft soil. But no. The walking stick had completely collapsed to its shortest length.

This was a slow, semicontrolled, downhill tipping-forward would-be fall with the walking stick's handle pressed firmly against my chest. Had it been a quick and forceful fall, or had I been using a short non-adjustable stick, I could easily have suffered injuries. How could I have prevented this? As far as the stick is concerned, I should have lengthened it before going down the steeper slope. From a movement perspective, with the slickened dead leaves covering the forest floor, I should have taken the path that wasn't as steep.

Be very careful using a short walking stick, especially one **without** a grip handle. When you're going downhill with a short walking stick, its usable length quickly becomes too short as the slope becomes steeper, and then it is useless to you.

■ ■ ■

CHAPTER 33

GOING UP STEPS AND STAIRS

The structure of the step is rarely the cause of the problem.

Curbs, steps, stairs, and anything that looks like them* are often scary, scary, scary when an individual's movement ability is impaired and posture is restrictive. For these people, steps are obstacles, places where accidents happen when these folks are forced to use them. Going up is often challenging. Coming down is frightening and filled with danger. A child's easy activity of adventure and achievement has become a complicated ordeal filled with humiliation for an adult with impaired movements.

Going up or down steps, the movement-impaired person with a restrictive posture often trips, tips, and stumbles while desperately clinging to the railing. When there is no handrail, most of them will avoid the steps at all costs.

MISTAKES

The most common errors people with impaired movements and a restrictive posture make when going up steps occur in three areas. As you should expect, these are repeats of movement mistakes we have discussed in many of the previous chapters.

1. Stiff shoulders that resist coming forward. If and when the shoulders finally do come forward, it is often not enough, and they commonly do not stay forward. Thus, the pushing pressure in the foot is not where it needs to be for the movement.

2. Stiffened knees that resist flexing. If and when the knees finally do flex, they tend not to stay flexed. And the non-flexing knees do not allow the body to move forward.

3. Stiffened feet that will not flex. This renders it difficult to lift a heel, making it very difficult to control or push the body through the movement.

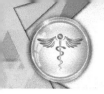

FALLING

For clarity: When people "fall" on steps, most commonly falling is *not* what has happened. Instead, they are typically forcing themselves off the step. For example, they push themselves backward off a step when going up. When they "fall" forward on steps, they are actually pushing too much with the back foot, pulling themselves forward too much with their hand on the handrail, or tripping themselves forward when their advancing foot catches on the step.

TINY HILLS AND LITTLE FLAT FLOORS

A hill is one flat floor on an angle. Stairs are actually a series of multiple little flat floors that are built into a hill, as shown in Figure 33.1. So, when walking up or down steps or stairs, we are actually continually walking on flat surfaces, while also walking up or down a hill.

Because they are separated by changes in elevation, these little flat floors are much scarier for many movement-impaired people. Thus, individually stairs appear impossibly more challenging and difficult than walking on one large flat floor. But stop right there. Even when the same little flat floors are on flat, level ground with spaces between them, they are still a challenge for these same people. So, is it the space between them and the elevation change that is scary stuff? In part, yes. But why? It is more because the little flat floors require the placement of the foot to be more accurate and consistent. It, therefore, comes back to their difficulties with supporting their bodies and controlling the movement using one foot, and specifically the forward part of that foot.

WALKING UP

How do we naturally walk **up** stairs, steps, or curbs? Essentially, we do it the same way we walk on anything, moving forward by taking one stride at a time from the ball area and toes of the pushing foot. The added factor here is the change in elevation we must push our body up to with each stride. This requires added coordination, control, and strength. But still, this simply means that moving up to the next step calls for the same postural adjustment and push that is required for walking up a hill, except we must do it better, with greater accuracy.

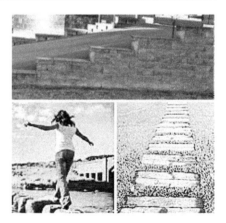

FIGURE 33.1: Stairs: multiple little flat floors cut into a hill. A hill: one large flat floor on an angle. Steps: little flat floors separated by spaces.

Imagine stepping up a four-inch-high curb to get onto a sidewalk at the edge of a parking lot. This distance is approximately half the height of the steps making up most of the stairs we commonly use. Still, for many movement-impaired people, this lower curb is just as scary as the higher step. However, when we dig deeper into the truth about the movement, a step up of less than one inch is frequently just as problematic for them as a step up of eight inches. Yes, the higher step up looks scarier. But, for the movement-impaired person with a restrictive posture, the act of doing *any* stepping-up movement activates the same type of inappropriate postural response.

Simplified to the basic components, any step up requires walking and pushing your body upward to move up to the next-higher little flat floor. So, for any obstacle on the ground, even a small twig, it is simply a matter of lifting the knee higher to move the foot over the obstacle. *But it is up*, and this is the part many movement-impaired people do not like. The question then is, is it really the knee going up that is the problem? No. *It is the unstable pushing foot they are not balanced on.*

SCARY CHANGE-IN-ELEVATION STUFF

A variation of the forward stride squat previously covered is the movement that is used to move up onto the next-higher step. The variation is in the increased height the knee must lift the advancing foot, and the distance the body must be pushed. The rest is the same. The movement requires a complete transfer of body weight and additional downward pressure into the pushing foot to stabilize and move the body forward and upward.

As the advanced foot makes contact with the upper step, the advanced leg pushes downward pressure into it to stabilize the body, and to complete the movement of lifting the body and the other leg and foot up onto the step. The pushing force required in the forward leg for this part of the movement is *the same as rising from a one-leg squat*, because that is exactly what it is.

When the transfer of body weight is not complete to either foot, stumbling and tipping instability on the steps is the result. Everything about movement on little flat floors requires that the movement be done *better*, not differently, with improved coordination and purpose, because there is less room for error. Understand this. The small errors made on a large, open floor will manifest as big mistakes on the little floors called steps.

Completing the weight transfer, especially on the upper step, is a routine struggle for many movement-impaired individuals. Because of this, remaining stable and balanced, pushing adequately, lifting the knee enough, placing the advancing foot appropriately, and then moving the body up onto the step is challenging in each stride. These challenges and problems largely stem from the person's inabilities and issues involving strength, flexibility, counterbalancing, and coordinating body movement in three basic functions:

1. Using only the forward ball area and toes of one foot to support and push the body.

2. Standing and squatting on one leg.

3. Positioning a foot on a small surface.

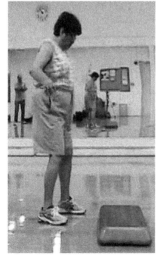

FIGURE 33.2: **So scary.**

What does this mean? These things describe the complexity of the movement. Any movement demanding improved control and ability will always highlight their dysfunction.

Consider these issues as you note what is happening in Figure 33.2. As she looks at the step, Rosemarie's mind is filled with doubt and fear. All she

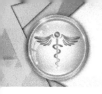

can see is a step that she knows she will have problems with, and there is nothing to grab to stop her from falling. The thoughts in her mind are "I don't like steps. I always have problems with them. It's too high for me. I don't like steps. There's no handrail. I'll fall again." Her mind is fixated on these thoughts and fears and essentially gives way to an all-consuming, all-controlling blankness that is blocking an otherwise useful and problem-solving mind.

This fear-driven blankness of thought and postural reaction to steps **will not** be weakened or washed away by helpful words of encouragement. It is too ingrained and too often relived. Such fear is real and founded in painful experiences. This is an important realization people who have never personally experienced this must come to understand.

This fear can only be weakened or washed away by the person living it. Before they will have the ability to quiet these psychological issues, they alone must learn and understand how to *physically* correct their physical problems. The intensity of their fear will only begin to diminish when they have gained improved stability and ability that they themselves create and trust. Anything short of this is, at best, wishful thinking.

HEIGHT OF THE STEP

To repeat an earlier comment, *any change in height* between two surfaces is too high for many people with a restrictive-posture movement impairment. Yes, higher steps are more intimidating, but it really doesn't matter if the difference is one inch or eight inches. Their psychological and physical reaction is the same to *any* change. It is their reaction that prevents them from adjusting their posture into the correct setup, to stand on the ball area and toes of one or both feet. It is their reaction that ensures that they will make the same mistakes and fail in the movement again and again. So, honestly, unless the step up is much higher than the typical height between steps on a staircase, *the height of it is NOT the problem.* If it were, many other people would also have issues with the increased height.

Another example: Many people who fear steps can walk comfortably on grass. They have the ability to relax and lift their feet over the top of the cut grass as they walk. However, many of these same people quickly balk when they see a small stick lying on the grass, even when it is not as high as the top of the grass. Just seeing the stick creates scary subconscious thoughts, causing them to guard and stiffen in mind and body. Suddenly, because of the stick they must walk over, they now have issues and problems walking on the grass.

Is their fear and posture change warranted in this situation? Absolutely not. But to them, it absolutely is! It comes from a deepened distrust of their abilities, and from past experiences. Realistically, they are confused by a conflict between what is real and what is perceived. Their conscious fears of the past join forces with a subconscious fear reaction that is again coming out in the present. Their fear is packed with frightening mental images and recalled physical harm. These are very difficult to forget and remove. They know it is simply a small stick on the grass, or a normal curb or step. But subconsciously, these register on the same magnitude as a high step without a handrail that is on the edge of a cliff.

This is why many adults with a movement impairment *fear anything on the floor or ground that is higher than the sole of their shoe.* Too many times they have lived through falls and embarrassment when trying to step over something. So, they avoid it.

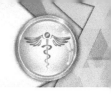

The fearful mind forces the body into a posture that induces failure.
The physical results of the failure support and intensify the psychological fear.
It becomes a self-serving cycle, feeding upon and reinforcing itself.

RELEASING FEAR

In Figure 33.3, Janette is casually walking up the stairs. The forward stride squat movement is seen in pictures 1 through 5. Her weight shifts are complete in pictures 1 and 7, and her knees are flexible in all the pictures. But just one month before this, she was terrified of walking up these steps or stepping over objects on the ground.

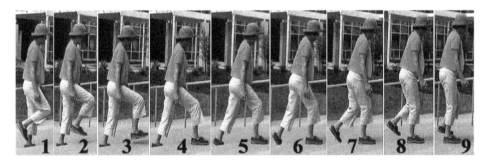

FIGURE 33.3: A month ago, Janette did not like doing this. A month ago, she had too much fear and postural stiffening to allow it. Today she shows her more natural abilities that had been hidden by the fear and stiffening.

One month of working on basic movement skills provided Janette with a renewed trust in her abilities, which she had thought were lost and unrecoverable. Now, she is stable and relaxed in her posture on the steps. She lifts the knee to place the advancing foot on the higher step as she pushes her body forward with a flexing foot. The clues in these pictures that indicate that she has a movement impairment are minimal and very subtle. She feels something she had thought she would never feel again. *Normal* is the word for that feeling.

Rosemarie's posture was very guarded in Figure 33.2, when she was looking at a step she needed to move onto, but then in Figure 33.4, her posture is much more relaxed than in her previous example. However, in picture 1, she is still not quite ready to begin moving up onto the step. Do you see why?

The movement she intends to do in both pictures is a forward stride squat, which requires the pushing pressure to be in the forward ball area and toes of the pushing foot. That *is not where the pushing pressure is* in her foot in picture 1. Instead, her right foot is close to being functionally flat, with slightly increased pressure toward the heel area. Note that her right knee is straight and her hips are back, while her upper body is slightly forward, and her head is down. In picture 1, she intends to move up onto the step. In picture 2, she is walking up a grassy hill. Her posture in picture 2 is correct, and what it should be in picture 1.

This setup in picture 1 is a very common mistake many movement-impaired people create when walking on steps. This is also why they have the same repetitive problems in their movements. For example, beginning the movement with a flattened foot or increased pressure toward the heel prepares the person for failure. They will customarily do one of three things because of it:

1. Without the forward push, they move their shoulders back and to the side to help transfer body weight to one foot and lift the other foot. The resulting increasing heel pressure pushes them backward and to the side.

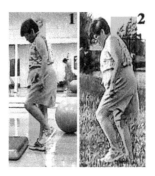

2. Without the forward push, they move their shoulders forward to start the movement. This quickly transfers pressure into the ball area and toes of the foot, which they commonly are not prepared for. This mistake causes them to tip and stumble forward. Why?

   The advancing foot goes to one of two places. One, it is not lifted high enough and hits the front of the step, resulting in a tip and stumble forward.

   Two, it *is* lifted high enough to clear the front of the step. However, because of the body's uncontrolled forward movement, the foot skids on the top of the step and/or hits the front of the next step. The result is a tip and stumble forward. This is how people "fall" up stairs.

FIGURE 33.4: Better posture, but not quite ready for the movement in picture 1. The pushing pressure in the right foot is not as far forward as it needs to be. In picture 2, the posture and pressure are correct.

3. Beginning with increased pressure in the heel, they push themselves backward, away from the step. When they are on a large surface about to move onto the first step, most of the time they catch themselves by stutter-stepping backward. But just as often, it is another person or a wall that stops their backward movement.

   The bigger problem is when they are on a step and push themselves backward. With their stiffened posture, there is limited possibility for a stutter-stepping recovery. So, either they stop the backward fall by clutching the handrail, or they push themselves backward off the step(s).

   All of these scenarios are why they will not begin or continue without their hand firmly grasping the handrail.

Remember this important fact. Beware of a movement-impaired person with a tendency to react with postural stiffening. When they begin a movement with a small pressure increase in or toward the heel, this invariably results in a strong tendency to move their upper body farther back. This is *the exact opposite of the reaction people with natural ability have* in this same situation.

For the movement-impaired person with a restrictive posture, when the knee comes up and the body hesitates to move, or there is a very small nudge of body movement backward, the habitual reaction is to move or jerk the shoulders backward. This is another reason they heavily depend on handrails.

Because of postural mistakes and incomplete transfers of body weight, these people truly and frequently enter into fights with themselves. For example, pressure in the heel of their foot pushes them backward. Their response: With hands and fingers tightly clutching the handrail, they frantically pull themselves forward against the heel pressure with their arm.

The other: Pressure too far forward in the foot pushes them stumbling forward. This forces them to lean heavily on the handrail, with their hands and fingers tightly clutching it in panic.

SHOULDERS FORWARD

To begin walking up steps, your posture should be somewhere between the postures for walking up a steep hill and for walking forward on a flat surface. The exact position varies with the individual and depends on their ability. The proper postural adjustment moves the pressure into the ball area and toes of the pushing foot, to the correct location so that *walking* and pushing the body up onto the next step happens easily, as shown in Janette's posture in Figure 33.3.

The lean toward the top of the hill must continue as you push to move up and onto each step. However, since you are always walking on little flat floors, you will *not* need to lean forward as far as you do when walking on a steep hill without steps. So, how will you know how much lean is correct? Your advanced foot on the top of the upper step and your overall stability will give you the exact answer.

With a forward-flexing and advancing knee moving your body forward, place the advanced foot on the upper step. Now adjust the lean of your upper body to make the advanced foot feel functionally flat on the step (Figure 33.5, pictures 1 through 5). This also moves the pressure forward in the pushing foot on the lower step to exactly where it needs to be to continue pushing your body up to the upper step. The advanced foot is now correctly positioned for pushing additional pressure straight downward into the upper step to stabilize your body and complete the movement of pushing your body up onto the step. To continue walking up any additional steps, simply hold this same posture (picture 6) and repeat the pushing process.

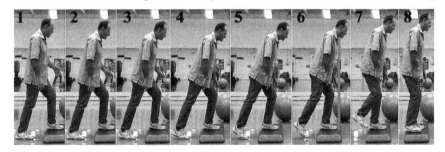

FIGURE 33.5: When walking on a flat floor or a hill, pushing from the ball area and toes of the foot is required. On a hill and steps, the force of the push must be increased to move your body up to the higher level. The movement-impaired person having difficulties should push the body forward to make the advanced foot functionally flat before moving up onto the next step. They will then be pushing into a stabilizing flat foot on the upper step when moving up onto it.

Recall the other mechanics of the movement. What moves my body forward from picture 1 to picture 5? The push from the ball area and toes of my right foot stabilizes the foot, and then the relaxed, flexing right foot (lifting heel) pushes the body. The distance the lifting heel moves adds the necessary length to the leg to move my body forward.

In picture 6, my body weight has been transferred onto a flattened left foot. The pressure directed straight down stabilizes me on the step and pushes my body up and out of the squat. In this example, my intent was to stop on the step. When the intent is to continue moving to the next step or walking forward on another surface, your upper body must remain forward to hold the pushing pressure in the correct location for both feet. This is frequently challenging for people with restrictive postures. Due to poorly controlled foot pressure and incomplete weight shifts, they lose stability, coordination, and balance to

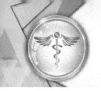

maintain the correct posture for multiple steps. The result: They intermittently stumble forward or tip backward while clutching the handrail.

Another important note: When people with *natural ability* walk up steps, the heel of the advancing foot is usually *not* the first part of the foot to contact the next step. Naturally, the first part to contact the step is most often the ball area and toes. They are prepared to continue the advancing movement.

In contrast, when *movement-impaired people with a restrictive posture* walk on steps, *the heel area of the advancing foot is* commonly the first part to contact the step (Figure 33.6). Their incorrect posture of shoulders held back causes this.

As with any stride, *the downward push into the forward foot should not begin until any increased pressure in the heel area has moved forward in the foot.* The only exception is when the person can easily compensate for and control it, and it causes no harm or deviation to the movement. But in general, movement-impaired people on steps have limited ability to compensate for and control the effects of heel pressure, so they should learn to avoid it. The easiest avoidance is adjusting the shoulders forward, and holding them there during the stride, to keep the advanced foot functionally flat on each step up. From experience, this is often very challenging to do.

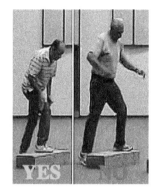

FIGURE 33.6: Your posture sets the forward foot. The YES posture creates a flat foot. The NO posture creates increased heel pressure in the foot.

In the picture on the right, Tom (with the label "NO" below the block) is attempting to move up onto the step. He has a weak push from his back foot, pressure in the heel of his front foot, and very little stabilization from either foot. Note his upright posture and significant guarding in his shoulders, hands, and arms.

In my setup (with the "YES"), my upper-body lean is forward and downward. The toe of my shoe, the forward knee, and my shoulders are in vertical alignment. With a strong push from my back foot, and pushing into the step with the advanced foot, this relaxed postural alignment is providing me with a functionally flat foot on the step. I am very stable, with strong support from both feet. As I increase the downward pressure into the foot on the step, my body moves straight up and onto the step. In contrast, when Tom pushed into his forward foot, he pushed his body backward off the step.

With natural ability, the forward-leaning posture I am showing is frequently *not* required. Those with natural ability have the strength, coordination, and flexibility to stand more upright while doing the same movement. The same will be true of a movement-impaired person who improves their strength, coordination, and flexibility to more easily do the movement correctly.

UP VERSUS DOWN

Walking up a step, the back leg does the forward stride, and then the forward leg does the squat.

Walking down a step, the back leg does the stride *and* the squat.

This is the added complexity and difficulty of the movement of walking down a step. It is the reason going down steps is the scariest and most difficult movement for movement-impaired people. This will be covered in detail in the next chapter.

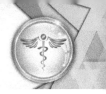

Nonflexing Foot

This is a fundamental problem for many movement-impaired people. When the pushing foot does not easily flex, the heel lift will be limited, and the body will not be adequately pushed through the movement. Therefore, the non-flexing foot and the inflexibility issues of the knee must be understood and at least partially corrected *before* the person practices walking on steps.

There are five important abilities needed to walk up steps. If the person does not have them, their movements on steps will always be challenging and sometimes difficult.

1. Trust standing comfortably on one foot and lifting the other knee much higher than when walking on other surfaces.

2. Trust using only the ball area and toes of one foot to support the body and push it up onto the next step, with or without a relaxed hand on the handrail.

3. Balance and hold the push in the back foot until the advanced foot removes the pressure from it by pushing downward into the upper step, to complete the transfer of weight to that foot.

4. Be comfortable moving onto and standing on a small, confining space.

5. Trust squatting on one foot and pushing up out of the squat while staying on that one foot, with or without a relaxed hand on the handrail.

Unknowingly, they create many of their own nightmares. *Their fear while on steps originates from the problems created by the instability and stiffness in their feet.* A reactive, restricted posture then frequently applies pressure in the wrong location in the stiff feet or foot, and compounds their problems. Holding shoulders back is a very, very common addition to these issues.

This *extremely* common mistake can be partially remedied by remembering two words before and during the movement:

1. Before starting to move up to the step, they need to say and position "*SHOULDERS FORWARD.*"

2. During the movement, they need to remind themselves "*SHOULDERS FORWARD.*"

3. At the end of the movement, they need to remind themselves "*SHOULDERS FORWARD.*"
    This will greatly help them keep pressure in the more correct location in the pushing foot for placing the advancing foot. Trust me. I know this through a great deal of personal experience. I still often remind myself of this when I am on steps, especially on days when my movements are challenging.

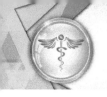

SHOULDERS TOO FAR FORWARD

In Figure 33.7, I am purposely holding a good amount of postural guarding and my shoulders are quite far back from the toe of the advanced foot's shoe in pictures 2 and 3. So, to move up onto the step, I use forward upper-body movement. I make it up on the step okay in picture 5. However, my upper body is now leading the movement and pulling me forward. This is seen in pictures 6 and 7, and then my upper body continues to move farther forward beyond the zone of stability.

The purpose of moving your shoulders forward is *not* to use them to spur the movement, as I'm doing in this example. Rather, it is only to correct the problem of holding your shoulders back, to move the pressure into the ball area of the pushing foot, where it needs to be. That is where the pressure is located here when I begin to step up, but the guarding I'm adding to my posture does things that prevent me from using it.

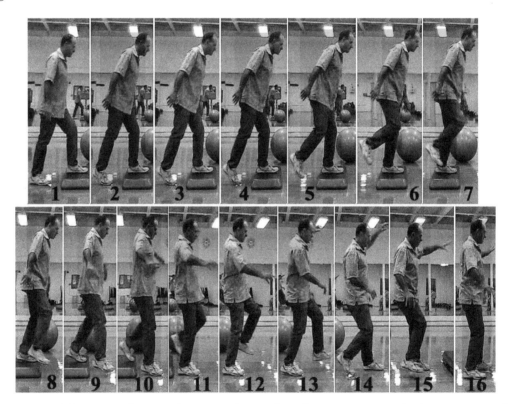

FIGURE 33.7: A guarded posture often results in a weaker push and excessive upper-body movement. This example begins with a push, but with the added postural guarding in picture 2, the movement changes into a pulling motion. The movement of my upper body quickly becomes faster than that of my legs and feet, forcing me off the step.

1. The pressure in my pushing foot is reduced when the muscles in that leg tense.

2. As muscles in the leg and foot tense, the flexing of the foot is restricted.

3. Then, as my upper body moves forward, pressure is pulled from the pushing foot, and further decreases the push from the foot.

4. The continuing upper-body movement pulls the remaining pressure and control out of my back foot (pictures 4 and 5). In picture 4, this is exactly the time the flexing pushing foot should be holding pushing pressure to the floor to help stabilize my body onto the advanced foot, as the pressure in the advanced foot is increasing.

5. Instead of using two feet to stabilize and control the movement, I'm standing on one unstable foot in picture 5. This allows the rest of the movement to proceed uncontrolled.

6. In pictures 1 through 4, there is increasing pressure in the heel area of the advanced foot. This is resisting the forward movement of the body from the pushing foot, and forces the upper-body movement to be stronger. That is why the pressure quickly moves forward in the advanced foot on the step, creating a forward push in pictures 6 through 10.

7. The result: My foot pushed and my upper body pulled me off the step in an uncontrolled movement. In this example, to stay on the step there is only one option. I must stop my upper body's forward movement to then stabilize the foot on the step. Immediately and without hesitation, in pictures 6 and 7, my shoulders must move backward just enough to move the pushing pressure back to a flattened and stabilizing foot. At the same time I also need to squat with the one knee I am standing on to quickly set the other foot down on the step, to squat with both knees on both flattened feet.

However, that corrective movement requires precise control of the upper body's alignment, to readjust the pressure in the foot to the correct recovery location, and also apply increasing downward pressure into the foot. In addition, the sudden squat and controlled upper-body movement are possible only when the body is relaxed enough to allow it.

Movement-impaired people with a guarded posture often do not do controlled movements quickly. However, their uncontrolled movements frequently do happen very quickly.

The movement and the recovery are that simple. Yet it is that complicated, but so very difficult for most people with a restrictive-posture movement impairment to do—even those with only a mild impairment. They require more time to respond and recover than the one second it took my body to go from picture 5 to picture 8. Therefore, their best "recovery" is based on prevention, on the proper setup before starting the movement.

In this example of tipping off a step, beginning in picture 5, most movement-impaired people are suddenly locked into a fear- and panic-driven nonresponse. Their mind and body quickly stiffen in anticipation of the coming fall. At that point, they are simply helpless to stop the movement, unable to logically attempt to respond. This is a recurring time-standing-still, mind-emptying episode of knowing the worst is seconds away. Sometimes, they get lucky and stumble into a fright-filled recovery instead of experiencing another painful disaster. Much of the time they go down.

These mishaps on steps are a common occurrence. In their minds, people struggling with this are left with only one realistic option: Stay off the steps! Avoiding steps and stairs is always their first choice. Curbs are on this no-go list, too, because typically there is nothing to hold on to. When a step up can't

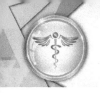

be avoided, paralyzing fear rules. The best they can hope for is to limit their injury and suffering. But they do not know how to do that either.

So how can they avoid an excessive-upper-body mishap like the one I demonstrated in Figure 33.7? In picture 1, before beginning the movement, stop to relax and reestablish increased pushing pressure in the ball area and toes of the pushing foot. Relax to allow the knees and feet to flex. Relax to allow both feet to control the body's movement on the step.

Now a question: How long does it take to do this preparation? A few seconds. A few seconds less than the time it takes to go through the forward-tipping movement, fall, and recovery. Many times, a few seconds of preparation and readjustment helps prevent embarrassment and painful mistakes.

HANDRAILS

The handrail is your very best friend when your movements are awkward on steps. However, many movement-impaired people are overly dependent on it, and they cause themselves added problems by misusing it.

Richie's impairment was moderate. In picture 1 in Figure 33.8, he stands with his advanced foot angled on the edge of the upper step (red arrow), and it remains this way through picture 4. With his mild postural guarding, that foot on the step causes a backward push, which he resists and overcomes by pulling himself forward with his right arm. In fact, in pictures 1 through 3, he pulls his upper body up and forward more than he pushes his body up and forward with his back foot, which should be doing the work of moving the body up to the step. Note that on the floor, the pushing foot is not flexing in pictures 2 and 3. This is because it is not doing much pushing.

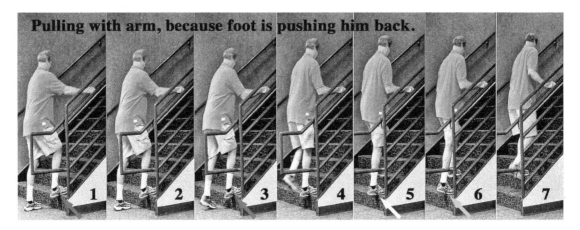

FIGURE 33.8: Fear of being on steps encourages tightly gripping the handrail. But that tight handhold also makes the movement more difficult, which triggers additional fear. With a strong pull by his right arm, Richie overcomes the back pressure from the angled foot on the upper step and moves up onto the edge of the first step.

Still holding the handrail tightly with his right hand, in picture 3 he begins using the advanced leg to push up onto the step. In pictures 4 through 7, he enters into a better posture and moves up to the next step with minimal pulling from the arm, while using a better push from the flexing foot on the bottom step. The green arrow points to the heel lifting.

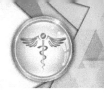

What does Richie forget to do in picture 1? He does not create a flattened advanced foot on the upper step. In this mistake, he doesn't adjust his posture appropriately to enable the push to move his body up and forward with the back foot on the floor, to keep the advanced foot flattened in pictures 2 through 4 as his body ascends onto the upper step.

But now, let's go farther back in this movement, to the setup. What happened there? Standing with both feet on the floor, his first focus was positioning his hand on the handrail. He needed that support to stabilize him so he could transfer onto his left foot, and then move his right foot up onto the step. Then he kept using his arm, forgot about pushing from the ball and toes of his left foot to push his body forward to place the foot. Instead, he only lifted his right knee to place his right foot on the step. This is why the foot only made it to the edge of the step. To get the foot on the top of the step, and flattened, his body would have needed to move forward to place it there. That requires a flexing pushing foot.

Now another question. Why didn't Richie use his arm to pull his body forward to move the foot on top of the step? He was unstable with a guarded posture in picture 1. If he had simply pulled himself forward, that would have caused a forward body lean that moved pressure into the ball areas and toes of his feet, and caused him to tip forward. Actually, this tipping themselves forward happens frequently with those with a restrictive-posture movement impairment. *Also, when these people are moving on stairs, the security of the tightly gripping hand on the handrail often becomes the cause of increasing insecurity and instability.*

In Figure 33.9, Richie (at right) and I are walking up the stairs. Take note that we are making the same movement with our feet in each picture. However, the movements of our upper bodies are different. The position of mine changes very little, while his changes in each picture. The main reason for his extra upper-body movement is his right hand tightly holding the handrail.

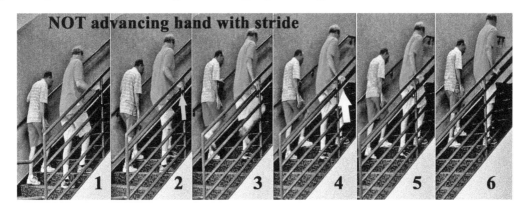

FIGURE 33.9: Richie has a tight grip on the handrail, so his hand will not move until he forces it to. When the hand doesn't move up the railing as the body moves up the steps, the upper body is pulled into rotation toward the rail. Compare my posture and upper-body movement (at left) with Richie's. My hand on the handrail moves along with the movement of my body.

As he moves up two steps in pictures 1 and 3, his hand stays in the same place on the handrail. He then moves the hand forward a small amount to take the stride seen in picture 4, and then moves it again in 5. Now take note of his right shoulder in these pictures. It rotates and moves backward toward the trailing hand on the handrail in pictures 2 through 4.

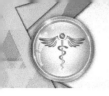

The trailing hand clinging to the rail is pulling his upper body in that direction and altering nearly everything about the movement. Think about it. One part of him (the foot and leg) is pushing forward while another part (hand and arm) is holding and pulling him backward. For people with a movement impairment, holding the railing tightly with the hand frequently complicates the movement and causes instability, and this happens while they are standing on the one place they dislike the most: The little flat floors called stairs.

Compare our upper-body postures again. Where is my left elbow? It is just barely seen in pictures 1, 2, and 4. What does this mean? It means my fingers were loosely on the handrail and the hand was constantly moving forward as I walked up the steps. With loose fingers on the rail and the hand sliding slightly in front of the body, it does not interfere with the movement of walking up the stairs. And yet, if I'd needed to use the handrail, I immediately could have.

When we use the handrail correctly while walking up steps, what moves the hand? Naturally, in controlled movements, the movement of the relaxed hand on the handrail is mostly accomplished by the feet. As the feet push the relaxed body, the arm simply rides along, pushing the relaxed hand the same distance. Any other movement of the hand is done with the elbow and shoulder. With natural ability, the purpose of the hand on the handrail is to provide momentary support to regain any lost stability on the feet. Then the hold is released to allow the hand to continue sliding forward with the body.

With a movement impairment, dependency on the hand increases as the impairment and instability situations become more problematic. Often only a mild impairment necessitates an intermittent to continuous use of the hand. As the mishaps and inadequate support by the feet become more frequent, it is challenging and difficult for these people to release their dependency on the stabilizing hand on the rail. This remains true even while they are improving their movement abilities. This is because they are still prone to making some of the same mistakes, albeit that the mistakes are smaller and less frequent. What does all of this mean for the movement of the hand on the handrail? Gradually the feet push the hand forward less, while the elbow and arm move the hand more.

In an effort to become less dependent on using the handrail, you must have a better supporting foundation. Work on these three issues. One, stop leaning on the handrail by increasing the use of your feet and legs. Two, relax your fingers (and elbow) to allow your hand to move on the handrail more easily with the movement of your body. Three, push a great deal more pressure into each foot on each step. Stomp on each step to practice this.

For those of you who feel unstable when walking on stairs or up curbs, use the "two-step" method. That is, stop and stand on both flattened feet as you move up onto each step, and then move your hand forward before ascending to the next step to repeat the process. This is what Richie is doing in Figure 33.10. Now go back and compare his posture in picture 1 here to his posture in picture 1 of Figure 33.8. In Figure 33.10, he is more relaxed and is stable on his feet. Now his posture is more cooperative. So, this time when he leans forward with his upper body to place his hand on the handrail, the rest of his body flexes and moves controllably with it. That keeps him stable, and then he moves his body and knee forward to place the foot. Note that his left foot is not flexing on the floor in picture 1 as he sets the foot on the step. It doesn't need to. With his hand on the handrail for support, the upper-body lean has tilted his hips forward enough to allow the knee to place the foot. Then, with the foot set on the step, he is in the correct setup posture to begin walking up the stairs using pushing and flexing feet.

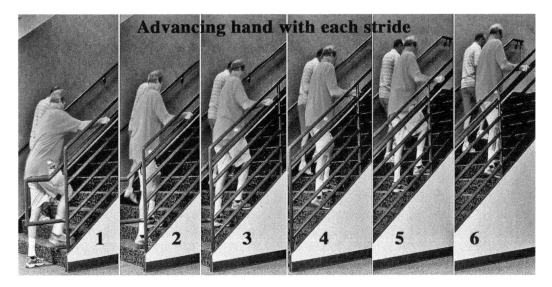

Advancing hand with each stride

FIGURE 33.10: Richie needs the stabilizing hand on the handrail to assist his movements on the steps. He begins by extending the hand forward on the railing, and then adjusts his posture to move up to the first step. When he completes moving to each step, standing with two flat feet on the step (not shown), he then moves his hand forward, and then proceeds to the next step. The hand is in the correct position for every stride, and the movement is better because the posture is better.

Now in the remaining pictures, check the location of his right hand on the handrail with respect to the movement of his body. From pictures 2 to 6, his right hand advances in every picture, and it stays in front of his body. Also, compare his upper-body posture here with that in Figure 33.9. In this example, he remains in the proper alignment for the continuing movement, providing him stability in his feet. And finally, note how his posture matches my posture, at Richie's left. This is a marked improvement from his prior attempts on the same day in Figures 33.8 and 33.9.

What else does this changed approach provide? A peaceful and quieter mind. It provides him with some clarity to focus on the basics and mechanics of the movement. Now his right hand is more relaxed. This means his posture is more relaxed and he is not restricting his movement ability as much. Suddenly, his movement impairment is less of an impairment. *This* is everyone's practice objective.

In Figure 33.11, Carole is walking up the steps using the handrail. However, the railing stops short of the last step. (The location of the post where it stops is marked with a red dot.) This situation is fairly common, and for those with a level of impairment that necessitates using the handrail, this example demonstrates how to deal with it. In picture 1, her hand (marked with a yellow arrow) is as far forward on the handrail as it can go. As she moves up onto the top step in pictures 2 through 7, she adjusts her posture to compensate for her hand staying in place behind her on the handrail. Her knees are flexed, her upper body is forward, and she holds the correct pressure in her feet. But still she does have some observable upper-body rotation to the left in pictures 3 through 7. This is due to her left elbow stiffening (indicated by the red arrow in picture 7) as she moves up onto the top step. Otherwise, she has good postural control and complete weight transfers, and she aligns her shoulder,

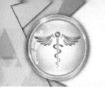
her knee, and the toe of her shoe in picture 7. This is very, very important to do, and with her moderate impairment, she did very well.

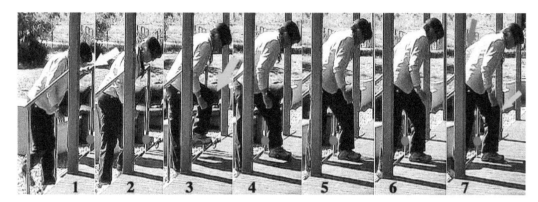

FIGURE 33.11: The handrail stops short of the last step (red dot), so Carole's hand stays behind on it as she moves up to the top step. Keeping a relaxed posture with flexing elbow and knees, she compensates for the hand and arm trailing behind her. She completes the movement on a very flat and stable foot.

Typically, a movement-impaired person, especially one with a restrictive posture, does not have this proper alignment coming off steps (up or down). Frequently, the trailing, gripping hand on the handrail prevents it, because that hand is pulling and rotating the upper body toward it. Then, when they are forced to let go of the handrail, their posture is backward leaning, and upper-body turning is holding increased pressure in the back and sides of their heels. The pressure is in the outside of the heel of the foot closer to the handrail, and in the inside of the heel of the other foot. The result is a tipping and pushing, spiraling-backward accident. So, what is the very first and last thing these people should remind themselves of *before* and *during* this last stride? Shoulders forward! Also,

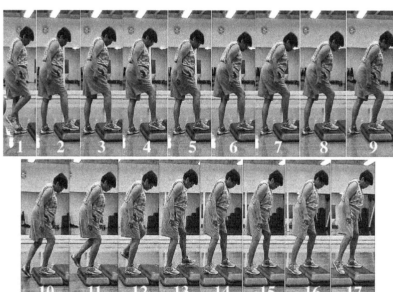

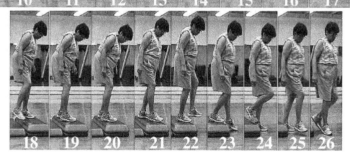

FIGURE 33.12: When you understand and apply the correct information, you give yourself a very good opportunity to rediscover your true potential. Negative issues change into positives. Good things happen, leading to an improved quality of life—according to your making and design.

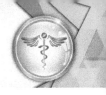

relax the elbow so the arm extends to allow the upper body to move where it needs to be, to adjust the pressure in the feet.

In Figure 33.12, Rosemarie now cautiously walks up and then down the steps while relaxed, stable, and in control. Formerly non-flexing, resistant feet and joints are now flexing, providing her with improved self-confidence and less fear as she moves. By correcting mistakes that led to inability, she earned the reemergence of hidden ability.

There are so many myths and misinterpretations that too many movement-impaired people are living and suffering with. For many of us, our disorders will continue to advance, causing us added problems and unpleasant moments throughout our lives. However, much of what is said about our disorders or conditions with respect to our movements do not need to occur. Through the many examples in this book, it has been repeatedly demonstrated that many of our problems and physical abilities are NOT strictly the direct effects of the advancement of our disorders. Some absolutely are, but the very important operative word here is *some*.

Proving to yourself the difference between what is and what is not:
This is your path to your truth.

■ ■ ■

CHAPTER 34

Walking Down Steps and Stairs

This is a very complicated movement for the movement impaired.

*I*n all movements, the pushing foot directs and controls the movement, and walking down steps is *not* an exception. Take the example of moving down one step. *The flexing foot pushes the body forward into the movement off the step*, and at the same time, the same leg's flexing (squatting) knee lowers the body down to the lower step. When the advancing foot has been placed on the lower step, the pushing foot, still on the edge of the upper step, holds and stabilizes the body, and continues this function until all of the body's support, stability, and control are transferred to the advanced foot on the lower surface. Then it is moved to the lower step beside the other foot.

When walking **down** steps, the first and most important focus needs to be on the pushing foot on the upper step, **and definitely NOT** on the foot advancing to the lower step or surface.

Likewise, when walking **up** steps, the first and most important focus needs to be on the pushing foot on the lower surface, **and definitely NOT** on the foot advancing to the upper step.

Walking down a step is *a forward "walking" stride movement*, with an added squat to lower your body down off the step to the lower surface. This tells you that your posture and the location of the pressure in your pushing foot must be very much the same as they are for walking up a step. The pressure in the pushing foot is also very close to the same location it's in for walking on a flat surface. *Both of these statements are exactly opposite to what most people think or have been told on this topic.*

The biggest and *most common problem* people with impaired movements have on steps is the improper positioning of their shoulders, especially when they are not relaxed. This is much more of a problem going down steps than it is going up.

The *scariest* part of walking down a step for movement-impaired people is *pushing forward off the step*.

The *second-scariest* part is *lowering* their body down to the lower step.

These issues are more problematic going down steps because their restrictive posture becomes more restrictive at the sight and/or thought of the step or steps they must use. At the first step, their primary reaction is to withdraw their shoulders, to hold themselves away from the danger. But what does this do? It has the opposite effect of creating more problems and a dangerous setup posture.

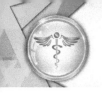

Intending to be more cautious, they make everything more difficult, unknowingly setting themselves up for failure.

THE UP AND THE DOWN

In pictures 1 through 7 of Figure 34.1, I walk up onto the step, and then in pictures 8 through 12, I walk down off the step. Compare them and note how the mechanics within the movements *are* different.

See this difference by comparing picture 4 with picture 10, paying close attention to what's happening with my knees.

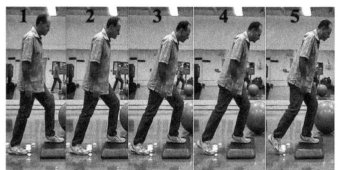
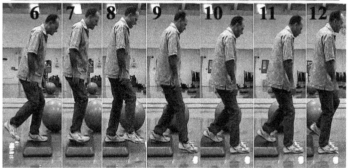

1. The difference in the mechanics of the movement is this: Going up, we push our body forward and upward with the back leg, and then push down on the step with the advanced leg, to move fully onto and stabilize on the step.

2. Coming down, we push forward *and* squat with the back leg (here the left).

What is the same? The posture for both is much the same, because the pushing pressure is from the same location in the foot for both going up and coming down. Therefore, the upper body must be forward to set the pressure in the ball area and toes, and the feet and knees must flex. This is *a huge problem for many people with a restrictive-posture movement impairment.*

FIGURE 34.1: Pictures 1 through 5: Pushing from the right foot to walk up onto the step, with the left knee flexing on the upper step to stabilize the body.

Pictures 6 through 12: Pushing the body forward from the left foot while the left knee flexes to lower the body down to the lower step.

Both movements, going up and down stairs or steps, are walking. Both movements are advancing forward movements that require the same stride length. Therefore, both movements require similar pushing pressure in the ball area and toes of the foot at the beginning of the stride. Yes, in Figure 34.1, my upper body is farther forward in picture 4 than it is in picture 10. The reason is I am going up, and that requires a stronger push. Coming down, the push can be less because gravity is doing part of the job. However, because the knee is flexing (squatting) to lower the body downward to the lower step, the pressure in the ball area and toes is higher to stabilize the body during the movement.

Of note: With natural ability, people's posture varies a great deal when they are walking up and down steps, as it does with other movements. Much of this is due to their varying strengths, abilities, balance, trust, and day-to-day variations in health issues. Thus, there is no absolute right or wrong posture, but there is an absolute right or wrong to the stability and performance of the movements.

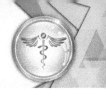

Now look at picture 7. All my body weight has been transferred to my left foot. In picture 8, my left foot is pushing my body into a forward stride. Note that my shoulders are forward in every picture during the stride. The upper body must be forward. Why? Because I am walking forward from one flat surface to another flat surface.

When going down a step, immediately following the beginning of the push into the stride, **the knee that you are standing on must flex into a "squat"** to move your body to the lower surface.

This is **not** the same squat we do in most other movements. This is a one-leg squat with the same leg you are pushing from while using only the forward portion of the ball area and toes of that foot, as shown in Figure 34.2. This is difficult to do when your movements are impaired, when your posture is not relaxed, and/or when your legs are weak.

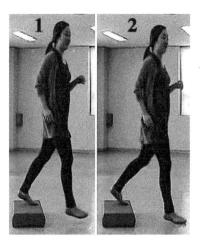

FIGURE 34.2: Natural movement: Squatting on only the ball area and toes of one foot to lower the body.

What else is this movement? This complex movement presents a huge psychological and physical problem for those with impaired movements and a restrictive posture. In a previous chapter I wrote, "When you can do a forward stride squat with ease and confidence, you will have the ability to do pretty much any other basic movement you want to do. The added qualification to this statement is, *your abilities are always limited by your physical capabilities.*" Well, walking down steps puts this stride-squat ability to its toughest test. It is a movement that demands adequate strength, with more precise and relaxed postural control.

SHOULDERS AND HANDRAIL, AGAIN

Overusing and tightly gripping the handrail creates another problem when walking on steps. With a firm grip, the hand is much more likely to NOT move with the body. Too often, as the body moves forward, the hand lags behind on the railing. Then, as they proceed, the hand fixed to the railing pulls the arm out behind them, which pulls their upper body backward and rotates it toward the handrail. This shifts the pressure in the pushing foot toward the outside of the heel and progressively shortens the stride length for the next step.

As he walks down two steps in Figure 34.3, Richie's right hand does not move on the handrail, and note that his stiffened arm moves farther behind his body. This process steadily pulls his upper body backward while rotating it (pictures 2 through 4). As he continues to move forward and down the steps with his legs in pictures 2 through 4, the pressure in his right foot moves farther into the heel area. This is why his stride length shortens. This is also why in picture 4 his left foot scrapes down the vertical face of the step.

But let's now go back to picture 1 and note that his shoulders are held back, and this is because his right hand gripping the handrail pulls and rotates his upper body backward. For those with this problem, you must learn to pay attention to what is happening. For example, any time your heel hits the top edge of the step (picture 3), or scrapes down its vertical face (picture 4), or becomes wedged between the vertical side and the lower step as Richie's foot is in picture 5, this is your alarm that YOUR SHOULDERS ARE TOO FAR BACK. *Stop.* Correct your hand and posture.

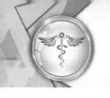

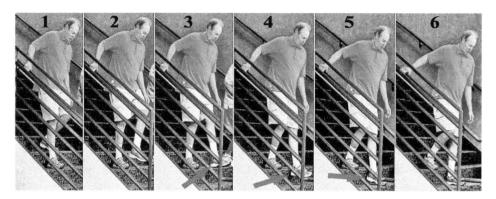

FIGURE 34.3: With a non-moving hand tightly gripping the handrail, the upper body rotates toward the handrail and is held back as the legs and feet continue. This moves the pressure toward the heel in the pushing foot, shortens the stride length, and causes the heel to hit the edge of the top step and vertical side of the lower step.

The heel-hitting and -scraping problems are very common, and they always cause instability. For many people with a restrictive-posture movement impairment, these heel problems happen *every time* they go down steps.

Test question: What is the only way the advancing foot will clear the edge of the top step and vertical side of the lower step?

1. The upper body must be forward enough.

2. The pressure in the pushing foot must be far enough forward in the ball area and toes so the pushing foot is capable of moving the body beyond the stair's edge.

3. The pushing foot must be flexible.

4. When one hand is tightly gripping the handrail as Richie's is, it holds the shoulders back and prevents all three of these things from happening.

The hand must move forward as your body moves forward, to keep the pressure in the correct location in each pushing foot. The other necessary factor is that the knee you are standing on must flex (bend) to lower your body down to the next step while keeping the pressure in the pushing foot's ball area and toes. Moving off this pressure is *the* mistake that creates the shoulders-back, heel-hitting problem. It is a tough one to correct and to keep corrected. So, again, why do these people continue to keep their shoulders back? They fear falling down the steps.

When the heel hits the edge or vertical face of the step, the person reflexively tightens their grip on the handrail and pulls their shoulders back even more. This reflexive reaction is in response to two things: tipping forward and instability. Remember, the advancing foot stops or slows when it hits or sticks on the step, but the advancing body does not. This happens more easily when you are going down a hill (steps). The continuing upper-body movement causing the forward tip is very scary and happens *frequently*. This is why these people quickly learn to hold postural guarding and/or stiffening with shoulders back before beginning the first step-down movement. They do this in hopes of avoiding pitching headfirst down the steps. But very often, the result is the complete opposite. Fear promptly causes their backward-leaning posture to become habitual. They use it in every step-down situation, even when the step down is very small and the area of the surface or step they are moving onto is very big.

But, for argument's sake, let's assume that a person with a restrictive posture did keep their upper body forward going down a step. Would they then make a better step down onto the lower step? NO! The outcome would be different, but not for the better. See the movement. Assume they push their body forward, and the advancing foot moves the distance to the middle of the lower step. This seems good. But NO, for them it is not. Remember, their knees are not flexing or are limited in how much they flex. Therefore, their pushing foot's knee typically does not flex enough to lower the body and the advanced foot to the lower step. This means the advanced foot is in the air over the lower step. So, how would they lower this foot when the other knee is not flexing into a squat? They would be forced to lean their upper body much farther forward, *and now they are falling down the steps.*

Our natural movements are highly dependent on a relaxed posture and easily flexing feet. The complexity of the movement of walking down steps accentuates this and quickly shows how problematic an unrelaxed (restrictive) posture and non-flexing feet actually are. Recall that *the distance our body and advancing foot travel is the distance our flexing foot and lifting heel push our body forward.* With feet that are not as flexible as they need to be, the stride length is shorter, and the body is not pushed far enough to make it to the next step.

On stairs, the distance between the steps determines how long the stride must be, and the space for foot placement is limited. Therefore, any person using the stairs must alter the length of their stride to match the distance between the steps, as well as be more precise in their foot placement. With natural ability, we adapt to this with a relaxed, cooperative posture and easily flexing knees and feet. With unnatural movements, we are challenged by a restrictive, uncooperative posture and limited flexing of the knees and feet. These greatly restrict stride length adjustments and foot "placement."

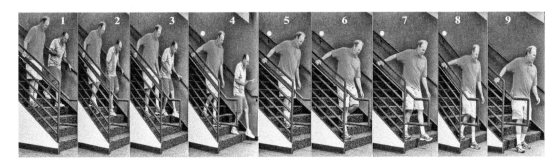

FIGURE 34.4: Contrasting posture and movements of a mildly movement-impaired individual (blue) with those of a person with a mildly moderate impairment (red).

Figure 34.4 is a good example to compare these issues; it's the more complete series of the previous example. My movement impairment is very mild (blue and white clothes), and Richie's is mildly moderate. In pictures 1 and 2, our beginning postures are close to the same. As I keep the same posture and

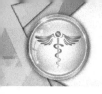
move easily down the steps, Richie changes his posture. The differences in his posture and movement show clearly in the remainder of the pictures. Where do Richie's problems begin? They begin between pictures 2 and 3 and continue to picture 8. The cause? His non-moving, tightly gripping hand on the handrail. From picture 1 to picture 8, it stays in the same place on the railing.

This will sound too simplistic. Your stability and trust on steps depend largely on how relaxed and controlled your posture is while you're using the small front area of one foot.

I cannot emphasize this enough, and it is a topic people frequently ask me about. After I explain the movement of descending stairs, a very common response is, "How can it be that simple? There has to be more to it. If it were that simple, I/they/we would not be having all these many problems."

Okay. But. If problems lie in the small surface area of the step, why do these same people have the same problems when the surface of the step is larger, or when they're on a big, open, flat, and smooth floor?

If the problem was due to the height of one step or multiple steps of a staircase, then everyone would be having a problem with them. And the small children going up and down adult-size steps—just look at the problems they have each time they use them. But they don't have these problems. It is only the adult thinking it's the steps' fault that is the issue.

Yes, when the surface of the step is small, the movement is more challenging. However, the step being too small or your foot being too big *is not* the cause of the majority of the problems. It merely creates an added challenge and highlights the non-flexing or limited flexing of the foot.

BOTH FEET

Naturally, whenever a foot comes in contact with the floor, we begin using it to help support our body and the movement while continuing to use the other. Naturally, in all continuing movements, we transition from supporting our bodies using one foot to two feet, and then back to one foot, and so on. Importantly, during this transition, the pushing foot becomes the anchoring foot, to hold the body in position and to prevent it from moving too far forward on the advanced foot, or backward toward the pushing foot.

Consistently using both feet in this natural manner is especially important when we are on steps (Figure 34.5). Walking down the step, as the advancing foot comes in contact with the lower step, the pressure in the pushing foot is held on the edge of the upper step. We don't release this anchoring pressure until we are stabilized and have completed the weight shift onto the foundation (advanced) foot on the lower surface. We do the same when walking up the stairs, as we do when walking on any surface.

Going up: The pushing foot on the lower step supports the movement until the advanced foot on the upper step takes over. Going down: The pushing foot on the upper step supports the movement until the advanced foot on the lower step takes over.

This is an *extremely important part of the movement*, but unfortunately many movement-impaired people don't do it very well. Instead, they have become overly focused on the foot moving onto the lower step, with their instability and restrictive postures making it difficult for them to transition between their feet or think of anything else.

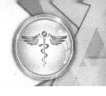

This natural part of our movements frequently goes unnoticed. Naturally, it happens without thought. Unnaturally, with a movement impairment, it slips away. Not holding that pushing and anchoring pressure in the back foot is a huge contributor to people's growing *inabilities*. And it is a huge contributor to their problems walking on steps.

But why is the ball area of my back foot on the front edge of the step in picture 1? This is because the back of my shoe is touching the front vertical surface of the

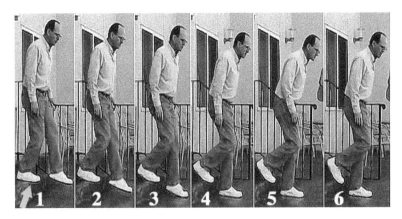

FIGURE 34.5: Slow down. Feel it. Hold the push on the edge of the step you are leaving until you are stable on the next step, and until that foot takes control.

step. So, yes, as shown in this example, sometimes the width of the step is too small for our foot. For this reason, when I started coming down the step in picture 1, the ball area of my foot on the edge of the step pivoted on the edge, and continued to pivot throughout the movement.

This situation of the front of the foot being near the front edge of the step tends to happen more often to the movement impaired. The reason is, they are typically coming down onto the step with a flattened foot. People with natural ability typically come down onto the lower step with the ball area of the foot first, because the foot is easily flexing and not taking up as much space (when that foot remains flexed with the heel up), especially as they continue down the stairs primarily using only the forward area of the foot.

The good of the foot on the front edge: Provided they continue to hold pressure in the foot, this actually helps them. How? The foot doesn't need to flex as much because the pivoting ball area lifts the heel.

The bad of it: When they *don't* hold pressure, the foot can easily slip off the step, particularly if the edge is slippery for any reason. This happens more often when their posture is not relaxed, and especially when their upper body is not held forward enough.

KICKING A BALL

Another natural remedy: To improve your ability to walk down steps, practice the playful movement of kicking a ball. The correlation is direct and simple. *If you do not have the ability to stay balanced while kicking a ball, even gently tapping the ball with your forward-moving foot, then you also do not—yet—have the movement skills for walking on stairs.*

In Figure 34.6, Rhoda is lightly kicking a ball on a thick, cushioning lawn. Compared with photos of her in Chapter 22 (Figure 22.6), this example shows how much trust in her movement ability she reclaimed during the month I worked with her. Here, she is stable and relaxed in her posture and movements while lightly tapping a ball with the toe of her shoe. This is the way to begin your practice. Get comfortable with a very light impact as the advancing foot lightly taps the ball during a walking stride— *before* practicing a more aggressive kick.

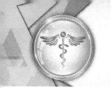

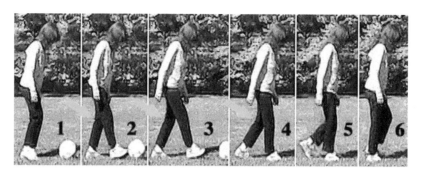

FIGURE 34.6: Begin by very lightly tapping the ball with the toe of the shoe as you walk "through" the ball. Flexing knees and shoulders staying forward are required.

This tap with the toe of your shoe on the ball is not a kick per se. It is simply the foot contacting the ball as the foot moves forward during the stride, and not allowing the tap to stop or pause the forward movement of the foot. For many people with a movement impairment, the foot stops moving forward when it contacts the ball. It takes practice *not* to allow that to happen. It takes practice to walk "through the ball," to continue walking as if the ball were not there. Another practice suggestion: If you are the least bit unstable when tapping the ball with your foot, practice the light kicking movement *with an imaginary ball*.

Focus on these things as you practice:

1. Have the pushing pressure in the back part of the ball areas of your feet as you walk, and relax your hands to relax your posture.

2. Complete the weight shift onto one foot *with shoulders forward*, keeping the pushing pressure the same in the foot that's on the ground.

3. As you lightly tap the ball with the toe of the advancing foot, remind yourself, **knee down. Shoulders forward.**

4. The most common problem is failure to stay balanced on the ball area of the foot on the ground.

5. The most common mistake that often turns this problem into a fall is allowing the shoulders to move up and back.

Be Careful

Light kicking practice *without* a ball will help many of you improve your setup, walking, and slight-kicking-movement posture. Why? Two reasons. One, for many, when the advancing foot taps the ball, it will pause or stop moving forward. Two, for many, when the advancing foot is about to tap the ball, their shoulders will move back. Pay attention to these things and the pressure in the foot on the ground. You'll need to have these aspects of the movement better controlled when you begin actually tapping or kicking a ball, because that is when your posture problems will happen more quickly and more often.

The following are things you can do to help stop these problems from happening:

1. Push *more* pressure into the foot as you transfer weight onto it, and keep pushing it down throughout the movement. This needs to be a great deal more pressure than you've been using in other movements.

2. Flex the knee of the pushing foot as you begin the kicking tap, and keep it flexed. Remind yourself: *Down! Remember, this will be the same movement as lowering yourself onto the lower step.*

3. As the advancing foot taps or kicks the ball, immediately remind yourself to squat with the advancing knee as the foot comes down. Go into the forward stride squat that you have been practicing.

When you are unstable, you **should not** be practicing a kicking movement. Instead, you should be practicing stabilizing on one foot when standing, and then remaining stable during simple movements. What else? Practice the heel-raise exercises on each foot to stregthen your calf muscles.

When you have the ability to stay balanced on the ball area and toes of the pushing foot and come down on the flattened advanced foot, and then squat with both knees in a forward stride squat, then you are ready to begin actually kicking the ball.

Use common sense. If you have the common problems described above, DO NOT begin kicking the ball as if you are playing soccer. DO NOT pretend you are at midfield about to score the winning goal with one skillfully placed kick, to the roar of the crowd. Instead, start the process as if you were teaching a small child how to kick a ball.

Practice walking "through the ball" to eliminate the hesitation of that foot. Practice this on short grass by only walking, NOT kicking. Simply walk into the ball, and the toe of your forward-moving foot will *lightly* tap the ball as you continue walking. Pay attention to the foot's movement after it contacts the ball *by continuing the strong push from the foot on the ground.* When the kicking foot hesitates at the ball, this nearly always means you did not have, or keep, enough pushing pressure in the ball area and toes of the pushing foot, with shoulders forward.

And again, be careful!

1. When the push from the back foot is weak, the kicking foot will slow or stop as it contacts the ball.

2. When the push from the back foot is weak, the shoulders will more likely move backward at the beginning of the movement, and more so when the kicking foot makes contact with the ball.

3. When the push from the back foot is weak, it's more likely that the kicking foot will touch the ground before striking the ball. This commonly happens when the transfer of body weight onto the foot on the ground is incomplete.

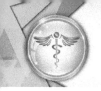

4. When the shoulders move backward during the kicking movement, the kicking foot will more likely make contact on the upper half of the ball, or may pass entirely over the top of it.

Be very careful of this. Often the foot will "stop" on the top of the ball, leading to a nasty twisting fall if the pushing foot is the slightest bit unstable.

Practice *lightly* kicking the ball with a focus first on remaining balanced and stable on the one foot on the ground. As this becomes easier, then focus on the **kicking knee** second. Yes, the kicking knee, because the knee controls the foot. Lightly kick the ball using the forward and extending movement of the knee to kick with the foot, as shown in Figure 34.7. Why? This will help many of you stop improperly trying to control, and overcontrol, the kicking foot.

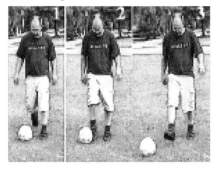

FIGURE 34.7: Aggressively push down into the ball area of the back foot and stabilize on it. Then kick with the forward knee to kick the ball with the foot.

Eliminating Foot Hesitation

Without hesitating or stopping, imagine you are walking through a spring-loaded swinging door. To do this you must aggressively push your body forward through and past the door in a continuous movement. The advancing knee cannot hesitate and the shoulders cannot move back, otherwise the door will push you back. Everything is forward.

This is precisely what you must also learn to do in all your movements. It is simply more critical when kicking a ball or walking up or down a step. So, practice this to know and feel it. Practice bracing and pushing so you control the door instead of letting the door pull and push you. You should be doing this with every door you open and close. And as for the doors you pull toward you, brace yourself with your legs and feet, with shoulders forward, so the door does not control you, and pull and push you around.

In taller grass and when using a heavier ball, a stronger kick is needed. No big deal. This only means that every part of the movement must be done better. It demands a stronger push on the pushing foot to enable the other foot to be lifted well above the grass to kick the heavier ball or move the ball farther forward. Hint: The required amount of pressure in the pushing foot for this is the same pressure you should be using in the pushing foot for walking up steps or a hill.

Coming down off the upper step, the flexing knee of the pushing foot's leg lowers our body down onto the lower surface. Kicking the ball, the flexing knee of the pushing foot's leg slightly lowers our body to stabilize the body, and the muscles in the leg are working much better to power the movement.

On steps: As the advancing foot contacts the lower surface, allow the advancing knee to flex slightly downward to absorb the force of your body coming down onto the lower step. The "hard landing" you experience when coming onto the step is due to non-flexing knees and feet, especially when increased pressure is in the heel area.

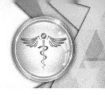

FLEXING FOOT

We take a forward stride when walking down off the upper step, but only a small *forward push* is needed to move the body and advancing foot beyond the front edge of the step. However, *a very strong downward push into the upper step is required for support and stability* as you lower yourself with a flexing knee. Why? It is needed to resist the effects of gravity and control the body's descent. For those with a movement impairment, very often both the push and the flexing knee are problematic. Often, the weaker push, combined with the limited flexing foot and knee, these stem from a restrictive posture, which is commonly due to the instability of using only the forward area of the pushing foot. The following are suggestions to help remedy this situation—when on wider steps.

When you're *starting* to come down the step, the pressure in the pushing foot does not need to be far out in the toes. In fact, for many with a movement impairment, having the pushing pressure in the forward ball area and toes weakens their support and inhibits flexing the knee. Therefore, as they begin practicing the movement, they should keep the pushing pressure back toward the center of the ball area of the foot. But when they do this, there is another thing they must do. The stride will be smaller, so keeping the shoulders forward helps prevent a stride that is too short.

The second part of this is, many people who have difficulty with steps begin with the pushing foot farther back from the edge of the upper step. Then, because the forward push is less with the pressure moved back in the ball area, to clear the edge of the upper step in the stride, the squatting knee and the advancing knee must move the advancing foot farther forward. But commonly this doesn't happen. The advancing foot hits the edge of the top step, and then the heel slides down the back vertical part of the step, and often wedges on it as the ball area of the foot contacts the lower step.

For this reason, begin with the ball area of the foot very near the front edge of the upper step. Then, as your body descends, the ball of the pushing foot will pivot on the edge of the upper step. Done properly, with the necessary pressure holding the foot in position, this makes the movement a bit easier and more user-friendly. As you become more relaxed in the movement and the foot becomes more flexible with a relaxing posture, you will begin moving pressure farther forward in the ball area and toes, to take more natural strides with a more natural foot placement on the step.

SIDESTEPPING

For those having a bad movement day, and for those with a *moderate or more significant impairment*, movement on stairs is frequently filled with peril, such that walking on them becomes all but impossible. However, there is a way to be safe and still successfully negotiate steps on a difficult movement day. Simply face the handrail at a slight angle in the direction you will be moving or face it squarely, holding it with both hands, and use a sidestepping movement to go up or down the steps one at a time. A common issue with the sideward movement is fitting both feet on the same step. This is the reason for the angled position of the body with respect to the handrail, as it also angles the feet on the step for easier placement and control.

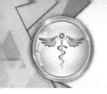

The rest of the movement is exactly the same as the sideward movement covered in previous chapters, Chapter 17 in particular, with the addition of continually moving the hands to have them where they're needed for support. So as not to be confusing, the mechanics of sideward movement going up and down stairs are the same as the mechanics of the forward-facing walking movements in this chapter. In other words, the same feet and knees do the same jobs. A complete transfer of body weight is required from foot to foot, and the movement to the next step comes from the pushing foot. The flexing knees do the same work, and the quality of the push and squats is the same. The *only* basic difference is in the direction of the movement and feet, and the feet do not need to be as flexible.

Many people in a more impaired condition will likely need to help the movement by pulling with an arm to move completely onto the next-higher step. But you need to be careful to limit how much you lean with your upper body while using your arms, because it's easy to overdo it. You must remember, when using your hands and arms, focus on pushing with your feet. Develop the habit of using your legs more to create added stability and ability, and using your arms less.

Anytime you have your hand or hands on the handrail, also try not to forget about moving it or them after you have moved onto each step. For this sidestepping routine, before you move your foot up to the next step, position the hand that's higher on the handrail at approximately the point where the advancing foot is to go on the step. Then, each time you move your body and other foot up to the step, move your other hand up the handrail in front of you. The objective is to keep your hands in front of you, spread a little farther apart than your shoulders. Practice with this to find what hand placement makes you feel the most comfortable and the most stable. Also pay attention to keeping a fairly relaxed grip on the handrail. With more relaxed hands, you'll have a better chance of relaxing your posture. And if your hands are more relaxed, that means your legs and feet are doing a better job.

Also, beware of hands spread too far apart on the railing. This limits your movements and often causes stiffening of your arms and the rest of your body. Always, the primary focus needs to be on the stabilizing pressure in your feet with complete transfers of body weight.

Leaning is also a problem when going up or down steps this way, and why do people lean? Inadequate use of the legs and feet. They lean to help lift the advancing foot to move it to the upper or lower step with a straighter knee. With these people's greater impairment, *non-flexing* feet and knees are a much bigger problem.

The upper-body lean used by these movement-impaired individuals is frequently to the side and toward the upper step when **going down**, which is opposite to their intended movement of moving down to the lower step. This sets up the same types of problems that occur when going forward down the steps with shoulders leaning backward. When **going up**, their lean is frequently to the side and toward the lower step.

THE FOOT ON THE NEXT STEP

In natural movement, while holding the correct posture and pressure in the pushing foot, *the ball area of your advancing foot will most often be the first to make contact with the next step.* However, even with a mild impairment, do not be overly alarmed if it is not. This takes practice and patience to relax enough to allow it to happen. So, if the foot is flattened when contacting the step and you are comfortable and stable, this is quite all right. The important thing is that you are comfortable and stable doing what you want to be doing.

But if the *heel* is first to contact the next step, that is not okay, and you have some corrections to work on.

You are not searching for perfect.
You are merely working to be better,
to feel more normal in your own skin with carefree movements.

■ ■ ■

CHAPTER 35

SPEECH

Victim of circumstance, or creator of opportunity?

Impaired speech is very common for people with degenerative neurological disorders. Many of them speak slowly and sluggishly. Others slur, garble, and run their words together in a fast and hurried, jumbled mess. Both are difficult for the casual listener to understand.

When our spoken words are unrecognizable to others, or it takes too much effort for the other person to understand them, people stop listening. Common reasons for this include:

- Often an immediate conclusion is, "This person has been drinking alcohol or is mentally impaired, or possibly both." Because of this assumption, many listeners automatically deduct points from the IQs of people with slurred and garbled speech.

- The impatient or intolerant listening person quickly becomes uncomfortable. They look for a way to move away from this person they cannot understand, to escape from someone they would rather not associate with.

Mixed with their personal feelings of embarrassment, humiliation, and self-rejection, these repeated public occurrences constantly remind the person with the neurological disorder of their deteriorating life and diminishing worth. Their response becomes a strong desire **not** to speak in public, and many will go to great lengths to avoid it. Then, when they must, they speak with less volume.

These reactions from both sides are part of our human nature, and they are not going to stop. Some people who don't respond well to their perception of this tortured speech simply are not interested in knowing anything more than what they wish to assume. Others actually do not have the time when the interaction happens. Some don't know how to cope with it. And there is another side to this situation that we, the affected people, need to be honest about. Not all of this is the fault of the listener. We share the blame.

When your speech reflects poorly on your character and intellect, it has a profoundly negative effect on your self-confidence, self-respect, and self-esteem. I know this well, because I lived that life. I lived

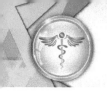

it until I found out how to reverse much of it. When I improved and corrected much of my degrading speech, these negative patterns and effects naturally resolved. Then, my speech improved so much that these public humiliations no longer happened.

Is my speech perfect? No. It simply is much better.

For most people with a degenerative neurological disorder affecting their speech, the process of transitioning from clear speaking to difficult-to-understand speaking occurs slowly. In the beginning, the change is subtle and noticeable only in certain words. Very often the affected person does not realize their speech is changing. This is typically followed by a phase of denial as they do become aware. Then gradually it becomes so undeniably obvious that they no longer attempt to conceal it. This is a common reaction for many. No one wants to admit they are losing their abilities and identity.

As their speech deteriorates and it sounds bad even to them, they speak less. When they must, most will then speak quietly in an attempt to avoid the looks and thoughts of others. Others need to realize, the speech-impaired very much dislike how their own speech sounds to them, so they try to select words they don't have as much difficulty pronouncing. With this avoidance, decreased volume, and selective word choices, their speech pattern also becomes slower. Then, as they attempt to speak selected words and pronounce them more clearly, they enter into what's referred to as "scanning speech." This is at the least a threefold process:

1. They are consciously pausing to select certain words and processing how to pronounce them properly.

2. While speaking, they often pause when they're having difficulty pronouncing a word and try to think of a word to replace it with.

3. As a direct *and indirect* effect of the disorder, they also have issues recalling some words, thoughts, or memories.

You Make It Worse

Because of these everyday realities, many affected people cast themselves into *self-imposed social isolation.* They spend more time alone and speak less. Their speech gets quieter and lazier, and all their speech issues and problems become worse.

Another factor that leads to more slurring and garbling of words occurs when they are advised to "slow down when you're speaking; that will help you improve your speech." No, mostly it does not. The basic problem with this is that they do not know how to improve their speech by slowing it down. Consequently, when they do slow the rate of their speech, they typically become lazier with their mouth and tongue movements. *The corrective action is **not** simply a matter of slowing down, and honestly this advise is directed more to helping the listener.*

Slurred, mumbled, and garbled speech is the result of the uncoordinated movement of the muscles that move the mouth (jaw), lips, and tongue. In its basic form, this is not different from any of the other movement problems we have previously discussed with regard to the rest of the body. Therefore, until the affected person learns how to better control and use their speaking muscles, their speaking voice will not change for the better.

Slowing down by forcing your mouth, lips, and tongue to work better, *to work more naturally*, is the key. Very importantly, this is not the person trying to "slow down" for the sake of slowing down. The importance of the difference lies in developing more deliberate speech patterns. So, to help yourself correct the garbled, slurred, and mumbled way of talking that you hate to hear, you must rehabilitate the responsible muscles to the best of your ability.

Use your muscles correctly or you will lose the proper use of them. It doesn't matter where the muscle is located. It doesn't matter what the function of that muscle is. It only matters that it is used and exercised correctly to do the natural function it is designed to do.

The following is the natural remedy that works for me.

THE SIMPLE BASICS

I focus on these three very basic and very simple things to substantially improve and maintain clearer speech:

1. **Animate** your mouth, lips, and tongue to form the correct sounds of every word.

2. **Enunciate** (properly pronounce) every syllable of every word.

3. **Project** your voice. Speak up and be heard.

Animate Your Mouth and Tongue

Begin doing this by *exaggerating the movement* of your lips, mouth, and tongue to form the sounds of each syllable in every word. Make the movements big. The goal is to make the sound of each syllable as close as you can to how it is normally spoken.

Pay close attention and practice speaking the words and sounds aloud. Not a whisper. Not hidden to yourself. The point is to be heard by others. Feel and hear what happens when you begin to open your mouth much wider and move your tongue and lips with much more expression. Make funny faces with the kids. Have some fun with it. Just remember, it doesn't matter what you look like when you're practicing. The only thing that matters is how clear the words and sounds are.

Because you are being more deliberate, doing this will naturally force the words you say to come out more slowly. With continued practice, they will gradually sound better and become easier to understand. You are working on *purposeful* movements to produce clarity of speech.

Enunciate Every Syllable

As you exaggerate and animate your mouth, lips, and tongue to form and speak the sounds of the syllables, the next logical thing you need to do is add the correct pronunciation of each syllable. Speak every syllable of every word, and hear them clearly.

As you enunciate (properly pronounce) each syllable, you will be adding another natural step to slowing the rate of and improving the clarity of your speech. With practice, your speech will improve while you consistently do only these two things, which means you won't have to repeat yourself as often. Why? People will understand what you're saying the first time. Imagine being able to let go of feeling embarrassed when speaking in public.

As you are coming out from under the embarrassment of slurred and garbled speech, many other aspects of your life will also improve. As you gradually pay less heed to the inner voice telling you to be quiet, your self-confidence will begin to reappear. This is a wonderfully amazing thing to have again.

It is up to you to insist on the clarity of the words coming out of your mouth. Say what you intend to say; be heard *and understood.*

There is another benefit this voice revival brings back into your life. As your speech improves, you begin regaining the lost social IQ points that your poor speech had squandered.

Project Your Voice

You need to add volume to your voice to be heard and more clearly understood.

However, this does not imply a yelling or screaming volume. All you need and want is the volume of authority and confidence (more social IQ points!). All you need and want is the ability to have the appropriate volume in your voice so that those you are speaking to can hear and understand it. When they are across the room, down the hall, across the street, or sitting across the table in a noisy restaurant, you want the ability to be heard and understood the first time you say the words.

You want and need a controlled, nonscreaming voice for the situation. For example, when you call out to the kids playing in the yard, you want them to clearly hear every word you say the first time you say them.

You can also practice these three things when singing, provided your family will allow it. My daughters would consistently tell me, "Dad, please stop!" Sigh. Even when my selection was a song they liked. Perhaps the issue had something to do with my changing the lyrics in my performance?

Do what you need to do. Rehearse your karaoke act when you're alone in the car, out walking, or sitting in the woods resting during a hike. It doesn't matter where. Just practice while carefully listening to yourself, or record your voice, to honestly critique *what you hear.*

Give yourself permission to try, to live, to enjoy being yourself again.

ONLY YOU

Only through your own personally directed efforts will you find the ability to release yourself from the strangling cocoon your inabilities and disabilities have wrapped you in.

It is your responsibility that others can only assist you with.

I know and understand this on a very personal level. Everything I have written in this book deals with what I have lived and done for myself. And much of it I will always need to continue doing.

Life with impaired speech and movement ability will not change for the better until you effectively apply the knowledge that actually shows you how to create the change. You now have that knowledge source. You are holding it in your hands. The choice of what to do with it is yours.

■ ■ ■

CHAPTER 36

What Will Motivate You
to Keep What You Gain?

To those with the idea:
"Sitting here, reading, I understand what you've written. It makes sense.
Now all I need to do is remember these things and my movement ability will improve":
You are gravely mistaken and will be bitterly disappointed.

Why did I begin this final chapter on such an apparently negative note? It is to highlight this truth. None of the information I have written in this book will help you *unless* you commit to understanding how to *physically* use it. Without understanding how to apply and use this information in the practical sense (physically), you will only gain intellectual information *you think you understand, but are confused how to use.*

IMAGINATION

Indeed, our imagination is the driving force within our ambition. We acquire knowledge and then use our imaginative thoughts to improve and expand on our basic knowledge even more. Imagination provides us with an ability to dream, see new possibilities, and reach higher goals. An active and healthy imagination enables us to wonder, ponder, and plan; to see beyond what is today. Imagination encourages doing, improving, discovering, and inventing new realities.

Without imagination, without our personal insights and questioning, everything would remain routine. Without imagination, there would be very few ripples on the pond of possibilities. Without imagination, the thought of anything different would not exist. Life would be stagnant. Without imagination, people sit and wait for someone to help them, to provide them with a better life. Many movement-impaired people are living stagnant lives, unaware of options to do otherwise; not knowing how to act on any imaginative thoughts of ways to reach for a better life.

Many people living the effects of a degenerative movement impairment, and similar problems, live consumed in negativity each and every day. They would love to have a reason to believe that pondering and exploring possibilities could change their predicament. But time has proved to them that having

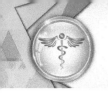

hope is futile. Too often they have become hopeful upon hearing of something that might help, only to become disappointed once again. For too many people, this is how their thoughts and dreams of a better life turned dormant; with all hope expelled through recurring disappointments.

However, the factual, practical, and useful information within this book does honestly offer them a realistic opportunity to rekindle some of their hopes and dreams. It provides them with much of the information and methods they can readily use to help themselves: To help them rebuild their reason to begin believing in possibilities once again.

MOTIVATION

You must find for yourself what motivates you. Why? This will be a major component that helps keep you on your path. Your hope, your trust, and living your successes are things only you can provide.

For me, my stubborn nature and hatred of being clumsy drove me to keep pressing on in the early stages. Then the pure joy of experiencing the steady improvements I was making kept me wanting more.

You *must* find yours. Whatever it is, put a candle under what motivates you and keep it burning by continuing to fuel the fire. Reaching your goals depends on it.

CAN YOU KEEP IT?

Many ask, "How do I know that any improvements I make will stay with me?" Stop! This question comes from a defeatist mind-set. Nip that negativity at the core, because it will only bring you down and give you an excuse to do little or nothing. To question is fine, and it is required. However, be careful of the mind-set you are in when you ask it. What if this same question were phrased, "What should I be doing to keep what I'm improving?" That turns a negative into a positive.

You either learn how to believe and trust in yourself again, or you don't. You either apply and use what you are learning every single day, or you don't. You either push your personal envelope to reclaim as much of your natural abilities as you are physically able to, or you don't. It's our choice.

I am often asked this question: "How many of the people you work with are doing better at the end of all the sessions?" My answer to that question is always, "All of them." *However*, the results any individual achieves depend on many variables. They depend on:

1. Each person's true physical abilities, and their not-so-true physical *disabilities*.

2. The level of fear the person lives with in their mind.

3. How much they work and play to process and use this information on their own, and how they bring their imagination and motivation into the mix.

4. How easy or difficult it is to get them out of their thinking minds.

The truth is, everyone has a greater potential for improvement than most imagine for themselves.

Now, you should rightfully be asking another question: "Of all the people you have worked with, how many of them have *kept* what they learned during their sessions with you?"

To that question, I wish the answer could again be all of them. However, that would be a huge lie. The truthful answer has four parts:

1. I *have not* had the ability to do an in-person follow-up review with most of the people I have worked with. Thus, I must rely on what they have written in follow-up correspondence to form guesstimates of their individual long-term outcomes.

2. Regarding those *with* degenerative disorders or conditions: I *have* had personal follow-up sessions with some, and the amount of improvement they have maintained has been widely split in two ways.

   ▪ These people had requested refresher sessions because they had lost part of the ability they had gained in the initial working sessions.

   ▪ When the time since last working with them had been fairly short, as in a year or two, most then quickly regained the ability they had previously achieved. Some of these people then also surpassed their initial level of ability and function in the refresher sessions.

   ▪ When the time since last working with them had been lengthy and their degenerative disorder had been rather aggressive, these people again showed improvement in the refresher sessions but were unable to recover the higher level of ability they had achieved the previous time.

   ▪ For others, the aggressive nature and progression of the *direct effects* of their disorder could not be undone or overcome. Thus, their abilities diminished in spite of their efforts.

3. Those who enthusiastically committed themselves to continue working independently on using and improving the abilities they gained during the initial working sessions reported better long-term outcomes. Some kept and often exceeded what they had initially gained, while others stated that they were maintaining what they had gained.

   The other part of this group reported that their abilities slowly declined. *However,* they also stated that the decline was much slower than it had previously been, and they had experienced better movement ability during the decline than others had, and relative to their former ability. This provided them with an improved quality of life for a longer duration.

4. Regarding those *without* degenerative disorders or conditions: None of the people in this group requested refresher sessions, and those who provided me with follow-up information reported that they were continuing with improved movement ability.

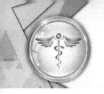

There is a common link among those who reverted to their previous inabilities after the initial sessions. Categorically, they did not work independently nearly as much after the sessions as they had during them, and they shared a common misconception. They thought that if they understood the information and remembered what I had told them, then they would know how to use it when they needed it. All who had this misunderstanding and attitude were disappointed. Some came to realize their mistake and then put forth more effort, and that was the reason they requested another chance to work with me.

Others blamed their disorder, while denying their mistake and lack of effort. In regard to their movements and disorder or condition, many of the people in this group have an issue of dependence on someone to motivate and guide them. Without this other person, they are easily lost. With someone reminding them what to do and encouraging them to keep on, they do better. What does this mean? It means they have the physical ability, but on their own they don't trust themselves to use it independently. Fear runs high in many of them and inhibits how they process, learn, and use the information. With fear and lack of trust, they doubt everything and use their ability less. As a result, much of the information they have attempted to memorize simply fades away.

For nearly everyone in any of these categories, the lack of a support program involving ongoing educational and movement therapy in this methodology is a key ingredient in their declining abilities. This guidance is crucial because of the nature of their problems and issues, and because they are attempting to change their behavior and developed habits. Changing personal behaviors and habits requires many months of personal commitment, and often requires the support of others who physically, emotionally, and intellectually understand the process involved for the particular behavior or habit. Those dealing with unnatural movement issues and problems commonly do not have this support, nor is there presently any program that is readily available to them—that understands the information presented in this book.

Still, the level of improvement any individual can achieve with or without an ongoing support system or program will always be a best guess. Why? The improvement for anyone is greatly dependent on that individual's participation and commitment.

Definitions

A definition of **inability** is *the state of being unable to do something.*

The definition of **disability** is *a physical or mental condition that limits a person's movements, senses, or activities.*

The operative word here is "limits." This word **does not** necessarily mean that the person is incapable of doing the movement. Rather, it means the person is unable to do the movement the same as a person without the "disability" can.

Yes, there are many people with a physical **dis**ability who definitely have the physical **in**ability to do certain movements. However, as a word, *disability* is frequently misused. In the context of movement, it is frequently used with the primary implication that the person physically *cannot* do the movement. Within this context, the word and the person are frequently negatively mislabeled and misunderstood by others, and themselves.

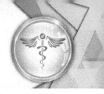

By definition, the prefix *dis-* references the negative of ability. Therefore, the meaning of the word *disability* is interpreted as the lack of ability (the inability of ability). The true definition of *disability*, which includes "limiting the ability," is lost, giving way to a common interpretation of "nonability."

This negative context highlights what the person with the disability is unable to do—and the accepted reason for this is their condition or disorder. Because of this, in many ways just the negativity of the word *disability* (referring to the disorder or condition) becomes the larger part of the perceived physical inabilities and psychological interpretation by the individual and society in general. Too often, then, the prefix *dis-* becomes the focus of the person's view, outlook, and criticism of themselves.

On the other end of the spectrum are the people with the resolve and commitment to do the best they can in spite of the disorder or condition. These people work diligently to destroy this imposed barrier, to do the best they can with what they have, and rid themselves of the disability label. They remove the *dis-* and replace it with "Yes, I can, so get out of my way." Yes, limitations in their ability continue, but *without* the disrespect and negative self-criticism of what they ambiguously should or should not do. Their focus flips to the positives of what they can do and how they can continue to do more. These people do better, yet still need this basic information that will allow them to do much better.

WHICH EXERCISE?

Is a certain exercise or activity better than another? Yes and no. Ask simple questions to know the difference:

1. Does this exercise or activity challenge me to work on my movement issues?

2. Does it test and develop my skills beyond what I thought I was capable of?

3. Am I stable and comfortable while doing it?

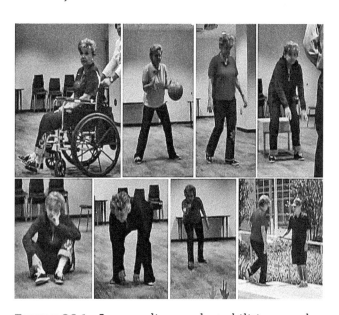

If the answers are yes, then it is a good exercise and activity for you to do.

If the answers are no, then move on to another activity that does meet these criteria, and possibly come back to this activity when you have improved. *Commonsense rules apply.*

Another note: It is very important to realize that your body will function in an apparently "lazy" manner if, for example, it is deficient in nutrients or sleep, you're in a toxic environment, or you have unaddressed medical issues or other health-altering situations or conditions. So, if any of this is affecting you, while you are embarking

FIGURE 36.1: As we rediscover lost abilities, we also rediscover the person who was lost within the disability.
Life is a dance. Choose your music to suit your style. Tamara, your walk is nothing more than the dance in your mind. Move to the music. Live your dance to enjoy every step of your life.

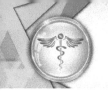

on such a big journey to improve your movements and ability, it is really important for you to seek remedies for your other troublesome issues as well. Doing so may substantially improve your overall health and outlook on life, provide you with a more fit body to meet your coming challenges, and take you ever closer to your goals and improving quality of life. (Figure 36.1)

It May Not Be "What It Is"

On John's T-shirt was the quote "It is what it is."

I would like to finish that quote with "*until it is changed from what it was.*"

What is the very important message here? Most people with a movement impairment are convinced that the unnatural movements they have developed cannot be changed, and that is because they believe they cannot change anything about their disorder or condition. Thus, they believe "It is what it is" is the only thing that applies to them. Too much of the time, they are reminding themselves, "I have accepted that I cannot change any of it."

What are they missing? They should NOT be attempting or believing they are working on the direct effects of the disorder or condition, because the individual person cannot change or modify them (with a very few exceptions). Thus, the direct effects are indeed a case of "it is what it is."

We are only working on the indirect effects, because we can remedy them. Therefore, reducing the indirect effects (maladaptive behaviors and bad habits) is the "until it is changed from what it was." Simply put, the indirect effects (maladaptive behaviors and bad habits) is the "*until it is changed from what it was.*" These *can be modified* (corrected and eliminated). Simply, when the indirect bad habits and behaviors are corrected, unnatural movements are transformed to more natural movements. This is how we create and enjoy improving movements that are increasingly more natural and safer to do, which, at the same time, creates an improving quality of life.

So, your responsibility is to work on your "*until I changed it from what it was.*"

Purposeful Movements

To improve and continue improving your movement skills and abilities, you must include purposeful movement activities and exercises in your daily routines. Purposeful movement activities are those that require more precise body and foot placement, which tells you they require improving relaxed postural control. Purposeful movements demand increased skill and fewer mistakes. Thus, they are more challenging to do.

What is the payoff? Better movement ability, and many purposeful movement activities also have a component of fun. Imagine the concept. You being able to take part in something fun that takes you out of your thinking mind, exactly how you learned advancing skills and abilities during your childhood. Thoughtless movements, simply for the fun of it. (Figure 36.2)

Finally, I suggest you heed this last piece of advice: Dig deep within yourself and allow the child hidden within to come out and play. You

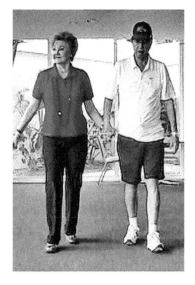

FIGURE 36.2: Yes, we can!

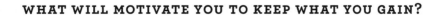

need that part of you to help the adult you are now with this transition. The more you can practice and play with a *childlike mind-set and fun-seeking attitude*, the easier it will be to work, practice, and play.

Yes, it is very okay for an adult with a movement impairment to have fun.

YES, *you can*!

■ ■ ■

ABOUT THE AUTHOR

In October 1997, Dr. Tom Clouse's world was forever changed when an evaluating neurologist informed him, "I'm sorry to tell you that you have a neurodegenerative disorder, and you will not be able to continue as a general surgeon. Also, as your symptoms and deteriorating movements progress, you will need to simplify your life to better cope with the changes. I wish there were something we could offer you in treatment or therapy, but there is nothing that seems to help." Dr. Clouse's productive life was thrown into a spiraling tailspin.

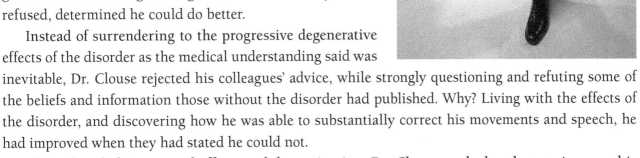

The neurodegenerative disorder is spinocerebellar atrophy, and the affected parts of his brain are the cerebellum and brain stem. The disorder causes these areas to slowly degenerate, to become smaller, and this negatively affects his speech and movements. Subsequently, due to his increasing movement difficulties and near-daily falling episodes, in 2003 a neurologist advised him to begin using a walker for his safety. But he refused, determined he could do better.

Instead of surrendering to the progressive degenerative effects of the disorder as the medical understanding said was inevitable, Dr. Clouse rejected his colleagues' advice, while strongly questioning and refuting some of the beliefs and information those without the disorder had published. Why? Living with the effects of the disorder, and discovering how he was able to substantially correct his movements and speech, he had improved when they had stated he could not.

Through only his personal efforts and determination, Dr. Clouse worked on how to improve his movements, and succeeded to such an extent that he regained and has retained his ability to function in a near-normal capacity. As a result, he has traveled extensively throughout the United States and internationally, working with other movement-impaired people to help them improve. His discoveries and techniques fill the pages of this book.

Printed in the USA
CPSIA information can be obtained
at www.ICGtesting.com
LVHW071927031023
760019LV00020B/564